What others are saying about S The New Power Eating...

*If you want to understand the impact that food can have on performance in power sports and learn how to design your own plan like a pro, there is no better resource than **The New Power Eating**.*

Jose Antonio, PhD, CSCS, FISSN, FNSCA

CEO and Cofounder of the International Society of Sports Nutrition

*Dr. Kleiner knocked it out of the park with **The New Power Eating**. It's science heavy, but it's also packed with practical, immediately actionable information. A perfect balance is struck between covering the fundamentals and providing cutting-edge research. This book is truly encyclopedic in terms of both its depth and breadth; it's a one-stop shop for virtually everything involved with nutrition and supplementation for optimizing sport performance, fitness, and health. The difficult feat of delivering academically rigorous yet highly readable material is also accomplished in outstanding fashion. I'm thrilled that practitioners, coaches, athletes, educators, and enthusiasts have this resource to turn to.*

Alan Aragon

*Dr. Kleiner's advice has made all the difference in helping me improve and extend my playing career. I've never felt, played, or looked better! **The New Power Eating** will also help you transform your physique and elevate your athletic performance.*

Sue Bird

Point Guard for the Seattle Storm (WNBA)

Member of Two WNBA Championship-Winning Teams (2004, 2010) and Four Olympic Gold Medal Teams (2004, 2008, 2012, 2016)

Member of Eleven WNBA All-Star Teams and Eight All-WNBA Teams

Fan Pick for the WNBA's Top 15 Players of All Time

*Dr. Kleiner showed me how to focus my food and fully fuel my body. I feel better, play better, and I know I'll be able to stay in the game longer. Add **The New Power Eating** to your training program and achieve your physique and performance goals.*

Megan Rapinoe

Midfielder/Winger for the Seattle Reign FC (National Women's Soccer League)

Member of the United States Women's National Soccer Team—Gold Medal in the 2015 FIFA Women's World Cup, Gold Medal in the 2012 Olympics, and Silver Medal in the 2011 FIFA Women's World Cup

Dr. Kleiner's athlete-first approach to sports nutrition makes all recommendations and guidelines practical and easy to customize for any athlete. Use **The New Power Eating** *to get all your sport nutrition questions answered by a pioneer and respected leader in the sport nutrition profession.*

Keenan Robinson
Director of Sports Medicine and Science for USA Swimming

Dr. Kleiner has decades of experience working with athletes of all levels to show them what works and what doesn't in their quest to develop power for their performance. With **The New Power Eating** *you can reap the benefits of that experience and take your game to a whole new level.*

Daniel Shapiro
Head Strength and Conditioning Coach for the Los Angeles Clippers (NBA)

The New Power Eating *is a MUST for every athlete. I have used Dr. Kleiner's information for years with the athletes I coach. In fact, I recommend her book to every high school athlete who reaches out to me. Athletes who want to get a leg up on their competition should study and apply Dr. Kleiner's principles. The book is written in a way that is easily understood, and the concepts are very simple to follow. Dr. Kleiner is simply the best sports nutritionist the United States has ever produced.*

Jed Smith, MS, CSCS
Head Strength and Conditioning Coach for University of Northern Iowa
USA Weightlifting National Coach
USA Track and Field Level 1 Track Coach

THE NEW POWER EATING

Susan M. Kleiner, PhD, RD

High Performance Nutrition, LLC
Mercer Island, Washington

with

Maggie Greenwood-Robinson, PhD

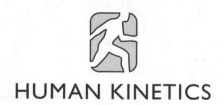

HUMAN KINETICS

Library of Congress Cataloging-in-Publication Data

Names: Kleiner, Susan M., author. | Greenwood-Robinson, Maggie, author.
Title: The new power eating / Susan M. Kleiner, PhD, RD, High Performance
    Nutrition, LLC, Mercer Island, Washington ; with Maggie
    Greenwood-Robinson, PhD.
Other titles: Power eating
Description: Champaign, IL : Human Kinetics, Inc., [2019] | New edition of:
    Power eating. | Includes bibliographical references and index. |
    Identifiers: LCCN 2018013651 (print) | LCCN 2018019989 (ebook) | ISBN
    9781492567271 (ebook) | ISBN 9781492567264 (print)
Subjects: LCSH: Athletes--Nutrition. | Bodybuilders--Nutrition.
Classification: LCC TX361.A8 (ebook) | LCC TX361.A8 K595 2018 (print) | DDC
    613.7/11--dc23
LC record available at https://lccn.loc.gov/2018013651

ISBN: 978-1-4925-6726-4 (paperback)

This publication is written and published to provide accurate and authoritative information relevant to the subject matter presented. It is published and sold with the understanding that the author and publisher are not engaged in rendering legal, medical, or other professional services by reason of their authorship or publication of this work. If medical or other expert assistance is required, the services of a competent professional person should be sought.

Notice: Permission to reproduce the following material is granted to instructors and agencies who have purchased *The New Power Eating*: pp. 283-288, 388-389. The reproduction of other parts of this book is expressly forbidden by the above copyright notice. Persons or agencies who have not purchased *The New Power Eating* may not reproduce any material.

This book is a revised edition of *Power Eating, Fourth Edition,* published in 2014 by Human Kinetics, Inc.

The web addresses cited in this text were current as of June 2018, unless otherwise noted.

Senior Acquisitions Editor: Michelle Maloney; **Managing Editor:** Anna Lan Seaman; **Copyeditor:** Pamela S. Johnson; **Indexer:** Andrea Hepner; **Permissions Manager:** Martha Gullo; **Graphic Designer:** Julie L. Denzer; **Cover Designer:** Keri Evans; **Cover Design Associate:** Susan Rothermel Allen; **Photograph (cover):** Vasyl Dolmayov/iStock/Getty Images; **Photographs (interior):** © Human Kinetics, unless otherwise noted; **Photo Production Manager:** Jason Allen; **Senior Art Manager:** Kelly Hendren; **Illustrations:** © Human Kinetics, unless otherwise noted; **Printer:** Data Reproductions Corporation

Printed in the United States of America   10 9 8 7 6 5 4 3 2 1

The paper in this book is certified under a sustainable forestry program.

Human Kinetics
P.O. Box 5076
Champaign, IL 61825-5076
Website: www.HumanKinetics.com

In the United States, email info@hkusa.com or call 800-747-4457.
In Canada, email info@hkcanada.com.
In the United Kingdom/Europe, email hk@hkeurope.com.

For information about Human Kinetics' coverage in other areas of the world, please visit our website: **www.HumanKinetics.com**

E7312

*In loving memory of Mom and Dad, who showed me
how to gracefully embrace strength and power.*

—Susan Kleiner

Contents

Preface

I have been working with strength athletes for more than 30 years. My work began with two major research studies: a 1989 seminal research study on the influence of diet on male championship bodybuilders who used anabolic steroids and those who did not, and another landmark study in 1994 on the diets of elite female and male championship bodybuilder competitors as they prepared for national competition. Back then, there was very little data on strength athletes and nutrition, so when I published the first edition of *Power Eating* in 1998, there was very little scientific information on how to fuel the body for strength sports. Since then, science has rocketed forward and my fifth edition of *Power Eating, The New Power Eating*, is packed with cutting-edge research on strength-training nutrition.

This new edition is not only longer than previous editions but also contains remarkably different information, even compared to the previous edition. Along with tweaks to the amounts and timing of macronutrient and micronutrient intake so that you can more precisely align your diet and supplements with your goals and genetic potential, I have added a full chapter, chapter 7, on the different nutritional needs of female athletes. Research on sport nutrition in female athletes has long been neglected, but now there is breakthrough scientific knowledge that is changing the game of female athletes, including young girls. Their passion to be the best they can be has inspired me to include this new chapter.

There is also a new chapter, chapter 8, on brain fitness as it relates to athletes. From the student athlete to the master athlete, the health of the brain and central nervous system is the foundation to lasting health and superior performance. Because it is rarely discussed within the confines of sport nutrition, I have included in this edition more in-depth guidance on the effect of food on neurobiology. The new chapter leads you through the current and emerging evidence of how food and nutrients affect your mental energy, focus, cognitive performance, memory, mood, coordination, and ability to cope with stress and anxiety and to rest, relax, and sleep. Chapter 11 is a third new chapter that addresses supplements for the brain and nervous system.

The field of sport nutrition practice is both a science and an art. Telling athletes about the science is the more straightforward part. Guiding and motivating them to trust the data, try your suggestions, and develop the internal drive to develop sustainable habits—even when life happens—is the trickier, more artistic part. Throughout this edition, I have included many in-depth discussions about the science and the art of developing sustainable nutrition habits that promote foundational health and high performance.

Part III of *The New Power Eating* is rich with the tools to create a nutrition plan that fits any athlete's body and needs. Since the first edition in 1998, athletes have depended upon the Power Eating menus and recipes to periodize their diets with their training protocols. The New Power Eating menus are unsurpassed in their level of detail yet are practical enough to customize and follow in a busy life. Whether you are trying to maintain, build, cross-train, lose fat, or cut, the New Power Eating diet plans will get your body where you want it to be when you want it to be there, and keep you healthy, safe, and legal. You *can* have it all! Train hard and POWER EAT!

Acknowledgments

Like Charles Darwin's Galapagos finches, *Power Eating* has evolved so much through the last 20 years that it has become a new species: *The New Power Eating*. (Unlike the finches, natural selection was not the influential force!) Since the beginning of this evolution, Maggie Greenwood-Robinson has been at my side—organizing and reformatting content, contributing insights, and sculpting my thoughts and words into an educational and motivational resource that is easy to navigate and fun to read. If writing scientific books for the public were a competitive event, Maggie would be an Olympian. Thank you, Maggie.

The growth of both athletic participation and the body of research in sport nutrition and exercise science has advanced exponentially in 20 years. The thoughtful work of scientists has established a greater collection of data, and the growing desire for evidence-based information and guidance for athletes, trainers, and coaches has created demand for every new edition of the book. I've been able to take *Power Eating* in new directions because of the great contributions of scientists and their subjects and thanks to the interesting questions and comments from my clients, colleagues, and growing community of loyal readers. You are an inspirational force.

Every person at Human Kinetics who interacted with *The New Power Eating* improved the book. We have sometimes struggled to come to an agreement about what the final product will contain and look like, but the expertise and professional wisdom of your team always create a better book, both inside and out. Many thanks to Senior Acquisitions Editor Michelle Maloney, Managing Editor Anna Lan Seaman, Permissions Manager Martha Gullo, Assistant Marketing Director/Publicity Manager Sue Outlaw, Marketing Implementation Manager Jenny Lokshin, and everyone else who contributes so much to this team effort.

Thank you to Savannah Hunt, my intern during part of the research and preparation for writing *The New Power Eating*. Your keen ability to find and catalog research articles was a tremendous stress reducer and time saver. Thank you to superb graphic designer Bernie Wooster, my friend and occasional business partner; the design of the Success Tracker resulted in an artful and useful tool. Everyone who uses it loves it.

To my dear husband, Jeff, who has been my partner and friend for 37 years, thank you for everything. When I was in my PhD program, you inspired me to deeply understand that excellence is a worthwhile goal. As we have continued on our path, taking many unexpected journeys with a sense of adventure, it has been with great love for the challenges that we face, the joy we can create, and the difference that we can make in the world. Your influence on me and support of who I am have made all the difference in my life. To my wonderful daughters, Danielle and Ilana, thank you for continuing to teach me new things, carefully listening and thoughtfully responding to my random ideas and brainstorms, laughing with me, and keeping me in the moment. I am so proud of you. To my one and only brother, Chuck, who loves to imagine and create as much as I do, thank you for always being in my corner. It's a magical place.

PART I

Foundation

The foundation of our knowledge in sport nutrition and exercise science does not change dramatically because the basics of human physiology have been well understood for decades. What motivated me to write this new edition is the accumulation of new evidence regarding mechanisms of physiological and neurological responses and the nuances of dietary genetic signaling, as well as updates to the art of sport nutrition guidance. In *The New Power Eating*, I share all that and more.

While I have included guidance for females in every book that I've written, this edition is robust with new research data, published within the last few years, for active and athletic women and girls, and state-of-the-art guidance that I have developed working with elite, Olympian, and everyday female athletes at all ages and stages of life. Additionally, as gender-specific research has advanced, there is greater recognition of male-centric issues in relation to body shape, physical performance, and emotional well-being. The more advanced science becomes, the greater the clarity about individual metabolic variance and response to diet and exercise training. I have added an amazing amount of new information and two brand new chapters to this section, chapter 7 on female nutrition and chapter 8 on the brain, to this landmark edition of *The New Power Eating*. My goal is to give you the knowledge and understanding to develop a Power Eating plan that adapts and evolves within your training cycles, and the tools to tweak it to make it your own. Chapters 1 through 8 are the foundation to creating your personalized Power Eating plan.

1

Eating for Strength, Power, and Speed

Muscle is strong, and knowledge is power. No matter who you are or where you are in life, having a body that is fit and strong is the most successful life strategy you can pursue, physically and mentally. It's not just about how you look. It's also about how you feel. By knowing how to personalize your workouts, you gain the joy of high strength, energy, and the power to perform, day in and day out.

Keep those images in your mind's eye. This book will show you how to achieve them with a few nips and tucks in one of the most important fitness factors of all—nutrition. But we're not talking about just any type of nutrition. This is a book for people who strength train to stay in shape, compete in strength-training sports, or want to improve their athletic ability. In other words, you're a strength trainer if you lift weights a few times a week or train for any competition. As a strength trainer, you have specific nutritional needs that overlap with your other athletic goals, and depend on your type and level of activity.

So, what kind of strength trainer are you? Are you a bodybuilder, a powerlifter, an Olympic weightlifter, an athlete who strength trains for conditioning and cross-training, or someone who works out with weights to stay in shape? These activities have different physical demands and different nutritional requirements, which is why you will find several individualized strength-training diets in chapters 15 through 19. But the common denominator is that all strength trainers, from competitors to recreational exercisers, are interested in the same thing: building lean muscle.

What Builds Muscle?

Most certainly, strength training builds muscle. But for this construction to take place, you have to supply the construction material: protein, carbohydrate, and fat. In a process called metabolism, the body breaks down these nutrients and uses the products to generate the energy required for growth and life.

During metabolism, proteins are broken down into amino acids. Cells use amino acids to make new proteins based on instructions supplied by DNA, our genetic management system. Through a complex system of translation, DNA provides information on how amino acids are to be lined up and strung together. Once these instructions have been carried out, the cell has synthesized a new protein.

On the basis of this process, logic would tell you that the more protein you eat, the more muscle your body can construct. Sometimes it works that way, and sometimes it doesn't. I will guide you through when and how to put protein to work for you. Too much can also work against your goals, when excess protein is converted to carbohydrate to be used as expensive energy or converted to fat for storage.

The way to make muscles grow is by a special synergy between your body's response to exercise stress and all the nutritional components supplied by your diet. When you place high demands on your muscles, you can make protein work harder. The muscles respond by taking up the nutrients they need, including amino acids from protein metabolism, so they can grow. If you work your muscles hard and give them comprehensive nutritional support, your muscle cells will continue to synthesize the protein required for muscle growth.

What Fuels Muscle?

To work your muscles hard, you have to provide the right kind of fuel. Muscle cells, like all cells, run on a high-energy compound known as adenosine triphosphate (ATP). ATP makes muscles contract, conducts nerve impulses, and promotes other cellular energy processes. Muscle cells create ATP by metabolizing components from food. Carbohydrate is unique among muscle fuel components because it can be utilized for energy with or without adequate oxygen. Fat is also used for fuel by muscles, but fat can be broken down only when oxygen is present, which takes more time. Therefore, it serves as primary fuel for low- to moderate-intensity exercise. When it comes to training intensely for strength, power, and speed, muscle cells prefer to burn fast carbohydrate, use fat for low-intensity exercise, and ideally use protein for growth and repair.

To be clear, carbohydrate and fat fuel muscles under most conditions, with lower and higher proportions of each nutrient based on the intensity (or lack of intensity) of exercise. Our fueling systems can be trained to adjust the proportions of fuel based on what is available from our diets, but this creates only a small margin of change within the extremes of exercise intensity. At one end of the extremes, when you are moving but not exercising, muscle depends primarily on fat for fuel. At the other end, when you are ready to puke or pass out from the high intensity of exercise, your muscles burn virtually all carbohydrate.

Your cells generate ATP through any one of three energy systems: the phosphagen system, the glycolytic system, and mitochondrial respiration, also called the oxidative system.

The Phosphagen System

The phosphagen system creates energy by breaking down and rebuilding ATP through a compound called creatine phosphate (CP), which supplies inorganic phosphate to the metabolic process and allows for the recycling of the high-energy compound. Energy is available for a period of 5 to 10 seconds. Once ATP is used up, it takes less than 5 minutes or up to 15 minutes, depending on depletion, for it to be replenished from the metabolism of additional food components and probably oxygen. During short, intense bursts of exercise such as weight training and sprinting, the working muscles do not have access to adequate oxygen. At this point, CP kicks in to supply energy for a few short seconds of work. CP can help create ATP when ATP is depleted. Any intense exercise lasting for up to 10 seconds rapidly depletes ATP and CP in a muscle; these compounds must then be recycled and replaced. Part of the job of the other two energy systems is replenishing ATP and CP.

The Glycolytic System

As ATP is broken down and exercise lasts longer than 10 seconds, the glycolytic system produces energy. Muscle cells nearly spontaneously begin to take in glucose from the bloodstream, and the glycolytic system makes glucose available to the muscles, either from the breakdown of dietary carbohydrate during digestion or from the breakdown of muscle and liver glycogen, the stored form of carbohydrate. This very rapid process is called glycolysis. During glycolysis, glycogen is disassembled into glucose in the muscles and, through a series of chemical reactions, is ultimately converted into more ATP.

The glycogen reserve in your muscles can supply enough energy for about two to three minutes of short-burst exercise at a time. If sufficient oxygen is available, a lot of ATP will be made from glucose. If oxygen is in short supply, energy metabolism wanes and begins to produce a by-product from glycolysis called lactic acid. Contrary to previous theories on fatigue, the buildup of lactic acid in a working muscle actually allows for the removal of a chemical, pyruvate. Pyruvate can lead to more rapid deterioration of ATP production. Lactate also reduces the buildup of metabolic acidosis (too much acid in the body). However, the ultimate rise in acidosis leads to the reduction of recycling of ATP and an increase in the cellular levels of the components of ATP. The net effect is fatigue. Lactate exits the muscle when oxygen is available to replenish CP and ATP. A brief rest period gives your body time to deliver sufficient oxygen to the muscles, and you can continue exercising.

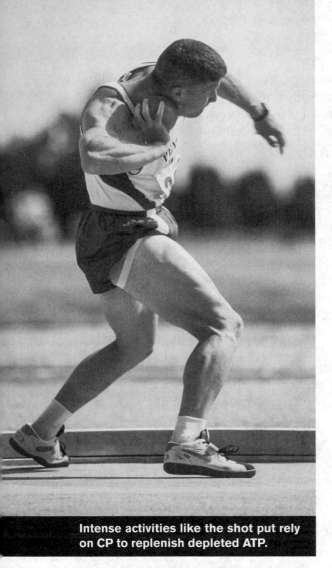

Intense activities like the shot put rely on CP to replenish depleted ATP.

Mitochondrial Respiration: The Oxidative System

The third energy system is mitochondrial respiration, or the oxidative system, in which the oxidation of the food we eat leads to the generation of volts of energy. This system helps fuel aerobic exercise and other endurance activities. Although the oxidative system can handle the energy needs of endurance exercise, all three energy systems kick in to some degree during endurance exercise. The phosphagen and glycolytic energy systems dominate during strength training, with minimal contributions from mitochondrial respiration.

Oxygen is not a direct source of energy for exercise; it is used as an ingredient to produce large amounts of ATP from other energy sources. The oxidative system works as follows: You breathe in oxygen, which the blood subsequently takes from your lungs. Your heart pumps oxygen-rich blood to tissues, including muscle. Hemoglobin, an iron-containing protein of the blood, carries oxygen to the cells to enable them to produce energy. Myoglobin, another type of iron-containing protein, carries oxygen primarily to muscle cells. Inside mitochondria, the powerhouse organelles within muscle cells, carbohydrate and fat are both converted into energy through a series of energy-producing reactions.

Your body's ability to produce energy through any one of these three systems can be improved with the right training diet and exercise program. The result is a fat-burning, muscle-building metabolism.

Nutrition Principles for Strength Trainers

If you are serious about improving your physique and your strength-training performance, you'll do everything you can to achieve success. We have come a long way in understanding the science behind metabolism, and we are still gaining knowledge at an increasing rate. There is some great information available to those who take the time to read, think critically, and evaluate. Unfortunately, there is also advice given to strength trainers today that is a hodgepodge of fact and fiction. It becomes particularly difficult to separate one from the other when kernels of truth are scattered among a wide array of falsehoods. My goal is to help you decipher evidence-based information by sharing several principles with you—principles that all strength trainers can follow to get in shape and achieve their personal best in performance. These principles are the same ones I have advocated for world-class athletes, Olympic contenders, and recreational strength trainers for more than 30 years. Let's review them here.

Always Fuel Your Training

A key to feeling energized is to eat the right amounts of calories to power your body for hard training. In the United States, the terms *calorie* and *energy* are often used interchangeably. Elsewhere, the joule is used as a measurement of energy. Although this book refers to calories, you can convert to kilojoules by multiplying the number of calories by 4.1868. A lack of calories will definitely make you feel like a wet dishrag by the end of your workout. A diet that provides fewer than 1,600 calories per day, for example, generally does not contain all the vitamins and minerals you need to stay healthy, prevent disease, and perform well in an athletic challenge. Very low-calorie diets followed for longer than two weeks can be hazardous to your health, and they do not provide enough of the nutrients needed for basic health. We will discuss the specifics of these issues in later chapters.

Historically, the recommended dietary allowances (RDAs) were the national standard for the amount of carbohydrate, protein, fat, vitamins, and minerals we need in our diets to avoid deficiency diseases and to maintain growth and health. The dietary reference intakes (DRIs) were established to update the RDAs based on more functional criteria instead of criteria based on deficiency diseases. Rather than focusing on avoiding disease, the DRIs focus on optimal performance, both mentally and physically. But under certain conditions—stress, illness, malnutrition, and exercise—we may require a higher intake of certain nutrients. Studies have shown that athletes, in particular, may have to exceed the DRI of many nutrients. Some competitive male bodybuilders have estimated their caloric intake to be greater than 6,000 calories a day during the off-season—roughly three times the DRI for the average person (2,000 calories a day for women and 2,700 calories a day for men). Other studies have demonstrated needs beyond the DRIs for calories and certain vitamins and minerals in athletic females.

How much you need of each nutrient depends on a number of factors, including your age and sex, how hard you train, and whether you are a competitive or recreational strength trainer. Generally, strength trainers need to eat more protein, more of the right kinds of carbohydrate, and more of the right kinds of fat. What's more, you may be wise to supplement your diet with certain vitamins and minerals. As a strength athlete proceeding through the stress of different training cycles, you may benefit by nurturing your gut biome using specific foods and supplements. And certainly what, when, and how you choose to fuel your body affects your mind and emotional outlook. You'll learn more about these issues as you read this book.

If you are trying to gain muscle and lose body fat, eating enough calories and taking in enough nutrients makes the difference between success and failure. Timing, or choosing when during your day you take in your fuel and nutrients, also matters. Restricting fuel just before or after your training leads to a less-than-optimal workout and recovery, resulting in you not reaching your goals. Fueling before, during, and after training is a hallmark of Power Eating. Then, if burning fat is your goal, you will learn how to plan your nutrition for the parts of the day when you are not exercising in order to meet those goals.

Put Carbohydrate to Work for You

It's well known that most athletes, strength trainers included, don't eat enough carbohydrate, the primary fuel for high-intensity training. Most athletes follow diets in which less than half of the total daily calories come from carbohydrate, but during high levels of training at least 5 to 7 grams of carbohydrate per kilogram of body weight should be consumed daily. That's more than half of an athlete's total calories, so eating enough carbohydrate is extremely important for a heavyweight competitive bodybuilder or Olympic weightlifter. If you lift to support other sport goals such as swimming, skiing, or skating, your carbohydrate needs are just as high, or perhaps even higher.

Lots of bodybuilders practice very low-carbohydrate dieting because they believe it promotes faster weight loss. What's more, many athletic females believe that their bodies won't use carbohydrate to fuel their exercise but instead will turn it into body fat. As a result, they perpetually underfuel their training and may never reach their competitive potential.

The problem with low-carbohydrate diets is that they deplete glycogen, the body's storage form of carbohydrate. Once glycogen stores are emptied, you start to have less-than-maximum workouts, and the body starts burning protein from tissues, including muscle tissue, to meet its energy demands. You lose hard-earned muscle as a result. Furthermore, for both women and men, health may be compromised.

The real story on carbohydrate for weight control and muscle building is that you should select whole-food carbohydrate—natural, complex carbohydrate as close to its natural state as possible—instead of refined, processed carbohydrate. What's the difference? A blueberry is a whole-food carbohydrate; a blueberry toaster pastry is a processed carbohydrate. Even so, when used in a targeted way, starches and sugars can be an athlete's best friend by providing the right fuel at the right time around training. But keep in mind that eating processed carbohydrate without a plan and without a purpose can be unhealthy.

One important reason whole foods are better than processed foods has to do with their high fiber content. Fiber is the remnant of plant foods that remains undigested by the body. It's what keeps your bowel movements regular and your gut well populated with healthy bacteria. Fiber is also a proven fat fighter. Research shows that people who eat healthy, high-fiber diets have smaller waistlines, for example, and are able to better control their weight. The bottom line is that the right types of carbohydrate can help you manage your weight.

Sport Nutrition Fact Versus Fiction: Is Carbohydrate Fattening?

Much misinformation exists about whether carbohydrate is fattening. Here's the real deal: Eating too much food is fattening. Further, eating sugary foods and highly processed foods, plus consuming carbohydrate alone (without protein and fat), is what triggers fat gain. By contrast, the right kinds of carbohydrate—meaning natural, unprocessed carbohydrate—will help you build muscle and get lean. What's more, these foods are low in calories. The healthiest diet for weight loss, disease prevention, and physical performance is one that combines carbohydrate, protein, and high-performance fat. So the problem does not lie in high-carbohydrate foods; the problem is poor selection and mindless eating of carbohydrate, in particular, and food, in general.

You will learn more about carbohydrate in chapter 3, especially how to personalize the right types of carbohydrate in the right amounts at the right times to fuel your muscles and your training, enhance performance, and sculpt your body better than ever.

Vary Your Diet

One of the delicious benefits of training hard is that you get to eat well—with a variety of foods in your diet. This means more than just choosing foods from all different food groups, however. It means eating a variety of foods within all the food groups.

All foods contain key nutrients, such as micronutrients, phytochemicals, bioactive compounds, probiotics, prebiotics, fibers, and other food factors. But these can be remarkably different from one food to another. For instance, the total nutritional compounds in a banana are very different than those found in a strawberry or a mango. The fats and fibers in flaxseeds are very different than those found in almonds and cashews. Fermented yogurts are different than skim milk. Fish is different than beef or eggs. Oats are vastly different than quinoa or buckwheat. It is variety in our diets that ensures that we obtain the most wholesome and life-giving properties from the foods that we eat.

Sometimes athletes such as bodybuilders follow unvaried, unhealthy diets. The first study I ever conducted investigated the training diets of male competitive bodybuilders. What I found was that they ate a lot of calories, roughly 6,000 a day or more. The worrisome finding from this study was that they ate, on average, more than 200 grams of fat a day. That's almost as much fat as you'd find in two sticks of butter! In the short term, that's enough to make most people sick. Eaten habitually over time, such an enormous amount of unhealthy fat may lead to heart disease.

Bodybuilding diets, especially precontest diets, tend to be monotonous, with the same foods showing up on the plate day after day. The worst example I've ever seen was a bodybuilder who ate chicken, pepper, vinegar, and rice for three days straight while preparing for competition. This is a good example of a diet that lacks variety. Without a variety of foods, you miss out on nutrients essential for peak health. By contest day, you certainly are not the picture of health, despite your best intentions.

As bodybuilders prepare for contests, they frequently don't eat much fruit, red meat, or dairy products. Fruit, of course, is packed with disease-fighting, health-building antioxidants and phytochemicals. Red meat is an important source of vital minerals like iron and zinc. And dairy products supply important nutrients such as bone-building calcium and bioactive proteins that promote lean muscle growth.

When people limit or eliminate such foods from their diet, potentially serious deficiencies begin to show up. In studies conducted by myself and others, the most common deficiencies observed are those of calcium and zinc, particularly during the precompetition season. Many female bodybuilders have dangerous shortages of these minerals year round. A chronic short supply of calcium increases the risk of osteoporosis, a crippling bone-thinning disease. Although a woman's need for zinc is small (8 milligrams a day), adequate zinc is an impenetrable line of defense when it comes to protecting against disease and infection.

In short, deficits of these minerals can harm health and performance. But the good news is that skim milk, red meat, and dark-meat poultry help alleviate some of these problems. A 3-ounce (90 g) portion of lean sirloin beef, for example, has about 6 milligrams of zinc; nonfat, 1or 2 percent milk has about 1 milligram of zinc in one 8-ounce (240 ml) glass; and 3 ounces (90 g) of dark-meat turkey have about 4 milligrams of zinc.

Another nutritional problem among bodybuilders is fluid restriction. Just before a contest, bodybuilders don't drink much water, fearing it will inflate their physique to the point of blurring their muscular definition. Compounding the problem, many bodybuilders take diuretics and laxatives, a practice that flushes more water, as well as precious minerals called electrolytes, from the body. Generally, body-builders compete in a dehydrated state. At one contest, I saw two people pass out on stage—one because of severe dehydration, the other because of an electrolyte imbalance. This practice is also common in other weight-class sports such as boxing, mixed martial arts and ultimate fighting, rowing, and weightlifting, but in these sports athletes try to rehydrate and refuel after their weigh-ins.

After a competition, bodybuilders tend to go hog wild with food. There's nothing wrong with this, as long as it's a temporary splurge for a few days. But such dietary indulgence over a long time can lead to extra body fat. Even worse, there have been clinical reports of dangerously high levels of blood fats and oxidative stress due to one very high-fat and high-calorie food binge. So beware of going off the deep end with your diet.

Most bodybuilders, however, do a lot of things right, especially during the training season. For one thing, they eat several meals throughout the day—a practice that nutritionists recommend to the general public.

Time and Combine Your Food and Nutrients

To achieve superb shape and maximum performance, forgo the usual approach of three meals a day. Active people must fuel themselves throughout the day, eating small meals and snacks every two to four hours, preferably timed around their workout schedules. As we'll see, these meals don't include just any type of food.

When eating multiple meals, you always want to combine protein with carbohydrate and fat. Examples would be a turkey sandwich, a sprouted grain bread with peanut butter, or an apple with nuts. Eating multiple meals also promotes variety in your diet and keeps your blood sugar levels even so that you avoid peaks and valleys throughout the day (a cycle that may cause poor appetite control and promote fat storage).

By including small amounts of protein in meals and snacks, you can control your appetite, feed your muscles more efficiently, and maintain muscle while losing fat. You also may burn fat better because eating protein, as well as eating multiple small meals, has been shown to increase thermogenesis, the process by which your body converts ingested calories and stored fat into heat. Another advantage of multiple meals is mental performance. Eating regular, timed meals helps you think and process information more effectively, increases your attention span, and boosts your mood.

Some research is ambiguous regarding the impact of eating several small, frequent meals versus three large meals in a day. However, I have found that for the reasons stated above it is often a good strategic choice. The bottom line is that how you feel using your established habits is what matters. For many people who seek both better athletic performance and improved physiques, eating small, frequent meals throughout the day is the best fat-burning, muscle-building strategy to pursue. Table 1.1 provides a look at how to time your meals properly and the benefits of doing so. The supplements listed in the table are discussed in detail elsewhere in this book.

Use a Food Plan

Any nutritional program aimed at losing body fat and building muscle should be based on a food plan that emphasizes lean protein, natural carbohydrate, and good fat. It should also include sample menus and recipes as well as information on how to make healthy selections that are personalized to your lifestyle. It should be neither so restrictive that it invites failure nor so unstructured that it causes confusion. These are precisely the guidelines for food planning that you will find here. More specifically, if your goals are to develop lean muscle while reducing body fat, then your plan should take into consideration several factors, including balancing protein, carbohydrate, and fat; increasing your water intake; organizing your food into multiple meals; timing your intake; and incorporating certain dietary supplements into the mix.

TABLE 1.1 Timing Meals

Throughout the day

Fluids: 8-12 cups (2-3 L) a day; at least 5 cups (1 L) should be water.

Breakfast: Never skip this meal! It improves physical and mental performance and helps regulate weight.

Meals: Small, frequent protein–carbohydrate (+fat) meals and snacks every 2-4 h.

Before exercise

Fluids: At least 8 oz (240 ml) before exercise.

Preexercise meal: At least 4 h before exercise so that the body properly assimilates carbohydrate for use by muscles.

Preexercise fuel: 30-90 min before exercise. Fuel should consist of 200-400 calories, including 30-70 g carbohydrate, 10-20 g protein, and no more than 5-7 g fat. Snack can be food or sport fuel supplement. This snack will provide additional energy for prolonged stamina and help decrease exercise-induced breakdown of muscle protein. If stomach emptying is slow, remove protein and use carbohydrate only.

Optional preexercise supplements: Consume these with your preexercise fuel: creatine (2-5 g); beta-alanine (amount depends on daily dosing); beetroot juice (dose according to product label); MSM; probiotic; cinnamon; cayenne; green tea; black tea; caffeine (3mg/kg); theacrine.

During exercise

Fluids: According to thirst or 7-10 oz (210-300 ml) every 10-20 min.

Carbohydrate sport drinks with or without electrolyte, as needed; sipping these during a long workout has been shown to extend endurance. Use them during phases when you're trying to build muscle but not when you're trying to lose fat.

After exercise

Fluids: Replace each pound (0.5 kg) of fluid lost with 16-24 oz (480-720 ml) of water or other beverage.

Carbohydrate: Consume 0.5-1.2 g/kg depending on what phase you're in.

Protein: Consume 0.5 g/kg protein with carbohydrate to encourage muscle growth. Postexercise snacks can be in the form of meal-replacement beverages with 0.5-1.2 g/kg of rapid carbohydrate and 0.5 g/kg high-quality protein. Solid food is also acceptable.

Follow this within 2 h of exercise with a meal containing lots of unprocessed carbohydrate and high-quality protein sources (e.g., fish, lean meats, low-fat dairy products, eggs, high-quality plant proteins).

Optional recovery supplements: Consume these with your meal replacement: creatine (2-5 g); glutamine (4-10 g); beta-alanine (amount depends on daily dosing); probiotic; cinnamon; turmeric/curcumin; ginger; tart cherry juice.

You have to be mindful about what you eat, and you need to make the right choices. Each decision about the calories that you put into your mouth has to be results oriented. To drive your fat-burning machinery and lose weight, for example, specific foods can go to work for you. These include dairy foods, whey protein, fish, soy, nuts, olives and olive oil, and green tea, to name a few. With the information you'll learn here, you can create a healthy diet that promotes fat loss and muscle gain.

Protein, Strength, and Muscle Building

For generations, athletes have believed that a high-protein diet will increase strength. This belief can be traced to a famous Greek athlete, Milo of Crotona, in the sixth century BCE. One of the strongest men in Greece, Milo was the wrestling victor in five Olympic Games and many other festivals. As the legend goes, he applied progressive resistance training by lifting a growing calf daily. When the calf was four years old, he carried it the length of the Olympian stadium, killed it, roasted it, and ate it. It is written that his normal daily intake of meat was about 20 pounds (9 kg).

While this may sound like a great idea to some people, Milo's dietary intake was quite monotonous, and protein alone does not build muscle. However, by cooking the meat, Milo did his body a favor. Cooking makes protein more readily available to your body. A protein molecule is a string of amino acids connected like a strand of pearls. If two strands of pearls were wound together and then twisted to double up on each other, they would resemble a protein molecule. Heating or cooking the protein molecule unwinds the string of amino acids, straightens it out, and separates it into smaller pieces. This is the process of heat denaturing, which is similar to the process of chemical denaturing, otherwise known as digestion. Cooking foods with protein can begin the digestive process and can actually decrease the net energy that the body must expend during digestion.

Protein is extremely vital in your diet, but by itself it is not the magic bullet for muscle gain. Instead, protein and carbohydrate together are the magic bullet, especially in combination with the right kinds of fat. In other words, you must place equal emphasis on the right types of protein, carbohydrate, and fat in your diet. These nutrients work in concert to give you the edge on building body-firming muscle.

Boost Recovery With
Anti-Inflammatory Foods

To build lean, quality muscle, there are two requirements: First, strength train to trigger muscle growth. Second, follow my recommended diet, which includes lean protein to repair damaged tissue and carbohydrate and fat to fuel the training and rebuilding process. Beyond those critical factors, your ultimate success or failure boils down to your ability to recover—that is, how fast and effectively you can bounce back from your training efforts. This is where anti-inflammatory foods make their entrance.

Training promotes inflammation in the body. The two main types of inflammation are classic and systemic. Classic inflammation, which accompanies physical injuries, results in swelling and pain; this is part of the protection and repair process and is considered relatively benign. Once the injury is healed, classic inflammation subsides.

Systemic inflammation, on the other hand, continues and is chronic. It can't be seen by the naked eye but can increase the risk for a number of diseases, including allergies, cancer, joint pain, heart disease, Alzheimer's disease, periodontal disease, and irritable bowel syndrome. Recent research suggests that systemic inflammation of systems or tissues may be the root of the fastest-growing preventable diseases: type 2 diabetes and obesity. These are generally considered lifestyle diseases because of their linked risk factors and the habits that have been proven to help prevent and reverse them (diet and exercise).

POWER PROFILE: Calorie Sources

Calories are certainly important in building muscle mass; however, the source of those calories is crucial if you want to be healthy, maximize muscle, and minimize body fat. A case in point is a professional rookie football player who wanted to lose weight to improve his speed on the field. Unless he trimmed down, his chance to be on the team was in jeopardy, so he needed a dramatic nutritional rescue.

This football player was eating slightly more than 7,000 calories a day. Broken down, those calories figured out to about 17 percent protein, 32 percent fat, and 49 percent carbohydrate. In daily fat grams, he was consuming a whopping 250 grams a day. The composition of his calories was an impediment to losing fat. I reconfigured his diet to 5,680 calories a day; 15 percent of those calories came from protein, 25 percent from fat, and 60 percent from carbohydrate. That mix slashed his fat grams to a healthier 142 grams a day.

He had been eating a lot of unhealthy fat in foods such as fried chicken, whole milk, and fast foods. These foods are full of pro-inflammatory fats, and inflammation can stall fat loss. For the high-fat foods, we substituted fish and skinless chicken breasts, 1 percent milk, and fast-food choices such as salads and frozen yogurt that were lower in fat. In addition, we modified some of his favorite dishes such as sweet potato pie into healthier versions. He also began to load up on anti-inflammatory foods containing complex carbohydrate, such as brown rice, whole-wheat bread, fruits, and vegetables. Plus, he began using leaner protein sources with a wider variety of choices.

The upshot of these dietary changes was that he lost the weight, made the team, and had a great season. He completed a full professional career on the gridiron and remains a healthy athlete into retirement.

Both types of inflammation exist throughout your body in various degrees and are influenced by external factors such as the food you eat, your workouts, and even the air you breathe. Researchers in South Korea found that eating large quantities of sugar and fat, even from just a few meals, causes an increased concentration of free radicals in the bloodstream, which creates inflammation in the body.

While the best sources of anti-inflammatory compounds are always foods, it is oftentimes difficult for athletes who are in hard training to eat enough food throughout the day to consume the nutrition they need and still feel empty enough to train. Because the goal of the Power Eating plan is to help you enhance your performance and achieve your goals, this is the time that I often recommend that my clients supplement their diets with anti-inflammatory compounds. As you read the micronutrient chapters, you will learn more about the best timing for eating and supplementing with these compounds to get the most out of your plan.

The Scoop on Supplements and Functional Foods

Many people ask me why we need to supplement if their diets are so complete. The answer goes back to the science of nutritional anthropology. According to investigations of early human life and lifestyles, our ancestors consumed and expended approximately 3,500 calories per day, on average. This number of calories was not necessarily consumed each day, but the foods they ate were very dense in nutrients and low in calories. Overall, their daily diets were composed of many nutrient-dense foods. When early humans exercised, it was in short bursts such as spearing a predator; in very long-duration, low-intensity activity such as tracking prey; or in long, moderate-intensity activity such as seeking new hunting grounds or foraging for roots and berries. At the same time, they also had long periods of recovery.

Today, most people can't consume 3,500 calories a day without gaining a lot of body fat. And anyone exercising to burn off 3,500 calories a day probably doesn't get enough recovery time. By consuming that many calories each day, our ancestors were taking in enough nutrients, fiber, and phytochemicals to maintain health, although they certainly did not live the long average life span that we have today. They had virtually the same bodies we have today, yet if we eat fewer than 3,500 calories daily in order to avoid gaining weight, we definitely don't get in the nutrition we need. On the other hand, if we consume 3,500 calories in order to replace our daily energy needs, we don't get the density of nutrients or the recovery time we need. The solution to this conundrum lies in supplementation. We need to supplement to achieve optimum performance and to continually enhance our performance and our health.

The supplement industry has finally recognized that consumers are looking for better-quality supplements. Some companies have pulled the supplement industry up by its bootstraps, conducting independent third-party laboratory testing for purity and potency and raising the bar of consumer expectations and quality guarantees. These companies have even conducted scientific studies on their products to ensure that they are pure and that they work. These are very promising developments in the supplement industry.

Another promising development is occurring in a category of foods called functional foods. These are foods or food ingredients that can prevent disease or improve health. Some well-known examples are calcium-fortified orange juice and fiber-enhanced cereal. But practically everything from milk to protein shakes to chocolate is being upgraded to functional food status through the addition of nutrient all-stars such as calcium, antioxidants, omega-3 essential fat, and probiotics. Other foods, such as Greek yogurt, green tea, berries, and most vegetables, are naturally functional. Functional foods provide extra nutrients, vitamins, minerals, protein, phytochemicals, enzymes, and other elements that give you energy, help fight disease and aging, and, for strength trainers, build muscle. Together, eating pure food, taking targeted, high-quality supplements, and enhancing your diet with functional foods most definitely gives you an edge.

How to Be a Power Eater if You're a Vegetarian

As I travel around the United States, one of the most common questions I'm asked is how to follow my Power Eating plan as a vegetarian. If you still eat fish, dairy, and eggs, the plan is really easy to follow. There is no need to eat meat or poultry. Whenever you see lean or very lean protein servings in the menu plan, just substitute fish or plant protein from such sources as beans or legumes. One-half cup of beans is equivalent to one very lean protein serving, plus one starch serving.

If you've eliminated fish, dairy, and eggs from your diet, or you are completely vegan (those who eat no animal products of any kind), you will have to put in a bit of extra effort to follow the Power Eating plan, but you probably already have noticed that about your diet. Substitute whole soy foods for eggs in the menu. They both contain the important phospholipids (a type of fat) from lecithin that are critical for brain health. Just make sure to eat soy foods that contain all the natural fat, such as soybeans, edamame, tofu, tempeh, and whole soy milk or yogurt with the fat still in it.

Substituting for dairy is just as easy as substituting for protein. Use soy milk or other plant-based milks such as rice milk or nut milks. Make sure they are fortified with calcium and vitamins A and D, all of which are very important for brain and body health. Milks other than soy milk are not really great substitutes for cow's milk because they are lower in protein and higher in fat and sugar. However, if you provide for that protein elsewhere in your diet, you will benefit from the fortification of calcium and vitamins that these milks provide.

Unfortunately, there is no easy substitute for fish. Only 5 percent of the type of omega-3 fat from flaxseed and other vegetable sources (alpha-linolenic acid, ALA) is converted into the two omega-3 fats found in fish (docosahexaenoic acid, DHA, and eicosapentaenoic acid, EPA). These are the two critical fats needed by the heart, brain, and central nervous system, and for all-around general health. Although the protein from fish is excellent, you can substitute other protein for a similar benefit. However, nothing that we currently know of substitutes as easily for marine oils.

If you don't eat fish because of taste preferences, then use a fish oil supplement. If you are allergic to fish, then you must consult your physician before using a supplement. Some of my vegan clients are using algal supplements of DHA and EPA with the understanding that they are much more expensive, and the recommended dosages on the labels are often much lower than what I recommend as a daily dose, so they need to double and triple the dose. Others have decided to use fish oil supplements because it is such an important health issue. Plus, they are less expensive and can be found more easily. Either way, you will certainly feel the difference when you consume optimal amounts of EPA and DHA. But this is certainly a personal choice.

If you have eliminated all animal products from your diet, you must add some important nutrients back in, such as vitamins B_{12} and D. You can purchase foods fortified with these vitamins, or you can take a multivitamin–mineral supplement that supplies them. Active women especially may have difficulty taking in enough iron and zinc. These nutrients can be in your supplement, too. Eat plenty of dark green leafy veggies, which contain calcium and iron. Also, choose calcium-fortified soy milk and orange juice. A supplement can also cover your calcium needs.

Adopting a plant-based vegetarian diet can be a great weight-loss strategy. One of the hardest things about losing weight is keeping it off. Several studies have identified many diet plans that can help you lose weight, but the problem is finding one you can stick with for longer than a few months. Some studies have shown that people on vegetarian weight-loss plans were able to stick with them longer than people who undertook some of the well-known diet fads. A study conducted at the University of North Carolina at Chapel Hill investigated the difference in weight-loss outcomes after one and two years between a group of postmenopausal women who followed a vegan diet and a group who followed a more moderate low-fat diet. The study also compared women who were offered support-group follow-up and those who were on their own. Vegans lost more weight and maintained a greater weight loss after one and two years. Those participants who received follow-up support maintained an even greater weight loss.

A study published in the *International Journal of Obesity* (2008) showed no greater weight loss or maintenance over 18 months in participants following a lacto-ovo vegetarian diet pattern than in those following a standard calorie- and fat-reduced diet. The authors noted, however, that those following the vegetarian diet pattern "had a significantly greater reduction in animal protein and greater increases in vegetable protein and in dietary fiber, all beneficial changes" (Burke et al., p 173).

You're doing your health a huge favor by emphasizing more fruits, vegetables, and whole grains in your diet. Plant-based diets appear to be protective against several types of cancer, including cancers of the breast, ovaries, lung, colon, esophagus, and stomach. Vegetarian-style eating may protect you from cardiovascular disease, diabetes, age-related macular degeneration, and overall mortality. That said, the conclusions from these and other studies raise a number of questions. Should athletes or people trying to increase muscle size, strength, and power restrict their intake of animal protein foods? Can they achieve their goals by adopting vegetarian diets or vegan diets? Or should they adopt a more varied diet following a more omnivorous

Sport Nutrition Fact Versus Fiction: Are Organic Foods Better for You?

With the amount of food strength trainers eat, many are opting to go organic to avoid the chemical fertilizers, pesticides, and additives used in many foods. Do you get an advantage in buying organic foods?

In general, organically grown foods are grown in soil-enriched with organic fertilizers rather than synthetic fertilizers and treated only with nonsynthetic pesticides. Organic farms use a soil-building program that promotes vibrant soil and healthy plants, usually including crop rotation and biological pest control.

In addition to plants, farmers can raise animals according to organic methods and produce organic meat, poultry, and egg products. These foods come from farms that have been inspected to verify that they meet rigorous standards mandating the use of organic feed, prohibiting the use of antibiotics, and giving animals access to the outdoors, fresh air, and sunlight.

You can tell the difference between organically produced food and conventionally produced food by looking at package labels. The United States Department of Agriculture (USDA) has developed strict labeling rules to help consumers know the exact organic content of the food they buy. Look for the USDA Organic seal; it tells you that a product is at least 95 percent organic.

Organic foods may have some advantages over conventionally produced foods. Here is what some of the latest research shows:

- Organic foods may be highly nutritious. According to a review of literature published in 2017 in the *Annual Review of Public Health*, organic food may be somewhat higher in vitamin C, beneficial fats, some minerals, antioxidants, phytochemicals, and bioactive compounds. Organic produce may be somewhat lower in protein and nitrogen, and organic milk may be lower in iodine and selenium.

- Organic foods have a lower risk of contamination from nitrates, the heavy metal cadmium, and pesticide residues. Mycotoxins may be lower in some organically raised cereals.

- Consuming organic food appears to lower concerns over the health hazards associated with pesticide contamination. In one study, children who ate organic produce and juice had only one-sixth the level of pesticide by-products in their urine, compared to children who ate conventionally produced food. Similar results have been found repeatedly when testing adults in various parts of the world. There are thus some important safety concerns for eating conventionally grown food. However, the crucial clinical evidence of adverse health consequences from low levels of exposure to pesticides has been limited. Studies have focused more on the amounts of exposure, and questions and concerns regarding the impact of exposure on long term health and development remain unanswered.

- Organic foods have little pesticide residue, and may be potentially safer than nonorganic foods. One study found that farmworkers who apply pesticides as part of conventional farming have higher concentrations of pesticides in their bodies. Conceivably, a continuation of the trend toward organic farming may help protect farmworkers from unhealthy exposures.

- Organic foods are not only good for you—they are also good for the planet. Organic farming methods are generally less harmful to the environment than conventional methods. The use of natural products helps to improve the soil. Organic pest control generally relies on preventive measures such as crop rotation and biological controls. These methods place little to no stress on the earth or its wildlife inhabitants. With organic agriculture now being embraced as environmentally sound and more sustainable than mainstream agriculture, consumers believe they are contributing to a better future and an improved environment, according to one survey.

Also, organic produce often tastes better than nonorganic produce. Here in Seattle, where I live, lots of organic food is grown locally. Consequently, the produce is very fresh because it hasn't been transported vast distances and therefore hasn't lost its flavor.

The most important move you can make healthwise is to eat more plant foods, organic or not. Much research shows that people can improve their health and the quality of their lives by consuming more fruits, vegetables, grains, nuts, and seeds. Despite the use of pesticides, populations that eat a wide variety and large amount of fruits and vegetables have lower rates of cancer and other life-threatening illnesses than populations that eat few fruits and vegetables.

In most cases you'll pay more for organic produce, so if your pocketbook is light, or if organic food is just not available nearby, buy fresh conventional produce and follow these guidelines for reducing pesticide residues in foods:

- Wash fresh produce in water. Use a scrub brush, and rinse the produce thoroughly under running water.

- Use a knife to peel an orange or grapefruit; do not bite into the peel.

- Discard the outer leaves of leafy vegetables such as cabbage and lettuce.

- Peel waxed fruit and vegetables; waxes don't wash off and can seal in pesticide residues.

- Peel vegetables such as carrots and fruits such as apples when appropriate. (Peeling not only removes pesticides that remain in or on the peel but also removes fiber, vitamins, and minerals.)

In the end, the choice is yours. Purchasing organic foods is not just a nutritional issue but a political, social, and personal issue as well. If you want to treat the earth well and potentially protect workers from pesticide exposure, speak with your pocketbook: Buy organic.

pattern, including both animal protein and plant protein? There has been quite a bit of research in this area, but the questions remain largely unanswered.

Studies do show that you can build muscle on both types of diets. What I have found in my own practice, however, is that it is very difficult to create a high-performance nutrition program if you are a vegan (i.e., you eat no animal products of any type). The time required to shop, plan, and prepare a vegan diet can be excessive if you are an athlete living on your own and are responsible for preparing your own meals. Additionally, vegan diets are high in fiber and that much fiber, even though it promotes health, is filling. If you fully fuel yourself on fiber-rich foods, you may always feel too full to train or exercise at peak capacity. The vegan concept may sound good philosophically and in theory but in practice can be very difficult to carry out. Of course, someone always points to a famous vegan athlete as the reason for wanting to follow a vegan diet, but it's no surprise that you can count the number of champion vegan athletes on one hand. There just aren't very many, and the reason is that it's simply too difficult to stay healthy and competitive on such a restrictive diet. Those vegan athletes who are successful typically are already genetically gifted in their sport, and they often have a support team to help them plan, shop, and cook. While it is getting easier to find more vegan convenience-style foods and supplements, making it easier to follow a vegan diet, the overall goal of Power Eating is to minimize the amount of prepared and processed foods in your diet. The bottom line is that athletes will find eating a vegan diet more time-consuming and possibly more filling, but it is certainly not impossible. To achieve nutritional wellness and peak performance, you really need to be mindful and knowledgeable about meeting your nutritional needs. Whenever possible, I encourage my clients to follow a mixed-protein diet that is plant centered but not exclusively plant based. There will be more on eating vegetarian and vegan style throughout the book.

Where Do You Stand Now?

Analyze your present diet now to see exactly what you're eating, particularly in terms of the three energy nutrients. You should also analyze how much water you're drinking, because water is a critical nutrient. This analysis will make the following chapters more relevant and interesting. For example, when you're reading about protein, you may wonder how much protein you're eating now. With this analysis handy, you can find out quickly.

Using the form provided in appendix A, record everything you eat over the course of three to seven days. Choose days that best represent your typical diet. Be as accurate as you can in terms of the amount of food you eat. Use the information in chapters 13 and 14 to help you figure out nutrients and calories.

Alternatively, you can use an online diet tracker with a nutrient database to help you record and analyze your macronutrient and energy intake. Nearly all free, online tools are full of ads and will try to upsell you to their fee-based, more professional tool. Beware that many databases contain missing data, and your diet analyses results are only as complete and accurate as the data contained in the database.

2
Manufacturing Muscle

Inside your body, a marvelous process of self-repair takes place day in and day out, and it all has to do with protein, the nutrient responsible for building and maintaining body tissues. Protein is present everywhere in the body—in muscles, bones, connective tissue, blood vessels, blood cells, brain cells, skin, hair, and fingernails. This protein is slowly but consistently being degraded or broken down at varying rates within different tissues as a result of normal physiological wear and tear and must be replaced. The younger you are the greater your protein turnover, meaning that your cells and tissues rejuvenate more frequently. Part of the aging process is the slowing of protein turnover and cellular rejuvenation. The good news is that exercise helps with cellular rejuvenation as long as you've got all the amino acids to support the ongoing rebuilding process.

The mechanism by which this repair occurs is really quite amazing. During digestion, protein in food is dismantled by other proteins (enzymes) into subunits called amino acids. Amino acids then enter cells, and other enzymes, nucleic compounds, and director proteins, acting on instructions translated from DNA, put them back together as the new proteins needed to build and repair tissue. Virtually no other system in the world repairs itself so wonderfully. Every day, this process goes on and life continues.

Under any condition of growth—childhood, pregnancy, muscle building—the body manufactures more cells than are lost. From an energy source such as carbohydrate or fat, the body can manufacture many of the materials needed to make new cells. But to replace and build new protein, the body must have protein from food in the form of the nitrogen-containing amino acids. Unlike carbohydrate and fat, protein contains nitrogen, and nitrogen is required to synthesize new protein.

Protein, therefore, is absolutely necessary for the maintenance, replacement, and growth of body tissue. But protein has other uses, too. The body uses protein to regulate hormone secretion, maintain the body's water balance, protect against disease, transport nutrients in and out of cells, carry oxygen, and regulate blood clotting.

Protein and Muscle Building

Protein is a key player in the repair and construction of muscle tissue, and we now know more about how to use protein to drive anabolic (tissue building or growth) machinery right down to the molecular level. Keep in mind that a balance is needed between protein synthesis and protein degradation; to build lean muscle, synthesis must be greater than degradation. With the right nutrition, muscle protein degradation is turned down and muscle protein synthesis is turned up.

A messaging system within your cells directly affects protein synthesis in your muscles. When you stress your muscles through resistance training, a cascade of biochemical events within your muscle cells responds to initiate the manufacture of new proteins, which ultimately leads to larger muscle tissue. However, enough amino acids must be available to jump-start this process. By supplying your body with protein and energy, particularly around exercise and for the next 48 hours afterward, you can keep yourself in an anabolic state.

A 2017 research study published in the journal *Cell Metabolism* pointed out that the muscle-building process can be maximized by performing high-intensity interval training (HIIT), in both young and older adults. HIIT involves resistance-type exercise performed at a very high intensity for a short duration with brief periods of rest between bouts. It induces rapid changes that initiate genetic responses and messages to ultimately alter muscle cell proteins and generate new proteins. The net effect is an increase in muscle size, strength, and power. HIIT should not replace your heavy lifting, however, but can be used in conjunction with it.

Along with building muscle when muscle cells are stressed through exercise, they increase their capacity to shore up their antioxidant systems as a protective reaction. Thus, it is vital to supply the body with antioxidant-rich foods along with protein. However, timing is important. According to recent data, after exercise may not be the optimal time to take antioxidant-rich supplements. I will give you the details on this in chapter 9. With this knowledge, you can target the protein and antioxidant needs of your muscles during and after training.

Protein and Fat Burning

Studies have suggested that, compared with diets high in carbohydrate and low in fat, diets high in protein and low in fat promote greater weight loss. One reason is that lean protein helps stoke your fat-burning fires. Its thermogenic (heat-producing) effect may be as high as 22 percent, compared with as low as 0.8 percent for carbohydrate. In other words, you burn more calories by doing nothing more than eating slightly more protein and less carbohydrate.

A research review position stand published in 2017 by the *International Society of Sports Nutrition* explains that, "Of the macronutrients, protein has the highest thermic effect and is the most metabolically expensive. Given this, it is not surprising that higher protein intakes have been seen to preserve resting energy expenditure while dieting. This is particularly true among active individuals" (7).

If you are an active woman taking oral contraceptive pills (OC), however, high-protein diets may not be as effective. Swiss researchers discovered that there was no thermic effect (a factor in fat-burning) of a high-protein diet when women were on the pill. Somehow, oral contraceptives interrupted the process of protein-induced thermogenesis—which means it becomes more challenging to burn body fat if you are a woman taking these drugs.

An increased sense of satiety (the feeling of fullness after eating) is associated with the thermogenic effect of protein. In one study, women on high-protein, moderate-carbohydrate meals had greater satiety during meals and for longer periods after meals compared with women on low-protein meals. The difference is associated with the thermogenic effect of the meal. Most people following a higher-protein, moderate-carbohydrate diet feel more satisfied and have greater control over what and how much they eat.

To capitalize on the thermogenic effect of high-protein meals, you should consume protein in frequent meals and snacks throughout the day. This allows for the most efficient absorption and use of protein. It also helps maintain higher levels of energy production to promote weight loss as well as promote additional strength and power.

As I stated in chapter 1, there is conflicting research regarding whether eating three large meals a day or multiple smaller meals a day has any advantage in supporting weight loss. Most of that weight-loss research didn't study athletes. What I have seen in my practice is that it really depends on what athletes can fit into their life, the timing during their off-season, and what strategy makes them feel the best and, of course, most effectively fuels their performance. Once they've experimented with both strategies, I find that in most cases multiple smaller daily meals win out.

Protein and Strength-Training Performance

It would seem that the more construction material (protein) you supply your body, the more muscle you'll build. If you are an active strength trainer and you do challenging workouts, along with consuming enough energy, this theory may be more true than many had previously thought. The key here, as discussed throughout this book, is that you need to continue rigorous training and give your body not only extra protein but also extra calories to fuel hard training and build more muscle.

To build muscle, you must maintain a positive nitrogen balance. Nitrogen leaves the body primarily in the urine and must be replaced by nitrogen taken in from food. Protein contains a fairly large concentration of nitrogen. Generally, healthy adults are in a state of nitrogen equilibrium, or zero balance—that is, their protein intake meets their protein requirement. A positive nitrogen balance means that the body is retaining dietary protein and using it to synthesize new tissue. If more nitrogen is excreted than consumed, the nitrogen balance is negative. The body has lost nitrogen—and therefore protein. A negative nitrogen balance over time is dangerous, leading to muscle wasting and disease.

Achieving a positive nitrogen balance doesn't necessarily mean that you have to eat more protein. Muscle cells take up the exact amount of nutrients (including amino acids from dietary protein) they need for growth, and strength training helps them make better use of the protein that's available. This fact was clearly demonstrated in 1995 by a group of Tufts University researchers led by Wayne W. Campbell. The researchers took a group of older men and women (aged 56 to 80) who had never lifted weights before, placed them on either a low-protein diet or a high-protein diet, and measured their nitrogen balance before and after participation in a 12-week strength-training program. The low-protein diet was actually based on the RDA for protein (0.8 g/kg of body weight daily). The high-protein diet was twice the RDA (1.6 g/kg of body weight daily). The researchers wanted to see what effects each diet had on nitrogen balance during strength training.

What they discovered was interesting. Strength training enhanced nitrogen retention in both groups—protein was being retained and used to synthesize new tissue. However, in the low-protein group, there was even better use of protein. Strength training caused the body to adapt and meet the demand for protein—even when the bare minimum requirement for protein was met each day. Although this low level of protein intake may not be optimal for building muscle, this study shows how marvelously the body adjusts to what is available and how strength training makes muscle cells more efficient at using available protein to synthesize new tissue.

So, exactly how much protein should you eat for maximum performance and results? That question has been hotly debated in science for more than 100 years and by athletes since the time of the ancient Greeks. Nutrition scientists have had difficulty reaching a consensus on protein intake for several reasons. One has to do with the type and frequency of exercise. In endurance exercise, for example, protein can act as kind of a spare fuel tank, kicking in amino acids to supply fuel. If protein is in short supply, endurance athletes can peter out quickly. In strength sports, additional dietary protein is needed to provide enough amino acids to synthesize protein in the muscles.

For generations, strength trainers have looked to protein as the nutritional panacea for muscle building. Is there any scientific basis to this belief? New research shows that as a strength trainer, you may benefit from eating some extra protein.

Age and Protein Intake

It's no secret that as you age, you can lose muscle mass, strength, and function, partly because of inactivity. One way to reverse the downhill slide is to strength train. Study after study has shown that you can make significant muscle gains well into your 90s if you strength train.

Scientific research indicates that senior strength trainers can get a real boost from additional protein. At Tufts University, researchers gave supplemental protein to a group of elderly strength trainers, while a control group took no supplements. Based on CAT scans of muscle, the supplement group gained much more muscle mass than the control group did.

The older we get, the more protein we need to eat. A 2015 review study noted that, "There is mounting evidence, as highlighted by multiple consensus statements, that the Recommended Dietary Allowance (0.8g/kg body weight) may be inadequate to promote optimal health in older adults" (248). This review also cited a long-term study in which middle-aged men and women (45-60 years old) who consumed high-protein meals more frequently (6 times a day) had lower abdominal fat and higher lean body mass as compared to subjects consuming a more traditional dietary protein intake.

But what if you're nowhere near your golden years? Can you get the same benefits from extra protein? Many studies say yes. Two groups of young bodybuilders following a four-week strength-training program followed the same diet but with one exception. One group ate 2.3 grams of protein per kilogram of body weight (much more than the dietary reference intake [DRI]), and the other group ate 1.3 grams of protein per kilogram of body weight. By the end of the study, both groups had gained muscle, but those eating the higher amount of protein had gained five times more!

And what about even more protein? Several studies on this issue have been conducted by Dr. Jose Antonio and colleagues at Nova Southeastern University in Florida. They have investigated strength-training young men and women who ate more than 3 grams of protein per kilogram of body weight per day. Dr. Antonio's lab has confirmed that just adding more protein but training with a maintenance program does not magically build more muscle. However, when extra protein (3.4 g/kg/day vs. 2.3 g/kg/day in the normal-protein group) was consumed along with the extra energy from the added protein (400 kcals/day), and a periodized resistance training program was performed exclusive of any aerobic exercise, favorable gains in fat-free mass were made, similar to the normal-protein group. In addition, the high-protein group had significantly greater fat-mass losses (-1.7 kg) compared to the normal-protein group (-0.3 kg). Neither group showed any negative health effects from the diets. Therefore, with the right training program, extra protein does not turn into extra fat. On the other hand, you don't need to consume this much protein to get the gains that you want.

Protein Requirements for Endurance: Sexual Inequality

Requirements for carbohydrate and protein differ among men and women involved in endurance exercise. Women don't use as much carbohydrate during exercise as men do, and they don't use as much carbohydrate after exercise for recovery, growth, and repair as men do. Contrary to popular belief, women are generally great fat burners; that's why they don't need as much carbohydrate to fuel endurance training exercise as men do.

Until only a few years ago, all the recommendations for protein needs for female endurance athletes were extrapolations from data collected on men. The theory was, and one indirect study on amateur female cyclists demonstrated, that women need approximately 25 percent less protein compared to men. That led to recommendations of 1.2 to 1.3 grams of protein per kilogram of body weight per day for female endurance athletes, with direct nitrogen balance data supporting the requirement for men of 1.8 to 2.0 grams of protein per kilogram of body weight per day.

In 2014, scientists from New Zealand finally carried out direct nitrogen balance studies on 10 female cyclists and triathletes who were training moderately during the midfollicular phase (first half of the cycle before ovulation) of their menstrual cycle. This direct measure resulted in data supporting a need for 1.6 grams of protein per kilogram of body weight per day to maintain nitrogen balance. During the study, 7 of 10 participants were in negative nitrogen balance while consuming 1.4 grams of protein per kilogram of body weight per day, an amount higher than previously recommended. Nine out of ten athletes consuming 2.7 grams of protein per kilogram of body weight per day were in positive nitrogen balance.

Your goal as an athlete is not to be in nitrogen balance but to achieve positive nitrogen balance so that you can continue to build muscle, strength, and speed. In addition, it is universally recognized that the majority of female, and some proportion of male, endurance athletes are frequently underfueled, meaning that they consume less energy than they burn. This is due to a number of reasons, including strategically maintaining lower body weights, time constraints, and controlling gut comfort during training. When calorie needs are not met, protein needs increase. So both female and male athletes need more protein when energy is chronically restricted. I like to see most of the serious endurance athletes that I work with consuming at least 2.0 grams of protein per kilogram of body weight daily.

Proper Protein Levels

There is now a large body of evidence, and quite a bit of consensus among sport nutrition scientists and professional societies, regarding protein intake. Depending on the competitive athlete's status, training regimen, and total dietary intake, the average endurance- or resistance-trained athlete requires 1.4 to 2.0 grams of protein per kilogram of body weight daily. The nutrition profession is moving away from very specific macronutrient guidelines and recommending more individualized guidance, with ranges that encompass an athlete's personal needs, nuances, and differences.

For instance, energy-restricted athletes have higher protein needs, whether the calorie restriction is intentional or not. However, endurance athletes depend on carbohydrate to fuel their high-intensity training, so it is important that protein intake not be taken so high that it takes up too much room in the diet to allow for optimal consumption of needed levels of carbohydrate and healthy levels of fat.

There is also evidence that healthy athletes undergoing progressive resistance training protocols may benefit from higher protein intakes, up to 3.4 grams per kilogram of body weight daily, without any negative health consequences. Determining how to target your own personal protein need will be discussed below and in part III.

Functions of Protein in Exercise
- Promotes growth and repair of tissue
- Provides bodily structure (muscle, connective tissue, bone, and organs)
- Supports metabolic and hormonal activities
- Enhances immunity
- Maintains bodily protein to prevent muscle tissue breakdown
- Minimizes fatigue by providing branched-chain amino acids as fuel

Your Individual Protein Requirements

As a strength trainer or bodybuilder, whether male or female, you need more protein than a less-active person does. Your requirement is higher than the current DRI of 0.8 gram of protein per kilogram of body weight a day, which is based on the needs of nonexercisers. Plus, individual protein requirements vary, depending on whether you're building muscle, doing aerobic exercise on a regular basis, cross-training, or dieting for competition. Here's a closer look.

Muscle Building

As you increase training intensity, you need additional protein to support muscle growth and increasing levels of certain blood compounds. We still lack direct protein research on strength-training females, but based on the latest research with strength trainers, I recommend that males and females eat a minimum of 2.0 to 2.2 grams of protein per kilogram of body weight a day while in the building phases. Here's how you would figure that requirement if you weigh 150 pounds, or 68 kilograms (a kilogram equals 2.2 pounds):

$$2 \text{ g of protein} \times 68 \text{ kg} = 136 \text{ g of protein a day}$$

Strength trainers living in high altitudes need even more protein: 2.2 grams per kilogram of body weight daily. If you're a vegan, your protein needs are also 10 percent higher to make sure your diet is providing all the necessary amino acids:

$$2.2 \text{ g of protein} \times 68 \text{ kg} = 150 \text{ g of protein a day}$$

If you are new to strength training, you may need to eat more protein than a veteran strength trainer typically consumes—as much as 40 percent more.

Aerobic Exercise

On average, most strength trainers and bodybuilders perform an hour or two of intense weight training daily, plus five or more hours a week of aerobic exercise. If you are in this category, your protein needs are further elevated. Here's why.

During aerobic exercise lasting 60 minutes or more, certain amino acids—the branched-chain amino acids (BCAAs)—are used for energy in small amounts,

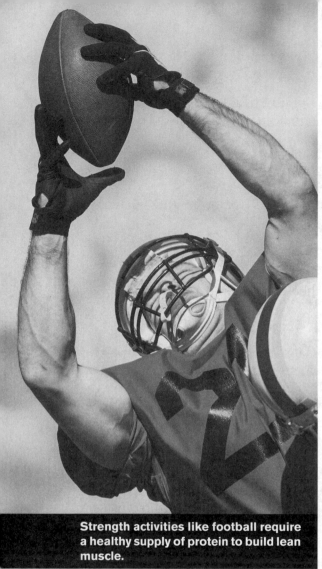

Strength activities like football require a healthy supply of protein to build lean muscle.

Comstock

particularly when the body is running low on carbohydrate, its preferred fuel source. One of the BCAAs, leucine, is broken down to make alanine, another amino acid, which is converted by the liver into blood sugar (glucose) for energy. This glucose is transported to the working muscles to be used for energy. The harder you work aerobically, the more leucine your body breaks down for extra fuel. In addition, studies show that availability of amino acids such as leucine stimulates muscle repair, as well as muscle development, in the period following exercise.

Given this special use of amino acids as an energy and recovery source, you should increase your protein intake if your training program includes more than five hours a week of an endurance program. Women may not need this increase, however, because it may be that females do not utilize as much protein, or BCAAs, for fuel during endurance or aerobic exercise as do males. Females are more efficient at burning fat during aerobic exercise and depend less on protein and carbohydrate for fuel. Generally, though, you may require as much as 2.2 grams of protein per kilogram of body weight during aerobic training. With the preceding example, you would calculate your requirements as follows:

$$2.2 \text{ g of protein} \times 68 \text{ kg} = 150 \text{ g of protein a day}$$

Cross-Training

If you're a marathoner, a triathlete, or even an ultramarathoner, you engage in cross-training, which consists of taking part in a variety of activities geared for your sport, including running, cycling, and long-distance swimming. And you may be lifting weights as a part of it all.

Years ago, cross-training athletes were encouraged to load up on carbohydrate. In more recent years, however, experts have contended that protein is equally essential for reaching new performance heights. However, protein intake is slightly lower than in strength trainers in order to leave room in the diet for increased carbohydrate, which is critical in the diet of an endurance athlete who is cross-training. A novice athlete at a lower training level will need less protein, and a more experienced athlete training more frequently will need more protein. Cross-training athletes thus need 1.5 to 1.8 grams of protein per kilogram of body weight a day, depending on the frequency and intensity of exercise:

$$1.5 \text{ to } 1.8 \text{ g of protein} \times 68 \text{ kg} = 102 \text{ to } 122 \text{ g of protein a day}$$

Cross-trainers, like endurance athletes, use more carbohydrate during training and competition than pure strength athletes do. Like endurance athletes, they need higher intakes of dietary carbohydrate than strength athletes do, and they may benefit from some carbohydrate loading before competition. Cross-trainers should use the updated, shorter version of carbohydrate loading. This entails long-duration training one week prior to the event to deplete muscle glycogen stores. Then they begin tapering their exercise and increase carbohydrate consumption three or four days prior to the event, reaching a preevent rest day during which they take in about 400 to 600 grams of dietary carbohydrate, based on body size and gender. Again, it seems female athletes use somewhat less carbohydrate during endurance exercise than male athletes do.

Competition Dieting or Trimming Fat

When cutting calories to get lean for looks or for competition, you risk losing body-firming muscle. Because muscle is the body's most metabolically active tissue, losing it compromises the ability of your body to burn fat. What's more, no bodybuilder wants to lose muscle prior to competition. One way to prevent diet-related muscle loss is to consume adequate protein while you're preparing for competition. Dieting bodybuilders need 2.2 to 2.5 grams of protein per kilogram of body weight a day or more, depending on how heavy you are lifting during this timeframe; if you are in a tapering, less heavy phase, I recommend starting at 2.2 grams per day:

$$2.2 \text{ g of protein} \times 68 \text{ kg} = 150 \text{ g of protein a day}$$

For more information on getting cut for competition, see chapter 19.

Benefits of Properly Timing Your Protein Intake

Let's say you've just finished an intense strength-training workout. If you could zoom in to the microscopic level of your muscles, you'd be astounded by the sight. There are tears in the tiny structures of your muscle fibers and leaks in your muscle cells. Over the next 24 to 48 hours, muscle protein will break down and additional muscle glycogen will be used.

These are some of the chief metabolic events that occur in the aftermath of a hard workout. And although these events might look like havoc, they are actually a necessary part of recovery—the repair and growth of muscle tissue that take place after every workout. During recovery, the body replenishes muscle glycogen and synthesizes new muscle protein. In the process, muscle fibers are made bigger and stronger to protect themselves against future trauma.

Feeding your body protein at specific times—such as after training—used to be a big issue in terms of promoting repair and recovery. However, it has been found to be less important than previously thought. What better enhances the recovery process is to consume protein throughout the day—including before and after your workout. That way, you are continually supplying your muscles with macronutrients. Not only do they serve as fuel and building material, they are also important activators of molecular signals that stimulate muscle protein synthesis (MPS) and halt muscle protein breakdown. As long as you continue to consume protein throughout the day, the immediacy around training is less of a factor.

As a practical matter though, many strength trainers and athletic individuals must time their fueling around training to allow for enough "feeding moments" throughout their day to accomplish their nutritional goals while still feeling comfortable enough in their gut to train hard. Depending on the time of day they train, they may schedule a meal an hour or two prior to exercise. This meal contains carbohydrate with protein in order to keep their protein pipeline running.

Many athletes are not hungry after an intense workout. If a snack or meal is not planned, they might let several hours pass before consuming protein and other food fuel. This can limit the magnitude and speed of recovery, repair, and growth. Having a readily available postworkout protein-carbohydrate shake or smoothie on hand is a good strategy.

Another food move is to eat a small meal immediately after exercise. Your body has already digested your preexercise protein, and it is working for you at the muscular level. Two or three hours later, as that effect wears off, your body begins to demand, and will benefit from, protein for the repair and recovery phase following a workout.

What would make a good meal? According to research, the most optimum strategy is to eat 0.5 gram of protein per kilogram of body weight, along with a rapidly digesting carbohydrate, such as dextrose, maltodextrin, fractionated starch, sucrose, or even honey, within 30 minutes of exercise. For example, if you weigh 150 pounds (68 kg), you should eat 34 grams of protein. We will discuss how to customize your carbohydrate recovery meal below and in detail in chapter 3.

When protein is consumed along with carbohydrate, there's a surge in insulin. Insulin is like an acceleration pedal. It races the body's glycogen-making motor in two ways. First, it speeds up the movement of glucose and amino acids into cells, and second, it activates a special enzyme crucial to glycogen synthesis. Additional research shows that a carbohydrate and protein supplement ingested after exercise triggers the release of growth hormone in addition to insulin. Both are conducive to muscle growth and recovery.

Also, the availability of essential amino acids (see table 2.1) after exercise boosts the rate of muscle protein resynthesis in the body. On the basis of these findings, I recommend that you consume 0.5 to 1 gram per kilogram of body weight of a fast-digesting carbohydrate (see table 3.3 in chapter 3) with 0.5 gram per kilogram of a protein food or a quality protein supplement—preferably one that contains all the essential amino acids.

TABLE 2.1   Essential, Conditionally Essential, and Nonessential Amino Acids

Essential	Conditionally essential	Nonessential
Isoleucine*	Arginine	Alanine
Leucine*	Cysteine (cystine)	Asparagine
Lysine	Glutamine	Aspartic acid
Methionine	Histidine	Citrulline
Phenylalanine	Proline	Glutamic acid
Threonine	Taurine	Glycine
Tryptophan	Tyrosine	Serine
Valine*		

*Branched-chain amino acid.

Adapted from M.G. Di Pasquale, "Proteins and Amino Acids in Exercise and Sport." In *Energy-Yielding Macronutrients and Energy Metabolism in Sports Nutrition*, edited by J.A. Driskell and I. Wolinsky (Philadelphia: CRC Press, 2000), 119-162.

Staying Anabolic All Day

Imagine walking around in an anabolic (growth) stage all day long, with your body in a tissue-building and fat-burning mode, continually. Is this possible? Yes—and I'll let you in on a few scientifically proven secrets.

The first secret to staying anabolic is planning regular meals with the right carbohydrate-protein combination. Your next secret weapon, though, is consuming optimal levels of leucine. Along with valine and isoleucine, leucine is one of the branched-chain amino acids (BCAAs). BCAAs are unique among amino acids in that they are used predominantly by muscle (most amino acids are processed and dismantled in the liver). Scientists have established that BCAAs produce energy during exercise, as well as promote protein synthesis. Other research further underscores the importance of leucine for both muscle growth and muscle maintenance while dieting.

A review of the role of leucine points out that leucine and insulin appear to work together to promote protein synthesis, more specifically by slowing down protein breakdown in skeletal muscle. This same review also noted that leucine taken alone after a workout is sufficient to "switch on" protein synthesis. Yet, although leucine alone is a potent activator of muscle growth, you still need a balanced consumption of the other essential amino acids to make those muscle proteins. In fact, there appears to be no advantage to resistance-trained athletes in supplementing with essential amino acids (EAAs) or BCAAs alone. Whole protein foods or supplements, such as whey protein, are the most ideal components for protein feedings around exercise and throughout the day since the ultimate nutrition goal is balanced intake. However, there may be occasions when the convenience of EAA or BCAA supplementation is preferable, such as for coordinating exercise timing or ensuring gut comfort.

Other research has pointed out the importance of leucine during dieting. To make a long story short, when calories are reduced, leucine in muscle is used to produce the amino acid alanine, which is used to manufacture glucose in the liver. It seems logical to hypothesize that high leucine intakes while dieting help spare protein and improve blood glucose control. The research has shown that 2.5 grams of leucine stimulates the metabolic pathways that catalyze muscle protein synthesis, thereby enhancing muscle growth and maintaining lean body mass.

This function of leucine, in addition to its anticatabolic function, may be critical in preventing overtraining. Although total energy intake is paramount, protein intake should not be ignored or limited during reduced training. If you have slowed training in an effort to prevent overtraining, don't drop your protein intake. Overtraining can be a result of and a state of catabolism. Optimal protein levels may decrease the risk of and enhance recovery from overtraining. In fact, it may even be more important at this time.

Of the commonly available dietary proteins, whey isolate has the highest leucine content (14 percent of its total protein content). Animal protein contains 10 percent leucine, whereas other proteins contain around 8 percent. Therefore, approximately 25 grams of animal or whey protein typically contains 2.5 grams of leucine. Strive to take in 10 grams of leucine per day from food and supplementation (see table 2.2). If you are consuming soy protein or other plant proteins, you would need slightly more. Eating protein at every meal and snacks throughout the day, approximately every three to four hours, allows for adequate energy and protein consumption to remain anabolic. This includes around exercise, both before and after.

Finally, while carbohydrate does not directly enhance muscle growth, it helps you replenish your glycogen stores for energy the next time you train.

TABLE 2.2   Leucine Content of Common Foods

Food	Leucine per 100 g of food
Meat, poultry, fish, shellfish	
Beef, ground, 85% lean meat, 15% fat, raw	1.450 g
Beef, ground, 93% lean meat, 7% fat, raw	1.627 g
Chicken, broiler or fryers, breast, skinless, boneless, meat only, raw	1.861 g
Chicken, broilers or fryers, thigh, meat and skin, raw	1.318 g
Crustaceans, crab, Dungeness, raw	1.381 g
Crustaceans, shrimp, mixed species, raw (may have been previously frozen)	1.165 g
Fish, cod, Pacific, raw (may have been previously frozen)	1.211 g
Fish, salmon, sockeye, raw	1.837 g
Fish, tilapia, raw	1.603 g
Fish, tuna, fresh, yellowfin, raw	1.900 g

Food	Leucine per 100 g of food
Fish, tuna, white, canned in water, without salt, drained solids	1.920 g
Mollusks, clam, mixed species, raw	1.200 g
Pork, cured, ham, boneless, regular (approximately 11% fat), roasted	1.574 g
Pork, fresh, loin, center loin (chops), bone-in, separable lean only, raw	1.873 g
Turkey, ground, 93% lean, 7% fat, raw	1.545 g
USDA Commodity Chicken, canned, meat only, drained	2.066 g
Dairy and eggs	
Cheese, cheddar	1.939 g
Cheese, cottage, low fat, 2% milkfat	1.049 g
Cheese, low fat, cheddar or Colby	2.145 g
Cheese, mozzarella, low moisture, part-skim	1.956 g
Egg, white, raw, fresh	1.016 g
Egg, whole, raw, fresh	1.086 g
Egg, yolk, raw, fresh	1.399 g
Milk, nonfat, fluid, with added vitamin A and vitamin D (fat free or skim)	0.319 g
Milk, reduced fat, fluid, 2% milkfat, with added vitamin A and vitamin D	0.313 g
Milk, whole, 3.25% milkfat, with added vitamin D	0.299 g
Yogurt, Greek, plain, low fat	0.529 g
Yogurt, plain, low fat, 12 g protein per 8 oz	0.529 g
Yogurt, plain, skim milk, 13 g protein per 8 oz	0.577 g
Yogurt, plain, whole milk, 8 g protein per 8 oz	0.350 g
Legumes, nuts, seeds	
Beans, black, mature seeds, cooked, boiled, without salt	0.708 g
Beans, kidney, all types, mature seeds, cooked, boiled, without salt	0.736 g
Chickpeas (garbanzo beans), mature seeds, cooked, boiled, without salt	0.631 g
Lentils, mature seeds, cooked, boiled, without salt	0.654 g
Nuts, almonds, dry roasted, without salt added	1.461 g
Nuts, cashew nuts, dry roasted, without salt added	1.285 g
Nuts, walnuts, English	1.170 g
Peanut butter, smooth style, with salt	1.546 g
Peanuts, all types, dry-roasted, with salt	1.535 g

> *continued*

TABLE 2.2 *> continued*

Food	Leucine per 100 g of food
Legumes, nuts, seeds (continued)	
Peas, split, mature seeds, cooked, boiled, without salt	0.598 g
Seeds, chia seeds, dried	1.371 g
Seeds, sunflower seed kernels, dry roasted, without salt	1.408 g
Soybeans, mature cooked, boiled, without salt	1.355 g
Soybeans, mature seeds, dry roasted	3.223 g
Soymilk, original and vanilla, unfortified	0.186 g
Tofu, firm, prepared with calcium sulfate and magnesium chloride (nigari)	0.728 g
Veggie burgers or soy burgers, unprepared	1.399 g
Grains	
Barley, pearled, cooked	0.154 g
Couscous, cooked	0.259 g
Oat bran, cooked	0.235 g
Pasta, whole-wheat, cooked	0.409 g
Quinoa, cooked	0.261 g
Rice, brown, medium-grain, cooked	0.191 g
Rice, white, medium-grain, enriched, cooked	0.197 g
Wheat bran, crude	0.928 g
Protein powders	
NutriBiotic Rice Protein Powder Raw Vegan Plain	
Olympian Labs Pea Protein Vanilla Bean	
Jarrow Formulas Whey Protein French Vanilla	
Simple Truth Organic Soy Protein Powder Natural Vanilla	

While In Training, Beware of High-Protein, Low-Carbohydrate Diets

The high-protein, low-carbohydrate diet approach is a defeatist strategy if you are a strength trainer or bodybuilder in training. Not eating enough carbohydrate constrains how much you can lift and how hard you can train and limits how much muscle you can build. Muscle is not built by protein alone; you actually have to stress your muscle tissue so that your body will kick in and do the work of rebuilding bigger, faster, and stronger. That's the point when protein does the heavy lifting, but you need carbohydrate to get you to that point. You might find that lowering your carbohydrate intake can help you drop weight, but that's not a building diet.

If you cut carbohydrate and lower your calorie intake to cut weight, your body will use protein from your diet to meet its energy demands. This reduces the amount of protein available for the physiological functions that only protein can perform.

Without enough protein or calories, more muscle is lost during weight loss, resulting in the undesirable effect of reduced strength, size, and metabolic rate.

When in a caloric deficit, you must add more protein to your diet, especially if you have cut carbohydrate. (Restricting carbohydrate, by the way, should be done for only a limited amount of time, or until you achieve your cutting goals). Although some studies have shown that resistance-trained men can achieve their body composition goals and maintain lean mass on a low-carbohydrate, high-fat diet with protein usually staying the same or higher, the time length of the studies has been relatively short.

Following a fat-loss diet that is 30 percent protein or at least 2.2 grams of protein per kilogram of body weight per day, which I recommended earlier in this chapter, is a win–win strategy. In this diet, you're lowering carbohydrate intake only slightly to make room for the extra protein, which will help drive fat burning. In chapters 3 and 8, you'll also learn why some carbohydrate and fiber from plant foods in your weight-loss plan will help you feel emotionally stronger and physically healthier while you're in your cutting phase.

The high-protein diets I object to are those that omit or drastically cut carbohydrate. Such diets promising quick weight loss continue to be the rage. These diets let you fill up on beef, chicken, fish, and eggs, with little emphasis on other foods such as vegetables and grains. What's wrong with such diets? To begin with, they're high in fat and nutritionally unbalanced. The mother lode of long-term diet data worldwide consistently points to plant-based diets, rich in vegetables, fruits, grains, beans, nuts, and seeds, with or without a small proportion of animal foods, as the healthiest strategies, regardless of the specific cultural food pattern. Low-carbohydrate, high-protein diets are out of balance with that equation. Most extreme protein diets are low in fiber, too. Without enough bulk to move things along, your whole digestive system slows to a crawl, which can lead to constipation, diverticulosis, and other intestinal disorders. Also, the fibers from plant foods function as prebiotics, which feed the healthy bacteria (probiotics) in your gut. Prebiotics and probiotics are other critical players in whole-body and mind health.

In addition, most protein diets are dehydrating. During the first week on a high-protein diet, you can lose a lot of weight, depending on your initial weight and body-fat percentage. You get on the scale, see an exhilarating weight loss, and feel wonderful, but most of this loss is water. You could be very dehydrated as a result, which spells trouble. If you weigh 150 pounds (68 kg), a mere 3-pound (1 kg) loss of water weight can make you feel draggy and hurt your exercise performance. The minute you go off this diet and eat some carbohydrate, water surges back into your tissues and you regain the lost water weight. Those fully hydrated, volumized muscle cells are also the most primed for muscle protein synthesis.

Clearly, your focus should not only be on protein but also be on a balance of nutrients. For an athlete, weight loss is an outcome of getting your diet and training dialed in; it is not a goal. Your goal is enhanced performance. Don't let the diet world fool you into believing that popular diet fads will put you on the podium. In fact, it's just the opposite. In chapters 15 through 19, you'll learn how to design your own personal eating plan, one that contains the right amount of protein, carbohydrate, and fat to help you build muscle and stay lean.

Fish Protein

Unless you've been stranded on a desert island, you know about the importance of fish oils and the omega-3 fat that comes from fish. But there is something else special about fish protein—it helps keep you lean.

The effect is partially from the omega-3 fat in fish, but scientists have learned that it may also be the fish protein that is making the difference. In a Canadian study, researchers found that when cod protein was fed to rats on a high-fat diet that had previously led to muscle insulin resistance, the cod protein protected against the insulin resistance. (Insulin resistance is a condition in which cells fail to let insulin usher glucose into cells to be burned for energy.)

The same researchers went back and looked into whether all fish had the same effect that cod had on insulin resistance. The goal of this new study was to determine whether other fish protein presented similar beneficial effects. So rats were put on a high-fat and high-sugar diet containing protein from casein or fish protein from bonito, herring, mackerel, or salmon. After 28 days, oral glucose tolerance tests were performed on the rats, and the tissues were biochemically analyzed. All the rats were fed diets of equal energy, but the salmon protein group had significantly less weight gain, which was associated with less fat gain. Whole-body insulin sensitivity for glucose improved also. In addition, the fish protein–fed group experienced a very powerful anticancer effect compared with the casein-fed control group. The anticancer effects were attributed to the anti-inflammatory properties that fish protein carries; the same protein may also protect against obesity-linked metabolic complications. Lastly, the salmon-fed group exhibited a rise in the circulating hormone calcitonin. This hormone plays a role in helping to control weight gain and may be the reason for the reduced weight gain in the salmon-fed rats. Although done in rats, this study sheds significant light on the role fish protein might play in human metabolism.

Researchers in Norway conducted a study to determine whether the amino acid content of various proteins may account for the ability of fish protein to enhance fat loss. It is understood that the amino acids taurine and glycine increase liver bile acid secretion and modulate bile acid metabolism, enhancing fecal bile acid excretion in rats. In this study, rats fed a diet containing fish protein hydrolysate from the saithe fish (pollack), which is high in taurine and glycine, experienced enhanced fat burning.

In addition to the studies on rats, we now have some excellent data that eating fish has a positive effect on body composition in humans. A 2009 study demonstrated that omega-3 fatty acids (found mostly in fish) are important for keeping body fat away. In that study, researchers from the University of Newcastle in Australia placed 124 men and women of varying weights into three categories based on their body mass indexes (BMIs): healthy weight, overweight, and obese. Blood samples were taken after subjects fasted for 10 hours and were measured for omega-3 concentration. The scientists found that the overweight and obese subjects had significantly lower levels of omega-3 fatty acids in their blood than those in the healthy-weight category. They also found that the lower the subjects' omega-3 levels were, the higher their BMIs, waist sizes, and hip circumferences were. This study tells us that eating fish and thus supplying the body with omega-3 fats is important in controlling weight.

I have watched the influence of fish in my clients' diets for decades. It is clear to me that when you eat fish five times a week, you get lean quickly. Of course, you have to do everything else right as well, but eating fish really helps spur the rate at which you can accomplish weight-loss goals.

Eating fish five times a week does not have to mean five fish dinners a week. You can have fish for breakfast in the form of smoked fish or a tuna melt on toast. It's easy to have canned salmon or canned tuna, or even fish tacos, for lunch. There are plenty of ways to vary the fish meals you eat during the week.

I am always asked about the safety of fish. How can we eat fish when there are so many problems with contamination? There are two primary concerns with fish safety: mercury and pesticide contamination. The mercury problem is a matter of contaminated waters and food chain hierarchy. Mercury is a by-product of heavy industry and manufacturing. It is released as pollution into the air, where it is trapped in the clouds and released in rainwater into the oceans, becoming methylmercury. Methylmercury is toxic to humans, and poisoning results in neurological disorders in adults. High levels of mercury will harm an unborn baby's or young child's developing nervous system. Because fish feed in these waters, the mercury builds up in them. The older and heavier the fish is, the greater the amount of smaller fish it has consumed. Over years, methylmercury builds up in large predatory fish and can reach relatively unsafe levels.

Nearly all fish contain trace amounts of mercury, as do all living things. However, large predatory fish such as swordfish, shark, tuna, king mackerel, and tilefish pose the greatest risks. Some shellfish can also be high in methylmercury based on their very small size in proportion to the contaminants they contain, the waters they feed in, and their key food sources.

The following advice from the U.S. Food and Drug Administration and the Environmental Protection Agency was updated in 2017 for women of childbearing age, pregnant women, and parents and caregivers of young children, to encourage them to include fish in their diets as a good source of very important nutrients (see figure 2.1). For adults not in these categories, I recommend a minimum of three fish meals per week from the "Best choices" category.

What the advisory doesn't tell you is that noncontaminated tuna is available from independently owned fishing vessels that sail out of the Pacific Northwest. These fishermen catch small tuna, weighing 7 to 12 pounds (3 to 5.4 kg), versus the fish, weighing 40 to 70 pounds (18 to 32 kg), caught by the longlining large commercial canneries. Rather than processing the tuna while the boats are still out in the ocean and boiling off the wonderful omega-3 fat only to throw it overboard into the ocean, these small tuna are flash frozen and canned with all their healthy fat intact. (The large canneries really do boil off omega-3 fat. At least one major cannery now sells its own omega-3 fat supplement; it takes it out of the fish and bottles it.) The fish caught by these independent fishermen are virtually mercury-free because of their size and the waters in which they are caught. These fishermen are

Advice about eating fish

What pregnant women and parents should know

Fish and other protein-rich foods have nutrients that can help your child's growth and development.

For women of childbearing age (about 16-49 years old), especially pregnant and breastfeeding women, and for parents and caregivers of young children.

- Eat 2 to 3 servings of fish a week from the "Best choices" list OR 1 serving from the "Good choices" list.
- Eat a variety of fish.
- Serve 1 to 2 servings of fish a week to children, starting at age 2.
- If you eat fish caught by family or friends, check for fish advisories. If there is no advisory, eat only one serving and no other fish that week.*

Use this chart!

You can use this chart to help you choose which fish to eat, and how often to eat them, based on their mercury levels. The "Best choices" have the lowest levels of mercury.

What is a serving?

To find out, use the palm of your hand!

For an adult
4 ounces

For children, ages 4 to 7
2 ounces

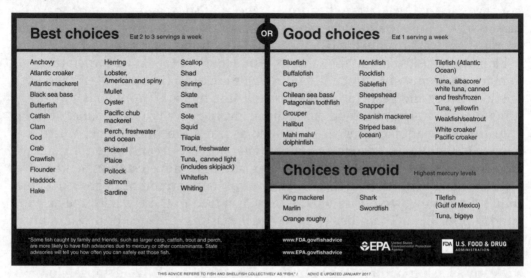

Best choices Eat 2 to 3 servings a week			OR	**Good choices** Eat 1 serving a week		
Anchovy	Herring	Scallop		Bluefish	Monkfish	Tilefish (Atlantic Ocean)
Atlantic croaker	Lobster, American and spiny	Shad		Buffalofish	Rockfish	Tuna, albacore/
Atlantic mackerel		Shrimp		Carp	Sablefish	white tuna, canned
Black sea bass	Mullet	Skate		Chilean sea bass/	Sheepshead	and fresh/frozen
Butterfish	Oyster	Smelt		Patagonian toothfish	Snapper	Tuna, yellowfin
Catfish	Pacific chub mackerel	Sole		Grouper	Spanish mackerel	Weakfish/seatrout
Clam	Perch, freshwater and ocean	Squid		Halibut	Striped bass (ocean)	White croaker/
Cod		Tilapia		Mahi mahi/		Pacific croaker
Crab	Pickerel	Trout, freshwater		dolphinfish		
Crawfish	Plaice	Tuna, canned light (includes skipjack)				
Flounder	Pollock	Whitefish		**Choices to avoid** Highest mercury levels		
Haddock	Salmon	Whiting				
Hake	Sardine			King mackerel	Shark	Tilefish (Gulf of Mexico)
				Marlin	Swordfish	Tuna, bigeye
				Orange roughy		

*Some fish caught by family and friends, such as larger carp, catfish, trout and perch, are more likely to have fish advisories due to mercury or other contaminants. State advisories will tell you how often you can safely eat those fish.

www.FDA.gov/fishadvice

www.EPA.gov/fishadvice

EPA United States Environmental Protection Agency

FDA U.S. FOOD & DRUG ADMINISTRATION

THIS ADVICE REFERS TO FISH AND SHELLFISH COLLECTIVELY AS "FISH." /   ADVICE UPDATED JANUARY 2017

Figure 2.1   Fish facts and advice for children and pregnant women.

also very environmentally responsible, catching only tuna (not sea turtles or other by-catch) and sticking to sustainable catch sizes. You get a delicious tuna with all the healthy fat and none of the mercury. The large nationwide canneries can't say that about their products. (See the sidebar for resources.)

The other major concern about fish is pesticide contamination. This is particularly a problem in the farmed salmon industry. Wild salmon are born in the cold rivers that run from Alaska to California. After hatching, they struggle their way to the ocean, where they grow into mature fish, returning to their natal rivers to spawn. Most wild salmon is caught in a short period in the late spring through the summer when the fish migrate back from the oceans to the rivers. This natural life process produces a lean, high-quality fish that is high in vitamins D and E and omega-3 fatty acids.

Contrary to wild salmon, farm-raised salmon are raised in an industrialized and contained habitat that allows for mass production. They are fed an artificial diet of small fish that are ground up into fishmeal. An artificial dye is added to the fishmeal to give the fish the pinkish hue that wild salmon develop naturally from their diet in the wild.

Pollutants get into farmed salmon through the small fish used in the fishmeal they are fed. Pollutants, such as factory runoff, enter the habitat of the small fish,

Tuna Safety Q&A

Q. What is the best and safest method for catching tuna?

A. The safest and most sustainable tuna is caught by hand poling or trolling.

Q. What about tuna steaks and sushi? Are those safe?

A. The most common method of catching these fish is longline fishing. All types of longline-caught albacore tuna, bigeye tuna (also known as ahi), and yellowfin tuna are considered high sources of mercury, regardless of whether they are canned or served as steaks or sushi. If you eat just a piece or two of tuna sushi every once in a while, this shouldn't be a problem. But if you make tuna sushi your meal twice a week, your mercury levels may be high.

Bluefin and skipjack tunas are considered safe for health, but the longline fishing technique is considered unsafe for the environment. Longline fishing leads to overfishing of the waters and high levels of by-catch (sea turtles, sea birds, sharks, and occasionally marine mammals). Hand poling and trolling are considered the most environmentally safe fishing methods.

"Light" canned tuna typically contains skipjack tuna, which is why it has been considered safer to eat than other tuna. However, a *Chicago Tribune* investigation discovered that "light" tuna sometimes contains yellowfin tuna without labeling it as such, and yellowfin is significantly higher in mercury than skipjack.

Q. Can sushi bars hide the fact that they serve fish of inferior quality?

A. One easy way to disguise less-than-top-quality tuna is to mix it with other ingredients. The spicy tuna roll is notorious in the sushi industry for using this method. There are also methods to make fish look fresher than it really is. "Gassing" or "smoking" tuna can make it look rosier than it is. Fish that is not processed using very high-quality methods can naturally lose its redness after death, even with freezing. After the tuna is butchered into loins or fillets and before it is frozen, it is exposed to carbon monoxide. The gas binds with hemoglobin to prevent any change in the flesh from red to brown or even to gray. This misrepresents the product to the consumer, making it difficult to evaluate the age of the fish based on the color of the flesh.

Although we hope that you get what you pay for, price is not always an indicator of the quality of the fish in a sushi restaurant. Here are a few tips to guide you:

- Fresh fish is rarely delivered on the weekend. Rule out Sundays and Mondays when considering a meal at a sushi restaurant unless you know the source.

- Fresh never means fishy. You should never know by walking in the door with your eyes closed that the restaurant serves fish. If there's a fishy smell, walk out.

- Fresh fish should be translucent and shiny. If the tuna looks as though it was painted red, it may have been gassed. Ask the chef if it has been smoked. If so, don't eat it.

- Busy is better. A busy restaurant will have higher customer turnover and fresher fish.

which absorb them. These pollutants are then highly concentrated in the fishmeal, which is fed to the farmed salmon; the pollutants are stored in the salmon's fat.

In the most current study, published in 2004, 700 salmon from around the world were analyzed for more than 50 contaminants. The greatest difference between farmed and wild salmon was in the presence of organochlorine compounds, and particularly the cancer-causing polychlorinated biphenyls (PCBs), dieldrin and toxaphene. Farmed salmon in Europe had the highest levels, followed by those from North America. Farm-raised Chilean salmon were the cleanest. And what about eating smoked salmon? Although smoked salmon probably has lower omega-3 fat levels and may contain some carcinogens as part of the smoking process (cold smoking may alleviate this), it is still a good choice if it is wild salmon.

The authors of the study stated that eating more than one meal of farmed salmon per month may increase the risk of cancer but presented specific recommendations by source. Table 2.3 lists the safe limits for salmon consumption.

These recommendations are for the average person. Recommendations for pregnant women are still under debate. These pollutants can damage the developing endocrine system, immune system, and brain. The compounds build up in body fat and linger there for decades—where they can be passed to a woman's fetus during pregnancy or fed to the baby through breast milk. Farmed salmon in the diets of women of childbearing age is a definite concern.

Isn't wild salmon expensive? Can you buy organic salmon instead? Wild salmon is definitely more expensive than farm-raised salmon, but it's well worth the price when you consider the risks involved and the benefits of eating salmon. But you do have some choices. During the salmon fishing season, you should be able to find half-fish fillets of wild salmon at large warehouse stores such as Costco. I recommend that you buy 5 pounds (2.3 kg) at a time, cut it into portions, and freeze it. Salmon will stay fresh in a frost-free freezer for at least six weeks as long as it is well sealed.

There is currently no definitive word on the organic labeling of fish. Any fish that you see that is labeled organic is not controlled by the U.S. government labeling standards the way other organic foods are. There is considerable speculation of fraud on the issue of organic fish labeling. The USDA organic certification program

TABLE 2.3   Safe Levels for Salmon Consumption

Source of salmon	Serving and frequency
Scotland and Faroe Islands farm raised	2 oz (60 g) per month
Canada and Maine farm raised	4 oz (120 g) per month
Chile and Washington State farm raised	8 oz (240 g) per month
Wild salmon	64 oz (1,920 g) per month (1 lb or 480 g per week)

Adapted from R.A. Hites, J.A. Foran, D.O. Carpenter, et al., "Global Assessment of Organic Contaminants in Farmed Salmon," *Science* 303 (2004): 226-229.

is considering adding fish, but stay informed about this program. Most likely the program will approve only farmed fish in the organic program. So stay closely tuned to any new regulations on the organic certification of fish.

Finally, remember that many fish besides tuna and salmon contain omega-3 fat. Sardines, mackerel, herring, black cod, catfish, and shrimp are all excellent sources of omega-3 fat. And any fish has more omega-3 fat than a hot dog does!

Red Meat

You may have shied away from red meat in the past because it tends to be high in fat and dietary cholesterol. Red meat, however, is a good source of protein, as well as iron, zinc, and other nutrients. Incidentally, so are dark-meat turkey and chicken.

Iron is necessary for manufacturing hemoglobin, which carries oxygen from the lungs to the tissues, and myoglobin, another transporter of oxygen found only in muscle tissue. The iron in red meat and other animal proteins is known as heme iron. The body absorbs heme iron better than it absorbs iron from plant foods, known as nonheme iron.

Zinc is a busy mineral. As one of the most widely distributed minerals in the body, zinc helps the body absorb vitamins, especially the B-complex vitamins. It is also involved in digestion and metabolism and is essential for growth. Like iron, zinc from animal protein is absorbed better than zinc from plant foods.

It may surprise you to learn that red meat can be very lean. In fact, 20 of the 29 lean beef cuts have, on average, only 1 more gram of saturated fat than a skinless chicken breast per 3-ounce (90 g) serving (see table 2.4).

Red meat clearly has some nutritional pluses. The key is to control the amount of fat you get from meat, especially saturated fat, which can promote inflammation. Here's how to control your intake of saturated fat from meat.

Serving Size

Keep the serving size moderate, because about 3 ounces (90 g) of lean beef contains just 8 grams of total fat and 21 grams of total protein. One such serving is about the size of a deck of cards or the palm of a woman's hand. To get 3 ounces (90 g) of cooked meat, start with 4 ounces (120 g) of uncooked, boneless meat.

Grade

Beef is graded according to fat marbling: prime, choice, and select. Select is the leanest grade. When choosing beef, look for lean cuts closely trimmed of fat, or trim them yourself at home before cooking them. Pork is also a leaner meat than it used to be. The leanest cuts of pork come from the loin and leg areas, and a 3-ounce (90 g) cooked and trimmed portion of any of these cuts contains fewer than 9 grams of fat and 180 calories. Lamb and veal are also lower in fat than beef. Follow the same guidelines for selecting lean cuts.

TABLE 2.4   The 20 Leanest Cuts of Beef*

Cut	Saturated fat (g)	Total fat (g)
Eye of round roast and steak	1.4	4.0
Sirloin tip side steak	1.6	4.1
Top round roast and steak	1.6	4.6
Bottom round roast and steak	1.7	4.9
Top sirloin steak	1.9	4.9
Brisket, flat half	1.9	5.1
95% lean ground beef	2.4	5.1
Round tip roast and steak	1.9	5.3
Round steak	1.9	5.3
Shank cross cuts	1.9	5.4
Chuck shoulder pot roast	1.8	5.7
Sirloin tip center roast and steak	2.1	5.8
Chuck shoulder steak	1.9	6.0
Bottom round steak	2.2	6.0
Top loin (strip) steak	2.3	6.0
Shoulder petite tender and medallions	2.4	6.1
Flank steak	2.6	6.3
Shoulder center (ranch) steak	2.4	6.5
Tri-tip roast and steak	2.6	7.1
Tenderloin roast and steak	2.7	7.1
T-bone steak	3.0	8.2

*Per 3 oz (85 g) cooked portion trimmed of visible fat.

Data from U.S. Department of Agriculture, Agricultural Research Service. 2008. USDA National Nutrient Database for Standard Reference, Release 21.

Preparation

To keep a lean cut tasty after cooking, you must handle and prepare it properly. Because leaner cuts have less fat to keep them moist and juicy, the method of preparation is important. More tender cuts, such as loin cuts, can be broiled or grilled and served immediately. Avoid overcooking. Beef can also be marinated to tenderize it. Because it is the acid in the marinade (vinegar, citrus juice, or wine) that tenderizes the meat, oil can be replaced with water without diminishing the tenderizing effect. To improve the tenderness of roasts, carve them into thin slices on the diagonal and across the grain when possible.

Beef Safety Tips

Consumer confidence in beef is fairly high despite concerns around the globe. Even so, you should take precautions to protect yourself against any meat-related disease, including food-borne illnesses. Here's what you can do to take charge of beef safety:

- Avoid ground beef as much as possible when you are not certain about the completeness of cooking. If you do eat ground beef, use a food thermometer to make sure it is cooked to 160 degrees Fahrenheit (71 degrees Celsius), eliminating any food-borne bacteria in the meat. Wash the thermometer immediately after using it.
- If you order ground beef in a restaurant, ask your server if it has been cooked to at least 155 degrees Fahrenheit (68 degrees Celsius) for 15 seconds (a safe option for restaurants).

How Great Is Grilling?

Let's get this out of the way right up front. Is the barbecue putting your health in danger? It might be. Does that mean you should trade in your grill for a stew pot? Not yet. For years nutritionists have been watching the research about the chemical changes that happen in foods when protein and fat are cooked at very high temperatures. Recent reports point to the production of a class of toxins, advanced glycation end products (AGEs), which develop during cooking and accelerate aging and serious chronic conditions such as diabetes, heart disease, and hypertension. While it sounds like a barbecued burger could do you in as quickly as a pack of cigarettes, the comparison isn't even close. When it comes to grilling, broiling, and even oven frying, moderation and variety are the keys to good food and good health.

AGEs are triggers of reactive oxygen species. A high production of reactive oxygen species plays a significant role in chronic diseases such as cardiovascular disease, renal disease, and diabetes. They also stimulate the inflammatory response and the systemic immune response that has been linked to instigation of arterial plaques in the development of cardiovascular disease, and they are often elevated in diabetic subjects. AGEs may be associated with Alzheimer's disease.

Although AGEs are produced as a normal part of metabolism, they have also been identified in food, especially in foods with significant protein and fat content that have been processed using high heat, such as grilling, roasting, and broiling. A diet low in processed foods and abundant in fruits and vegetables, with several daily servings of dairy, and that includes eggs, fish, poultry, and vegetable proteins as your major protein sources, is going to be low on the AGE scale.

How you prepare your foods on a regular basis is also important. Poaching fish and braising meats, along with stewing and microwaving, are the cooking techniques that produce the fewest AGEs. Stir frying would likely follow next on the

Marinade Tips for Taste and Health

Marinating meats in acidic compounds like vinegars, commonly part of Mediterranean and Asian cuisines, has been shown to reduce the production of AGEs from high-heat cooking. Certain herbs and spices contain natural antioxidants that may decrease the production of heterocyclic amines (HCAs), a class of carcinogenic compounds generated by cooking beef at high temperature. Research from Kansas State University shows that by marinating meats and fish with herbs from the mint family such as basil, mint, rosemary, sage, savory, marjoram, oregano, and thyme, HCAs are significantly reduced after grilling.

While the marinade with these herbs showed the greatest effect, two other marinades with different herbs were tested and found to be almost as effective. The rosemary/thyme marinade also contained pepper, allspice, and salt. Another marinade included oregano, thyme, garlic, and onion. A third marinade had oregano, garlic, basil, onion, and parsley.

Source: Food Safety Consortium, "Brush on the Marinade: Hold Off the Cancerous Compounds," *Newswise*, last modified June 4, 2007, http://www.newswise.com/articles/view/530543.

---

list. Meats that work best for braising include sliced turkey, veal, pork, and low-fat meats that can't be tenderized with dry heat.

It's what you do day in and day out that matters. So if you live in the sunbelt (or not) and use your grill every day, it's probably prudent to get out of the sun and use your indoor stovetop and oven more regularly. When you do grill or broil, stick with fish and vegetables most of the time. But when it comes to opening day at the ballpark, Memorial Day, Fourth of July, and Labor Day, a burger or steak on the grill can still be part of the celebration.

Going Meatless, Staying Muscular

Can you be a vegetarian and still build muscle? Absolutely—as long as you plan your diet properly. The key is to mix and match foods so that you get the right balance of amino acids.

You can think of amino acids as a construction crew building a house. Each crew member has a specific function, from framing to wiring. If just one crew member doesn't show up for work, then the construction job doesn't get finished. It's the same with amino acids. There are 22 amino acids, all of which combine to construct the proteins required for growth and tissue repair. For your body to build protein, all of these amino acids must be on the job. If just one amino acid is missing or even if the concentration of an amino acid is low, protein construction comes to a halt.

Of the 22 amino acids, 8 cannot be made by the body; they must be supplied by the food you eat. These eight amino acids are called the essential amino acids. Seven of the twenty-two amino acids are termed conditionally essential amino acids. This means that they are made by the body but, under certain conditions, are required in greater amounts. The remaining seven, which can be manufactured by the body, are known as the nonessential amino acids. Your body makes nonessential amino acids from carbohydrate and nitrogen and by chemically re-sorting essential and nonessential amino acids. (The essential, conditionally essential, and nonessential amino acids are listed in table 2.1.)

Foods that contain all the essential amino acids in the amounts required for health and growth are called complete proteins. Proteins found in dairy products, eggs, meat, poultry, fish, and other animal sources are complete proteins. Various plant foods typically provide incomplete proteins that either completely lack or are low in a particular essential amino acid. The essential amino acid that is missing or in short supply is called the limiting amino acid.

To get enough essential amino acids from a vegetarian diet, select foods that complement one another's limiting amino acids. In other words, mix and match foods during the day so that foods low in one essential amino acid are balanced by those that are higher in the same amino acid. It's not necessary to combine these proteins at one meal; you can simply eat a variety of protein sources throughout the day. For example, grains contain a limited amount of lysine but a higher amount of methionine. Legumes such as navy beans, kidney beans, and black beans are high in lysine but low in methionine. Thus, by combining grains and legumes, you create a complete protein meal. Soybeans are an exception and are considered a complete protein. Other fully nutritious protein combinations are as follows:

- Rice and beans
- Corn and beans
- Corn and lima beans
- Corn tortillas and refried beans
- Pasta and bean soup

If you are a vegetarian who chooses to eat milk and eggs, you needn't worry about combining foods. The protein in milk, eggs, cheeses, and other dairy products contains all the essential amino acids you need for tissue growth, repair, and maintenance. A word of caution, though: Dairy products can be high in fat, so be sure to choose low-fat or nonfat dairy foods such as milk, cheese, and yogurt, if these foods are a mainstay of your diet each day.

Whether you choose to include or exclude meat in your diet is a matter of personal choice. If you decide to go meatless, plan your diet carefully to avoid certain nutritional danger zones—namely, deficiencies in iron, zinc, vitamin B_{12}, vitamin D, calcium, creatine, and the omega-3 fats DHA and EPA. These deficiencies can hurt exercise performance and, if extreme, your general health. It is important to consider the following nutrients to help you avoid deficiencies if you're a vegetarian strength trainer.

- *Protein.* A challenge for vegetarian strength trainers is to obtain the 2 grams of high-quality protein per kilogram of body weight required daily to support muscle growth. You can do this by including plenty of low-fat dairy products and protein-rich plant sources in your diet. If you are a pure vegan (you eat no animal foods at all), increase your daily protein intake to at least 2.2 grams of protein per kilogram of body weight. Be conscious that you might easily fill up on fiber since all your protein sources (unless you use supplements) are high in fiber, so plan your meals and snacks carefully to allow yourself to be fully fueled, but feel empty enough to train. Having said this, you might consider plant protein supplementation to get in all the protein you need and avoid feeling overly full around training.

- *Heme iron.* Include some sources of heme iron in your diet. As noted, all types of animal protein contain the more easily absorbed form of iron, heme iron. If you're a semivegetarian—that is, still eating fish or chicken but no red meat—you're in luck, because chicken and fish contain heme iron. If you avoid animal protein, you won't be consuming heme iron. That means you have to work harder to get all the iron you need. No easy absorption tactics will be available to you.

- *MFP factor.* Meat, fish, and poultry (MFP) contain a special quality called the MFP factor that helps your body absorb more nonheme iron. When meat and vegetables are eaten together at the same meal, more nonheme iron is absorbed from the vegetables than if the vegetables had been eaten alone. If you're a semivegetarian, your slightly lower iron intake will signal your body to absorb extra iron from vegetables.

- *Vitamin C.* Fruits, vegetables, and other foods that contain vitamin C help the body absorb nonheme iron. For example, if you eat citrus fruits with an iron-fortified cereal, or tomato sauce with spinach, your body will absorb more iron from the cereal and the spinach than if either had been eaten alone.

- *Iron and zinc.* Some foods contain phytates, oxalates, or other substances that block the absorption of iron and zinc in the intestine. Coffee and tea (regular and decaffeinated), whole grains, bran, legumes, and spinach are a few examples of foods containing blockers. These foods are best eaten with sources of heme iron or vitamin C to help your body absorb more iron and zinc. In addition, consider iron and zinc supplements. Our bodies don't absorb the iron that comes from vegetables as easily as the iron that comes from animal foods. Those who don't eat meat, especially active people or menstruating women, must pay attention to their dietary iron needs. Animal flesh is the major source of zinc in most diets, so all vegetarians may be at greater risk of having low intakes of this mineral.

  Although dietary supplements are not replacements for food, it may be a good idea to supplement if iron and zinc are in short supply in your diet. Daily supplementation of iron and zinc at 100 percent of the DRI is insurance against harmful deficiencies. This is an important strategy for vegans. Female athletes in particular should consider iron and zinc supplementation along with the dietary strategies above.

- *Vitamin B_{12}.* Guard against a vitamin B_{12} deficiency. Vitamin B_{12} is one of the most significant nutrients typically missing from the diets of vegans. That's

POWER PROFILE: Vegetarianism

I once worked with a professional basketball player who, for philosophical reasons, was a lacto-ovo vegetarian (i.e., he ate no animal foods except dairy and egg products). He was determined to stick to his vegetarian game plan both on the road and at home.

Unexpectedly, this player's biggest problem was not protein. He was getting plenty of protein from dairy products. But he wasn't getting enough iron, selenium, and zinc—minerals that are plentiful in meat. In addition, his diet was high in fat because he was eating a lot of cheese-laden vegetable lasagna.

To solve the mineral problem, he began taking a mineral supplement containing the RDA of the minerals he was lacking. After basketball practice, he started drinking one or two meal-replacement beverages, which contain extra nutrients and fit perfectly into a lacto-ovo vegetarian diet.

With my help, he discovered several new low-fat recipes, such as vegetarian chili, that he could pack for road trips as long as he had a microwave oven in his hotel room. He took dried fruit on the road, too, which can be eaten anywhere and is loaded with minerals and energy-packed calories.

At home, he began to vary his diet using vegetarian staples such as beans, tofu, rice, and peanut butter. By varying his diet, he was also getting plenty of quality, nutrient-dense calories to fuel both training and competition. Equally important, he learned that he didn't have to sacrifice his beliefs for athletic performance.

because it is available only from animal products. Fortunately, the body needs only tiny daily amounts of this vitamin (the DRI is 2.4 mcg for adults), which is used in the manufacture of red blood cells and nerves. Even so, a deficiency is serious, potentially causing irreversible nerve damage.

Fermented foods, such as the soybean products miso and tempeh, supply some vitamin B_{12} from the bacterial culture that causes fermentation, but generally not enough. Vegans should eat foods fortified with B_{12} or take supplements to ensure a healthy diet.

- *Calcium and vitamin D.* Vegan diets are often low in calcium, and many indoor-sports athletes have low blood levels of vitamin D. Although dairy is the best source of calcium, if you are vegan, include a wide array of green leafy vegetables and legumes. Also, choose calcium and vitamin D–fortified foods when available. It is often very important to use supplements for these nutrients, as well.

- *DHA and EPA.* These are the two omega-3 fats that are found primarily in fish oils. If you do not eat any fish and will not supplement with fish oil, I strongly advise that you supplement with an algal source of DHA and EPA, as well as include fortified foods in your diet such as DHA-fortified eggs. These nutrients are critically important anti-inflammatory agents throughout our entire body.

- *Creatine.* Vegans and vegetarians have been found to have lower levels of muscle creatine compared to people who eat meat. Creatine is an energy-producing substance found primarily in animal tissue, particularly in red meat. If you are a strength trainer and train for power and speed, your performance will most likely be enhanced with creatine supplementation. Creatine monohydrate supplements are vegetarian.

Protein Quality and Type

As an exerciser or athlete, you should be concerned about the quality as well as the type of protein you eat. The bottom line is that you need either high-quality protein or a variety of protein sources to ensure adequate intake of all eight essential amino acids—particularly after exercise.

How Do You Rate Protein Quality?

Protein is rated on its quality, or the content of essential amino acids. To rate the quality of the protein in foods, scientists have developed a number of measurement methods. Here's a rundown of the three most common methods.

Protein Digestibility Corrected Amino Acid Score (PDCAAS)

The protein values you read on food labels are calculated using the PDCAAS. It describes the proportion of amino acids in a protein source, as well as its digestibility, or how well a protein is used by the body. In calculating the PDCAAS, the food is first assigned a score based on its amino acid composition. The score is then adjusted to reflect its digestibility.

Digestibility, which varies from food to food, is important. Generally, more than 90 percent of the protein in animal foods is digested and absorbed, whereas about 80 percent of the protein in legumes is used. Between 60 and 90 percent of the protein in fruits, vegetables, and grains is digested and absorbed. With the PDCAAS, the highest possible score is 100. For reference, egg whites, ground beef, milk powder, and tuna have scores of 100; soy protein has a score of 94.

Protein Efficiency Rating (PER)

The PER reflects a particular protein's ability to support weight gain in test animals and gives researchers a good indication of which foods best promote growth. The yardstick for comparison is the growth produced by the complete protein found in egg whites or milk. Egg protein, in particular, is considered the perfect protein, because it contains all eight essential amino acids in the ideal proportions and is the reservoir of nutrients to grow a bird. The standard value, set for casein, is 2.7. Anything greater than 2.7 is considered excellent.

Biological Value (BV)

The BV represents the percentage of protein absorbed from a particular food that your body can use for growth and repair rather than for energy production. As with the PER, the BV of egg whites serves as the yardstick by which other protein sources are compared. Complete proteins tend to have high biological values, whereas incomplete proteins have lower values. Lower BV foods are used mainly for fuel rather than for growth and repair.

What Type of Protein?

To bump up the protein in your diet, consider some additional sources of protein (besides lean choices such as fish, poultry, or meat) such as low-fat dairy and soy proteins. I am a major proponent of milk in the diets of athletes—for two important reasons. First, when taken after strength training, milk proteins have been shown in research to affect the development of muscle. Specifically, these proteins work by stimulating the uptake of amino acids by the muscle—a process that leads to the building of muscle. The two proteins found in milk are whey and casein; both have beneficial actions in producing muscle gains (see the following discussion). Also, research with animals hints that lactose, a sugar found in milk, may also be instrumental in stimulating muscle development. This is probably because lactose slightly elevates insulin, and insulin is necessary for pushing protein into muscle cells for energy, growth, and development.

The second reason I advocate that athletes drink milk is that milk is naturally high in the amino acid tryptophan. This amino acid elevates brain levels of serotonin, a natural chemical that makes you feel good mentally and emotionally. And milk has a small amount of natural carbohydrate, lactose. The protein-carbohydrate partnership supports the manufacture of serotonin in the brain. When you're in a good mood, you just feel more motivated to work out and achieve your fitness goals.

That said, what follows is a rundown on the benefits of various types of protein to consider as additions to your diet.

Whey

Whey is a natural, complete protein derived from cow's milk and is available in protein supplements; it provides numerous benefits if you strength train. Whey is considered a "fast protein" because it is digested and absorbed quickly, making amino acids readily available for muscle repair. Whey is thus ideal to consume immediately after exercise because of its rapid uptake. As noted earlier, whey is high in leucine—a branched-chain amino acid that can help you maintain an anabolic state. In recent years there has been a tremendous amount of research on whey protein and its influence on muscle protein synthesis and degradation. To briefly summarize this research, whey protein does the following:

- Enhances protein synthesis, outperforming most other sources of protein in this regard
- Limits the degradation or the damage that occurs from exercise

- Enhances recovery, repair, and growth
- Promotes cellular growth and immunity
- Is vital for a healthy nervous system and brain
- Is an abundant source of the amino acid leucine, which is directly involved in muscle growth
- Boasts an ideal proportion of essential amino acids to stimulate synthesis and enhance the training response
- Stimulates fat-burning mechanisms in the liver and muscle, as well as making more fat available for fuel during exercise

Of course, for anyone who is a vegan, whey protein is not an option. If you are lactose intolerant, however, whey protein isolate or soy protein is a very good option (discussed later).

Sport Nutrition Fact Versus Fiction: Do Supplemental Amino Acids Build Muscle?

For a long time, a debate has raged as to whether exercisers and athletes should take amino acid supplements such as EAAs and BCAAs as a natural way to enhance the muscle-building process. A mound of research validates the need to take protein prior to and after exercise to activate the repair and growth of lean muscle mass.

As for amino acids in particular, after years of research studies it appears that while BCAAs, and especially leucine, activate muscle protein synthesis, ongoing muscle protein synthesis (MPS) requires all the EAAs and a ready pool of all amino acids. So whatever small advantage there may be (and this is not conclusive) from BCAA supplementation, the full array of amino acids from whole protein sources are still required to capitalize on hard training.

Resistance trainers do not depend on BCAAs for fuel, but endurance athletes do use some proteins for fuel during long-distance exercise. Should they supplement with BCAAs? Consider these facts: Your body starts drawing on BCAAs for fuel during exercise primarily if you're not eating enough or taking in sufficient carbohydrate (carbohydrate keeps the body from burning up too much of its BCAA supply). However, some athletes report feeling better when they have a source of BCAAs either prior to or during endurance exercise.

Similarly, although there is no convincing data that BCAA or EAA supplementation enhances MPS, there are instances of convenience when this smallest, most significant, and easiest to digest of amino acid sources is the right choice for the athlete at the right time. However, supplementing with BCAAs and EAAs is an expensive choice with marginal evidence to support the strategy, and you should be able to easily get all that you need from food and whole protein supplements. Each of the following foods contains all the BCAAs you need daily to utilize during aerobic exercise and to promote recovery from resistance training:

- 3 ounces (90 g) of water-packed tuna
- 3 ounces (90 g) of chicken
- 1 cup (230 g) of nonfat yogurt
- 1 cup of cooked legumes

In addition, a great way to replace BCAAs lost during exercise is to consume dairy products or whey protein after your workout.

My clients know that I would rather see you get your amino acids naturally—from food or at least whole protein supplement sources. And just as important, time your protein intake by having a small mixed meal of protein and carbohydrate prior to and after your strength-training session.

Food remains the best protein source for your body. One of the main reasons has to do with absorption. All nutrients are absorbed better when they come from real food. There are substances in foods, which scientists have coined "food factors," that help the body absorb and use nutrients. We don't even know what many of these food factors are, but we do know that they aren't found in food supplements.

As for protein, it is one of the best-absorbed foods, particularly animal protein. Scientific research has found that 95 to 99 percent of animal protein is absorbed and used by the body. Even protein from plant sources is well absorbed: More than 90 percent of the protein from high-protein plants is taken up and put to use by the body.

If you eat a variety of protein sources (see table 2.5), you don't need to take protein or amino acid supplements. However, protein supplements are an important convenience in the diets of most active people.

Casein

Casein is another milk-derived protein that is also available in protein supplements. It is considered to be a "slow protein" because it generally forms into a solid in the stomach and is delivered to the muscles more slowly—in a timed-release fashion. Consuming 30 to 40 grams of casein prior to going to bed has been shown to be a good move in both young and older men because of this sustained action in feeding your muscles throughout the night while you sleep, enhancing muscle protein synthesis. In obese women, a presleep feeding of casein combined with an exercise program enhanced early morning satiety over whey protein or carbohydrate. Both milk proteins are high in glutamine, an amino acid that assists in muscle building and in fortifying your body's immune system.

Soy Protein

Soy protein is a complete protein extracted from soybeans that provides the essential amino acids to meet basic protein needs. However, a diet that is 100 percent dependent on soy protein may not be adequate to meet the needs of a person trying to gain muscle and strength. Soy, however, is a good substitute if you are a vegetarian or have a sensitivity to milk proteins. Soy protein also contains isoflavones, which have a number of potential health benefits.

TABLE 2.5 Good Sources of Protein

Food	Amount	Protein (g)	Calories
Animal foods			
Beef, lean, sirloin, broiled	3 oz (90 g)	26	172
Roasted chicken breast (boneless, no skin)	3 oz (90 g)	26	140
Sole or flounder, baked or broiled	3 oz (90 g)	21	100
Turkey	3 oz (90 g)	25	145
Dairy products			
Cheese	1 oz (30 g)	8	107
Cottage cheese, 2%	1/2 cup (105 g)	16	101
Egg, boiled	1 large	6	78
Egg white, cooked	1 large	4	78
Milk, dried nonfat, instant	1/2 cup (34 g)	12	122
Milk, low fat, 1%	1 cup (240 ml)	8	102
Milk, nonfat	1 cup (240 ml)	8	86
Yogurt, low fat, plain	8 oz (230 g)	13	155
Yogurt, low fat, fruit	8 oz (230 g)	11	250
Nuts, seeds, nut products			
Peanuts, dry roasted	1 oz (30 g)	7	166
Peanut butter	2 tbsp	8	190
Pumpkin seeds, dry roasted	1/2 cup (114 g)	6	143
Sunflower seeds, dry roasted, hulled	2 tbsp	3	93
Soy products			
Soybeans, cooked	1/2 cup (90 g)	15	149
Soy milk	1 cup (240 ml)	8	79
Tofu	1/2 cup (126 g)	10	94
Vegetables and high protein			
Black beans, boiled	1/2 cup (86 g)	8	114
Chickpeas (garbanzos), boiled	1/2 cup (82 g)	7	135
Lentils, boiled	1/2 cup (99 g)	9	115
Pinto beans	1/2 cup (86 g)	7	117

Research with strength trainers has investigated a blend of dairy and soy protein supplementation. One human study published in 2013 has shown a benefit to the blend of whey, casein, and soy in extending muscle protein synthesis post-training. No follow-up studies have been conducted.

Several studies of the influence of soy protein in weight-loss diets appear to conclude that soy protein doesn't confer an advantage. This doesn't mean that soy protein should not be used. The biggest advantage of soy protein is that it is an alternative protein supplement when whey protein can't be used, isn't available, or is unpalatable to an athlete. As a food source, it offers important nutrients and phytochemicals and is an excellent source of plant protein, giving variety to the diet. As a supplement, soy protein also offers variety. It is still a good protein source, nurturing the body and providing the essential amino acids required for muscle repair, recovery, and growth.

Egg Protein

Egg (ovalbumin) protein was once considered the best source of protein, especially in supplements. But because egg protein is fairly expensive compared with other forms of quality protein, its popularity has decreased.

The Bottom Line on Protein

Protein is definitely a key to manufacturing muscle, and the latest research shows that strength trainers who are building muscle, are vegetarians, or do cross-training require at least slightly elevated amounts of protein, and sometimes even more. You don't have to go overboard, but do make sure that you get what you need. By following the recommendations here, you'll get the optimal amount of protein to build muscle and maintain strength.

3

Fueling Workouts

From the oatmeal you eat for breakfast to the baked potato you eat for dinner, carbohydrate is the leading nutrient fuel for your body. During digestion, carbohydrate is broken down into glucose. Glucose circulates in the blood, where it is known as blood sugar, to be used by the brain and nervous system for energy. If your brain cells are deprived of glucose, your mental power will suffer, and because your brain controls your muscles, you might even feel weak and shaky.

Glucose from the breakdown of carbohydrate is also converted to glycogen for storage in either the liver or muscle. Two thirds of your body's glycogen is stored in the muscles and about one third is stored in the liver. When muscles use glycogen, they break it back down into glucose through a series of energy-producing steps.

It is no surprise that vegetables, fruit, cereal, pasta, grains, sport drinks, energy bars, and other forms of carbohydrate are the foods of choice for most endurance athletes, who load up on carbohydrate to improve their performance in competition. But carbohydrate is just as necessary for strength trainers as it is for endurance athletes—in the right amounts—and combined with protein and fat. The glycogen provided by carbohydrate is the major source of fuel for working muscles. When carbohydrate is in short supply, your muscles get tired and heavy. Carbohydrate, particularly in combination with protein and fat, is thus a vital nutrient that keeps your mind and muscles powered up for hard training and muscle building.

The amount of carbohydrate you need in your diet each day varies, depending on your training goals, how frequently and intensively you train, your gender, and your own individual needs. After decades of working with athletes at all levels and in all kinds of sports, I have noted that carbohydrate is needed in highly variable amounts from one individual to another even doing the same level of exercise. In general, to fuel performance, athletes need from 4.5 to 10 grams of carbohydrate per kilogram of body weight every day. This very large range depends on the factors noted earlier, including the type of exercise; exercise goals; the frequency, intensity, and duration of exercise; gender; and the weight requirements of the sport. Carbohydrate needs are different still when the goal of the diet and training program is to lose fat. That discussion can be found in chapters 4 and 5 of this book.

The Force Behind Muscle Building and Fat Burning

Among the nutrients, carbohydrate is the most powerful in affecting your energy levels. But it also influences your muscle-building and fat-burning power. It takes about 2,500 calories to build just 1 pound (0.5 kg) of muscle. That's a lot of energy! The best source of that energy is carbohydrate. It provides the cleanest, most immediate source of energy for body cells. In fact, your body prefers to burn carbohydrate over fat or protein. As your body's favored fuel source, carbohydrate spares protein from being used as energy. Protein is thus free to do its main job—building and repairing body tissue, including muscle.

Carbohydrate is a must for efficient fat burning, too. Your body burns fat for energy in a series of complex chemical reactions that take place inside cells. Think of fat as a log on a hearth waiting to be ignited. Even when athletes choose to eat low-carbohydrate, high-fat diets, carbohydrate remains the metabolic match that ignites fat at the cellular level. Unless enough carbohydrate is available in key stages of the energy-producing process, fat will just smolder—in other words, not burn as cleanly or completely.

Carbohydrate is also important because it affects carnitine levels in muscle cells. Carnitine is an amino acid–like nutrient that carries fat into the mitochondria of cells (the machinery that burns fat for fuel). The human body requires carnitine for fat metabolism. Researchers at the University of Nottingham gave healthy young men carnitine, as well as insulin and glucose, intravenously at the same time. The researchers supplied just enough glucose to keep the blood sugar levels of their subjects constant. The treatment lasted for five hours. The more insulin that circulated in the body, the higher the level of carnitine in the muscles following carnitine supplementation. This suggested that carnitine probably works best when taken with carbohydrate, and their follow-up feeding study proved the theory that you don't have to live in a lab to make it work.

Through your diet, you can increase the carnitine in your muscle cells, which can improve your exercise performance. A 2011 study found that men experienced a significant increase in athletic performance when they combined 2 grams of carnitine with 80 grams of a carbohydrate supplement; less muscle glycogen was burned during exercises and lactate production was significantly lower.

The implication here is that endurance athletes who load up on carbohydrate before a race might be further helped by carnitine supplements. The same may be true for high-power athletes such as downhill mountain bike racers, who operate in the anaerobic zone almost exclusively. These athletes may even be helped more by carnitine supplementation. Strength trainers who want to give their muscles a glycogen boost before training may also find a benefit. Keep in mind that the research in this area is very young, and we don't know whether the results from dietary consumption are specific to the type of carnitine and carbohydrate used in the study, or it is a generalized effect. Clearly, the insulin spike is a key component to getting carnitine into muscle cells.

Increase Carbohydrate Calories

The most important nutritional factor affecting muscle gain is calories—specifically, calories from carbohydrate. Building muscle requires a rigorous strength-training program. A tremendous amount of energy is required to fuel this type of exercise— energy that is best supplied by carbohydrate. A carbohydrate-dense diet allows for the greatest recovery of muscle glycogen stores on a daily basis. This ongoing replenishment lets your muscles work equally hard on successive days. Studies continue to show that carbohydrate-dense diets give strength-training athletes an edge in their workouts. The bottom line is: The harder you train, the more muscle you can build.

To build 1 pound (0.5 kg) of muscle, you need to add about 2,500 calories a week. This means introducing extra calories into your diet. Through the many years of my career, I have found that the oft-cited magical number of 500 calories per day—a little less to lose weight or a little more to gain weight—is not the best number to use. Often it removes more calories than is sustainable for athletes who are trying to lose weight, or increases the fat-to-muscle ratio too much on the gain side. Ideally, I prefer that women increase their calorie intake by 300 a day and men by 400.

You should increase your calorie consumption gradually so that you don't gain too much fat. What I suggest to strength trainers in a building phase is to start by introducing only 300 to 350 more calories per day. Then after a week or two, add another 300 to 400 calories a day. As long as you're not gaining significant amounts of fat, start introducing extra calories into your diet weekly, again at the same rate of 300 to 400 calories. Incidentally, for losing fat, you can drop calories by the same amount—300 calories a day for women and 400 calories a day for men.

But back to increasing calories: Most of these additional calories should come from carbohydrate in the form of food and liquid carbohydrate supplements. An example of 300 to 400 calories worth of carbohydrate from food is 1/2 cup (70 g) of whole-grain pasta, 1/2 cup of yams (68 g), and 1 banana. It just doesn't take that much additional food to increase your carbohydrate intake. Later in the book, I'll show you how to time your carbohydrate intake properly and how to combine the additional carbohydrate with the right foods to enhance muscle building. You might also find that your extra calories are fueling your more intense training or increased training volumes. You can put your fuel to work for you by getting your extra carbohydrate from eating easy-to-digest foods and supplements before, during, and after your training.

When I'm working with athletes, first I make sure their protein and fat needs are taken care of; then I look at their carbohydrate intake. I adjust calories by increasing or decreasing carbohydrate calories because the ups and downs are completely related to their exercise programming. Carbohydrate calories are the fuel, so if someone wants to gain weight, carbohydrate calories go up to fuel building training goals. To lose fat, carbohydrate calories go down because typically training volumes and intensities adjust downward with a nod to fewer calories. Remember, you should always eat carbohydrate in combination with the right amounts of protein and fat; it should not be consumed alone except perhaps in a sport drink when you just can't eat any additional solid food. (In most cases, sport drinks should only be consumed around and during exercise, not as a beverage during the rest of the day.)

To be really exact, you can match your carbohydrate intake to your weight. If you are a strength trainer and want to build muscle, you should take in about 4.5 to 7 grams of carbohydrate per kilogram of body weight a day, depending on whether you are female or male and the stage of your training. An athlete who cross-trains with strength training, wants to build, and does any type of endurance activity needs anywhere from 5 to more than 10 grams per kilogram of body weight a day based on the same factors.

Supplementing with liquid carbohydrate, including smoothies, is an excellent way to increase those calories, boost carbohydrate and protein consumption, and take in nutrients conveniently. It's also a great way to consume nutrients when you don't feel like eating, particularly after a heavy weight-training session. In addition, liquid nutrition is absorbed faster than nutrition from solid foods is. Liquid supplementation certainly supports muscle growth.

In a landmark experiment, competitive weightlifters took a liquid high-calorie supplement for 15 weeks. The goal of the study was to see how the supplement affected the athletes' weight gain, body composition, and strength. The weightlifters were divided into three groups: those using the supplement and no anabolic steroids, those using the supplement plus anabolic steroids, and a control group taking no supplements or steroids but participating in exercise. (This study was conducted many years ago and obviously could not be repeated today because of the drug use.) The supplement contained 540 calories and 70.5 grams of carbohydrate, plus other nutrients.

All of the participants followed their usual diets. The steroid group and the control group ate most of their calories in the form of fat rather than carbohydrate (45 percent fat, 37 percent carbohydrate). The supplement group ate more carbohydrate and less fat (34 percent fat, 47 percent carbohydrate). What's more, the supplement group ate about 830 more calories a day than the control group and 1,300 more calories a day than the steroid group.

Here's what happened: The weight gain in both supplemented groups was significantly greater than in the control group. Those in the supplement-only group gained an average of 7 pounds (3 kg); those in the supplement and steroid group, 10 pounds (4.5 kg); and those in the control group, 3.5 pounds (1.6 kg). Lean mass in both the supplement and steroid groups more than doubled compared with the control group. The supplement group lost 0.91 percent body fat, whereas the steroid group gained 0.5 percent body fat. Both the supplement and steroid groups gained strength—equally.

These results are amazing. They prove that ample calories and carbohydrate are essential for a successful strength-training and muscle-building program. Even more astounding is the fact that you can potentially attain the same results with diet alone as you can with drugs. That's powerful news for drug-free strength trainers everywhere. In chapter 16, you'll learn how to plan your own carbohydrate-dense diet to support muscle growth.

POWER PROFILE: Carbohydrate Supplementation in a Professional Basketball Player

Sue Bird, one of the WNBA Greatest of All Time point guards and four-time Team USA Gold Medal Olympian had never worried too much about her nutrition. Although she basically selected healthy foods, she focused on her training much more than on her diet. At 34 years old, with numerous orthopedic injuries and repairs, Sue wondered if working on her diet might help her stay in the game a while longer. My answer was a resounding *yes!*

Sue was an incredible client and very diligent. She kept a 10-day diet record so that we could get a very good snapshot of her overall food intake. It revealed that she was underfueling her body 1,000 to 1,500 calories a day, depending on the day's training protocol. She was taking in only about 100 calories above her resting metabolic rate, with a very slight increase on game days. Few things would tear her body down faster than that large an energy deficit.

To begin, I added 170 grams of carbohydrate, 20 grams of fat, and 50 grams of protein. She periodized her carbohydrate intake, as can all my clients, by adjusting her carbohydrate supplementation around training. High-intensity training days and game days got more carbohydrate, including carbohydrate supplementation before, during, and after training. Rest days didn't require carbohydrate supplementation. Easy!

Well, try telling an elite-caliber athlete that she needs to eat at least another 1,000 calories a day! But Sue was a model client. We took it in steps to get her mind and body used to the extra food, but the minute she saw, and felt, the results, she was all in. And despite the fact that Sue had always been very fit, her extra ripped abs were a nice added benefit!

Sue has put her own stamp on her food choices but sticks with the Power Eating program template that we designed 3 years ago. At first, she was skeptical of all the carbohydrate supplementation around training, but today she has added more Vitargo for half-time refueling and encourages her teammates to use it as well. And that talk about retirement? No way! Sue is still fully in the game, and I get to watch her championship play all season as the Floor General of the Seattle Storm.

Choose the Best Carbohydrate

Not just any type of carbohydrate is appropriate for building lean mass and developing a fit, streamlined physique, or for staying healthy. The best types of carbohydrate come from unrefined, whole foods such as vegetables, fruits, legumes, and whole grains. There is also some carbohydrate in milk and dairy from lactose, the milk sugar. By contrast, the typically unhealthy types of carbohydrate come from processed foods, including all kinds of simple and refined sugars and syrups, white flour, white rice, commercial baked goods, many packaged foods and snack foods, and alcohol. Processed foods have been stripped of their important nutritional factors, including fiber. Because they lack fiber and phytochemicals, and have engineered flavors added, it is easy to eat huge quantities of calories without feeling full. Foods with processed carbohydrate are the ones you should mostly avoid.

Not surprisingly, people who eat the best types of carbohydrate tend to weigh less and have better control of blood lipids and carbohydrate metabolism when compared with those who eat predominantly simple sugars and refined starches. Increased whole-grain intake in particular is associated with decreased risks of obesity, coronary heart disease, type 2 diabetes, insulin resistance, and many causes of illness. Thus, by replacing nutritionally poor types of carbohydrate with the best, nutritionally rich ones, you gain better control over most of the physiological and metabolic risk factors associated with the development of obesity and chronic disease.

High in Fiber

The right carbohydrate is rich in fiber, which is found only in plant foods, primarily whole foods and largely unprocessed foods. Fiber is a structural and storage form of carbohydrate and is mostly undigested as it passes through the human digestive system. It is classified by its ability to dissolve in water into two types: water soluble and water insoluble. Soluble fibers, which come primarily from beans, fruits, and whole grains, can be dissolved in water and include plant material such as gums, mucilages, pectin, and some hemicelluloses. Insoluble fibers, which come primarily from vegetables, beans, whole wheat, and fruit skins, do not dissolve in water and include lignins, cellulose, and some hemicelluloses. Both types of fiber improve the work of the intestines, although in different ways. Water-soluble fiber is generally sticky and viscous and slows down the movement of food through the digestive tract. Water-insoluble fiber acts like a stool softener and bulk former and keeps things moving through the system.

We used to think of fiber more or less as a cleaning aid for the intestinal wall and a transit aid for excrement, as well as a filler in the diet, taking up space but not giving us many calories. Everything about that kind of thinking has changed with our expanding understanding of the bacteria in the gut, technically known as the *biome*. Bacteria and yeasts live symbiotically in and on our bodies, and are called probiotics and mycobiotics, respectively. They are essential to our physical and mental health and well-being. Many of the fibers from the plant foods that we eat are nourishment for these living cultures, and they are called prebiotics.

Sport Nutrition Fact Versus Fiction: Does Carbohydrate Make You Fat?

The media continues to beat the drum about carbohydrate-dense diets making people fat and therefore being bad. This is based on the fact that overweight and obesity are risk factors for the development of insulin resistance, a condition in which the pancreas oversecretes insulin to maintain normal blood levels of glucose after a carbohydrate-dense meal. This oversecretion causes carbohydrate to be converted to stored body fat, leading to more overweight and obesity, and ultimately landing people on the pathway to the development of type 2 diabetes. Although this may be true for a sedentary population, it's just not the same case with athletes and other active people. In fact, for bodybuilders, insulin is an anabolic hormone that helps build muscle mass by fueling the muscles.

As someone who's active, you're already keeping your insulin levels in line. Although the exact mechanism isn't clear, exercise makes muscle cells more sensitive to insulin. For glucose to enter muscle cells, it has to have help from insulin. Once insulin gets to the outer surface of the cell, it acts like a key and unlocks tiny receptors surrounding the cell. The cell opens and lets glucose in for use as fuel. Maintaining muscle tissue through strength training helps normalize the flow of glucose from the blood into muscle cells, where it can be properly used for energy.

What may be even more surprising is that during exercise you don't need insulin for glucose to enter muscle cells. In fact, as exercise intensity increases, insulin secretion decreases. Instead, a transporter protein named GLUT-4 facilitates diffusion of glucose across skeletal muscle tissue into muscle cells. That way, glucose can target muscles during exercise, and not be delivered to all the other body tissues that require insulin for transport. In addition, since insulin secretion suppresses fat-burning, the more insulin circulating during exercise would limit the ability to use fat as fuel. This would be a biologically inefficient strategy. But the more well trained you are, the more readily you can move glucose into your muscle cells without insulin during exercise.

Should you be worried about eating pasta and bread? No! But you should concentrate on a variety of whole-carbohydrate foods such as beans, whole grains, fruits, and vegetables in addition to whole-grain bread and pasta. Too much emphasis on refined starches nudges out more nutritionally dense foods from your diet. Even in the unlikely event that you are insulin resistant, the variety minimizes the effects, as does mixing carbohydrate with protein and fat. Also, staying active helps control body weight and builds muscle tissue, which helps regulate the body's use of glucose.

Insulin and carbohydrate are not the bad guys when it comes to fat—calories, poor diet planning, and a sedentary lifestyle are. You gain body fat when you remain inactive, make poor choices, and eat more calories than you burn. It's just that simple.

Research studies regarding everything about our biome are vast and growing daily, and there is no way to discuss the wide array of issues that overlap with diet and health here. What is important to convey is that high-fat, low-carbohydrate diets may upset the balance of good bacteria to harmful bacteria in the biome. This imbalance can affect not only your gut health but also your entire body and brain.

The fibrous prebiotics that act as food for the probiotic and mycobiotic cultures are only found in plant foods, which tend to be sparse in a low-carbohydrate diet. Studies show that animals and humans who must follow a low-carbohydrate or ketogenic diet long term for health reasons have altered gut linings and poor populations of healthy bacteria. This internal environment sets the stage for obesity, inflammatory bowel disease, other chronic diseases, and even depression. During low-carbohydrate eating, it is thus essential to eat fiber-rich plant foods in order to maintain a healthy gut biome.

Interestingly, probiotics are currently under study for performance-enhancing potential in athletes. Also, if certain strains of probiotics can help keep athletes healthier and fight off respiratory, intestinal, and other infections, then athletes can train more regularly and compete at higher levels. It is still way too early to tell whether any of these studies will reach significant results, but it is really fun to watch the science evolve.

Another benefit of fiber is that it can help keep you lean. Add 5 more grams of fiber to your diet every day. This small amount will reduce your chances of experiencing an expanding waistline and becoming overweight. French researchers found that a 5-gram increase in total dietary fiber can reduce the risk of becoming overweight by almost 11 percent and reduce the risk of an expanding waistline by nearly 15 percent. This relationship was particularly strong with insoluble fiber from fruit, dried fruit, nuts, and seeds.

Another study published by a research group from Harvard showed that women who increased fiber intake by about 8 grams per day ate 150 fewer calories per day than those who decreased their fiber intake by 3 grams per day during the study. During the 12 years of the study, the women with the highest fiber consumption lost about 8 pounds (3.6 kg), compared with a nearly 20-pound (9 kg) weight gain for those who cut their fiber intake during those years.

How does fiber work its weight-controlling wonders? First, high-fiber foods take longer to eat and they expand in your stomach, resulting in a full, satisfied feeling. Second, they lower levels of insulin, a hormone that stimulates appetite. Third, more energy (calories) is used up during the digestion and absorption of high-fiber foods. Fourth, high-fiber diets are lower in calories and help you naturally manage your weight. Studies report that one of the primary ways people succeed at keeping weight off is sticking to a high-fiber diet over time.

One more important point: By avoiding obesity through a high-fiber diet, you lower your risks for the development and progression of cardiovascular disease, cancer, hypertension, and diabetes. And last but not least, those living cultures in your gut may actually alter the amount of calories that you extract from the food you eat, thereby influencing energy balance. So keep eating fiber to keep you and your biome healthy. Table 3.1 provides a list of the best high-fiber foods for strength trainers, bodybuilders, exercisers, and other athletes.

Here's a question a lot of my clients ask me when I advise upping their fiber intake: How do you get a lot of fiber in your diet without feeling bloated or going

TABLE 3.1 Good Food Sources of Dietary Fiber Ranked

Food, amount	Dietary fiber (g)	Calories
Navy beans, cooked, 1/2 cup (91 g)	9.5	128
Bran ready-to-eat cereal (100%), 1/2 cup (30 g)	8.8	78
Kidney beans, canned, 1/2 cup (89 g)	8.2	109
Split peas, cooked, 1/2 cup (98 g)	8.1	116
Lentils, cooked, 1/2 cup (99 g)	7.8	115
Black beans, cooked, 1/2 cup (86 g)	7.5	114
Pinto beans, cooked, 1/2 cup (86 g)	7.7	122
Lima beans, cooked, 1/2 cup (85 g)	6.6	108
Artichoke, globe, cooked, 1 each	6.5	60
White beans, canned, 1/2 cup (90 g)	6.3	154
Chickpeas, cooked, 1/2 cup (82 g)	6.2	135
Great northern beans, cooked, 1/2 cup (89 g)	6.2	105
Cowpeas, cooked, 1/2 cup (83 g)	5.6	100
Soybeans, mature, cooked, 1/2 cup (90 g)	5.2	149
Bran ready-to-eat cereals, various, ~1 oz (~30 g)	2.6-5.0	90-108
Crackers, rye wafers, plain, 2 wafers	5.0	74
Sweet potato, baked, with peel, 1 medium	4.8	131
Asian pear, raw, 1 small	4.4	51
Green peas, cooked, 1/2 cup (80 g)	4.4	67
Whole-wheat English muffin	4.4	134
Pear, raw, 1 small	4.3	81
Bulgur, cooked, 1/2 cup (91 g)	4.1	76
Mixed vegetables, cooked, 1/2 cup (82 g)	4.0	59
Raspberries, raw, 1/2 cup (62 g)	4.0	32
Sweet potato, boiled, no peel, 1 medium	3.9	119
Blackberries, raw, 1/2 cup (72 g)	3.8	31
Potato, baked, with skin, 1 medium	3.8	161
Soybeans, green, cooked, 1/2 cup (90 g)	3.8	127
Stewed prunes, 1/2 cup (124 g)	3.8	133
Figs, dried, 1/4 cup (37 g)	3.7	93
Dates, 1/4 cup (45 g)	3.6	126
Oat bran, raw, 1/4 cup (18 g)	3.6	58
Pumpkin, canned, 1/2 cup (123 g)	3.6	42
Spinach, frozen, cooked, 1/2 cup (95 g)	3.5	30
Shredded wheat ready-to-eat cereals, various, ~1 oz (~30 g)	2.8-3.4	96

Food, amount	Dietary fiber (g)	Calories
Almonds, 1 oz (30 g)	3.3	164
Apple with skin, raw, 1 medium	3.3	72
Brussels sprouts, frozen, cooked, 1/2 cup (78 g)	3.2	33
Whole-wheat spaghetti, cooked, 1/2 cup (70 g)	3.1	87
Banana, 1 medium	3.1	105
Orange, raw, 1 medium	3.1	62
Oat bran muffin, 1 small	3.0	178
Guava, 1 medium	3.0	37
Pearled barley, cooked, 1/2 cup (79 g)	3.0	97
Sauerkraut, canned, solids and liquids, 1/2 cup (71 g)	3.0	23
Tomato paste, 1/4 cup (131 g)	2.9	54
Winter squash, cooked, 1/2 cup (103 g)	2.9	38
Broccoli, cooked, 1/2 cup (78 g)	2.8	26
Parsnips, cooked, chopped, 1/2 cup (78 g)	2.8	55
Turnip greens, cooked, 1/2 cup (72 g)	2.5	15
Collards, cooked, 1/2 cup (95 g)	2.7	25
Okra, frozen, cooked, 1/2 cup (92 g)	2.6	26
Peas, edible pod, cooked, 1/2 cup (80 g)	2.5	42

Source: ARS Nutrient Database for Standard Reference, Release 17. From the U.S. Department of Health and Human Services and the U.S. Department of Agriculture, *Dietary Guidelines for Americans 2005*, http://www.health.gov/dietaryguidelines/dga2005/document/html/appendixB.htm.

to the bathroom all the time? The answer is to stick to your regimen of smaller multiple meals that include carbohydrate, protein, and fat. These small, frequent meals give you timed-release energy while lowering the total volume of fiber you take in at any one time. You'll also experience less gas with smaller, more frequent meals. When the friendly bacteria in your gut feeds off fiber, a by-product of bacterial digestion can be gas, but if you take in fiber in smaller amounts, less gas is produced. Start out slowly and add more fiber over several weeks; don't make a big change all at once. Also, the natural enzyme product Beano is a great addition to decreasing gas production from high-fiber foods. If you have trouble with bloating, the following list includes the high-fiber foods that form the least gas:

- Fresh fruits with skin, dried fruits, and fruit juices with pulp
- Potatoes, sweet potatoes, and yams with skin
- Peas
- Carrots
- Winter squash

- Tomatoes
- Romaine, leaf, Boston, and Bibb lettuces
- Whole grains and cereals

The Glycemic Index: Three Myths

Sport nutrition is full of half-baked truths and urban legends that often prevent athletes and exercisers from figuring out just how to eat to maximize muscle gains or fat loss or both. A good example is the glycemic index (GI), which rates carbohydrate sources by the effect they have on blood sugar. Originally, it was designed to help diabetics control their blood sugar, but over time, it was applied to diets as a tool to differentiate between good carbohydrate and bad carbohydrate and slow-digesting carbohydrate versus fast-digesting carbohydrate.

Three major myths have thus arisen regarding the GI and its use in nutrition and sport nutrition.

Myth #1: The glycemic index is a measure of how fast carbohydrate from a food, beverage, or supplement is digested and absorbed after consuming a specific amount.

Fact: The GI is not a measure of how fast ingested carbohydrate gets into the blood. Rather, it's a measure of the total rise in blood sugar over time. The difference is that nearly everyone (including myself, at one time) made the assumption that a total rise in blood sugar represents speed of entry into the bloodstream. However, making assumptions in science, unless it's part of a study design, is not a good thing. We should never assume that because we know fact A, it automatically translates to fact B.

Research conducted by two different laboratories has shown the rate of glucose entry into the bloodstream, called glucose kinetics, for two high-GI carbohydrate sources can be remarkably different. In fact, a low-GI carbohydrate source may possibly enter the bloodstream more rapidly than a high-GI carbohydrate-rich food.

Which brings us to the next myth . . .

Myth #2: Simple, refined carbohydrate sources raise glucose levels quickly but more complex carbohydrate sources raise glucose slowly.

Fact: A 2003 study demonstrated that the interpreted concept of what the GI represents is substantially incorrect. In that study, scientists compared the glucose kinetics of a low-GI breakfast cereal (bran cereal) and a high-GI breakfast cereal (corn flakes) that each contained 50 grams of available carbohydrate. The GI of corn flakes was more than twice as high as the GI of bran cereal, despite the fact that there was no significant difference in the rate of appearance of glucose in the bloodstream between the two foods during the 180-minute test. In other words, the rate of entry of glucose into the bloodstream was the same for corn flakes and bran cereal.

A major difference, however, was that the increase in the level of insulin in the bloodstream after the consumption of bran cereal was significantly faster and higher compared to the corn flakes. Insulin release is not part of GI testing, yet it is the job of insulin to remove extra glucose from the bloodstream and transport it to muscle and liver cells. Twenty minutes after consuming bran cereal, participants' insulin concentration was 76 percent greater, leading to a 31 percent greater rate of disappearance of glucose from the bloodstream compared to after eating corn flakes. Therefore, it appears that the lower GI of bran cereal is not due to the slower rise of glucose in the bloodstream. On the contrary, the rate of the increase in the level of glucose in the bloodstream between the two foods is the same. The difference is that the glucose from the bran cereal was being removed from the bloodstream more rapidly, and therefore, the total rise in glucose concentration was lower compared to that from corn flakes.

This is so mind-blowing that I'm going to repeat it with a more visual example. Think of your bloodstream as a bathtub with a faucet pouring water (blood sugar) into the tub and a drain where the water drains out of the tub (the more open the drain, the higher the insulin concentration). Now imagine two tubs side by side. The water is pouring out of the faucet into the tub at the identical rate for both tubs. In the first tub, the drain is mostly closed, but in the second tub the drain is wide open. The total rise of the water level in the first tub keeps going up and up as long as the faucet is pouring water in and only a small amount trickles out the drain. In the second tub, the water is draining out rapidly from the bottom at the same time that the water is pouring in from the faucet, and the water level never goes as high. By measuring only the total rise of the water level, you never see that the rate of water entry into the tub is identical, only that the total rise is much higher for the first tub versus the second.

The total rise in the water level (blood glucose) is what the GI actually measures. In the case of this study, the high-fiber bran cereal stimulated a more profound insulin response, draining glucose from the bloodstream more rapidly, creating a lower total blood sugar rise; thus the low GI designation. This has nothing to do with the speed of digestion, absorption or glucose entry into the blood. Glucose from the more refined and simple sugar–sweetened corn flakes entered the bloodstream at the same rate as glucose from the more complex bran cereal.

This data cannot be translated to apply to all foods, unless we conduct glucose kinetics studies on all foods. However, the examples from these studies completely disprove the assumption that GI represents speed of entry into the bloodstream. Moreover, it is absolutely an untruth that simple carbohydrate ingredients are automatically high-GI foods that are more rapidly absorbed into the bloodstream compared to more complex carbohydrate, low-GI foods.

Which undeniably leads us to . . .

Myth #3: Choose all your foods and supplements based on GI rating.

Fact: You might think that because a low-GI food was shown in research to stimulate a better insulin response and faster movement of glucose out of the bloodstream and into the cells that using GI is a smart way to design a healthy diet. Unfortunately, that is jumping the gun yet again. Knowing this data about one food, or even several foods, does not give us license to assume that this is what happens with all foods. Additionally, we cannot assign a health benefit to an observed function until it is tested and proven to result in a healthier outcome. When it comes to GI, many tests have actually been done, yet there is no consensus on whether GI truly makes a difference in long-term health outcomes.

OmniCarb Randomized Clinical Trial is one of the most recent large-scale trials to test the effects of high versus low GI on cardiovascular risk factors and insulin sensitivity. For five weeks, subjects followed either a low-GI or high-GI DASH-type diet, which is a plant-rich diet plan that has been shown to be very healthy in multiple international studies. After five weeks, they had a washout period and then crossed over to the opposite GI plan. There were no significant differences or improvements in insulin sensitivity, lipid levels, or systolic blood pressure levels between the subjects on the different GI diets. In this study, following a low-GI diet did not result in a healthier cardiovascular risk or insulin sensitivity clinical outcome.

There are many claims that the GI is a factor in successful weight loss. While many diet approaches have been shown to be helpful in facilitating weight loss, there are very few dietary plans proven to support weight-loss maintenance. In a multicenter trial, researchers tested the effects of dietary composition on energy expenditure during weight-loss maintenance. Three diet styles were tested—low-carbohydrate, low-GI, and low-fat—in a four-week crossover design with a washout period in between each diet.

The low-carbohydrate diet not only created the highest resting energy expenditure (REE) and total energy expenditure (TEE) but also resulted in the greatest release of the stress-related hormones and markers, cortisol and C-reactive protein (CRP). The low-fat diet led to the lowest REE and TEE , but the lowest cortisol release with a moderate CRP measurement. In this study, the low-GI diet may be the better choice for a maintenance plan, resulting in only a moderate drop in REE and TEE, and a moderate response of cortisol and CRP.

When it comes to athletic performance, there is absolutely no data to support that any specific GI translates to enhanced performance. Any claim regarding the effects of certain foods, diets, beverages, or supplements on athletic performance should be backed up by scientific research data—not simply the GI of the food or product. Remember: A muscle biopsy study is required to show that carbohydrate is entering the muscle cell for fueling and recovery. Therefore, only when solid, well-designed research has demonstrated an association between a food or product and enhanced performance can a reliable claim be made about the food or product.

With what you now understand about the variability of foods, their transport in the body, and their GI, the only way you can know if something enhances performances is to see data that it actually enhances performance. If manufacturers are talking about speed of digestion, absorption, and transport to muscle cells, you now know that you need to see that data from the testing of that product, not simply rely on the GI of the product.

If Not the Glycemic Index, Then What?

The GI by itself is not a bad thing. It was designed as an experiment to see if the data could actually provide dietary guidance and, in some cases, it may. The unveiling of these myths doesn't take away from what the GI actually represents, but it illuminates the fact that we are giving the relatively abstract number of the GI more dietary credence than it deserves.

Moreover, the packaged food industry has presented the GI as a badge of goodness or healthiness for foods that are highly processed and engineered. While processing and engineering of foods is not inherently bad or unhealthy, a diet abundant in these foods is generally higher in salt, sugar, and disease-promoting fats, and lower in micronutrients, fibers, phytochemicals, and other food factors that are widely known to promote health. Our misunderstanding of the three GI myths outlined here, combined with the labeling of packaged foods with a GI rating, has led to a misplaced notion of the contents of a healthy diet. Because fresh foods like produce, meats, breads, and dairy do not typically have GI ratings attached to them at the store, you may place a higher health value on packaged foods because the GI rating is clearly labeled. The intent of the labeling is to say that the food is low GI, and low GI is healthy; therefore, the food is healthy, regardless of the ingredients in the package.

My recommendation is that you learn about the food, not the GI, which has not held up to the assumptions first made about it. The GI is an abstract set of numbers that do not necessarily relate to the factors that we had hoped it would. Instead, focus on the food, ensuring it is as fresh as possible, and that you include a variety of foods from all the food groups, with the purpose of fueling your body and feeding your mind.

Nibbling, or eating smaller meals more frequently, allows you to eat smaller portions and thereby reduce the amount, or load, of carbohydrate you eat at one time. Because carbohydrate is digested more rapidly than protein or fat, when you eat combinations of foods such as an apple with peanut butter or bread with cheese, you mimic the whole-food response and slow down stomach-emptying and digestion, which some research shows may help to prevent weight gain. Rather than having to follow a diet devoid of carbohydrate, you can still enjoy carbohydrate and get the same weight-loss benefit.

Here are a few pointers to help you organize or create a system of how you can best manage carbohydrate-rich foods in your diet to maximize fueling and health promotion, as well as feel best in body and mind.

- Whole, unprocessed foods in their natural state are always your first choice.
- Raw, uncooked foods take longer to eat and longer to digest, and may help you feel fuller for longer.
- Solid foods will keep you feeling more satisfied for longer than liquid foods.
- Foods higher in fiber, fat, and protein are slower to digest, give you a nutritionally balanced meal, and keep you feeling fuller for longer.
- A smaller portion of carbohydrate-rich food provides a lower load and allows you to eat carbohydrate multiple times throughout the day, creating greater nutritional balance each time you eat.

Sugar and Your Health

So what's the scoop on sugar? Should you eat it or not eat it? If you're active, there is certainly a place for sugar in your diet—a small place. Anyone who is consuming at least 2,000 calories a day can tolerate some added sugar, as long as exercise is part of the program.

What do I mean by *added sugar*? It's the sugar not found naturally in foods that is added either by you (such as the table sugar you add to your coffee or tea) or the food manufacturer (to sweeten foods). Although it's fine to eat a tiny bit of sugar, your goal should always be to eat as much whole food as possible to support your training and your health. Downplay processed foods, which tend to be loaded with added sugar.

You can, however, put sugar to work for you. Sugars and refined starches are the mainstays of sport drinks that you can use before, during, or after your workouts. That's when it is best used as fuel, and you will burn it off quickly. But you pay for too much added sugar with calories allotted from your diet that could otherwise have been spent on whole foods.

If eaten too frequently, not burned off, or not used to replenish muscle glycogen, sugar becomes an empty food that causes health problems and decreases physical and mental performance. Studies have shown that high-sugar diets trigger systemic inflammation in your intestines and intestinal lining. This not only alters the health of your gut biome, but it also can weaken the integrity of your intestinal lining, allowing the inflammatory substances to leak out into the rest of your body. Chronic systemic inflammation is detrimental to your current and future health. It is linked to periodontal disease, obesity, heart disease, type 2 diabetes, cancer, poor pregnancy outcomes, and poor mental health. It increases the stress response in your body, and together stress and inflammation ultimately diminish both physical and mental performance.

How much sugar should, or can, you eat and still achieve your goals? If you look at the building diet in chapter 16, you'll see that on a 2,000-calorie diet, you can have 3 teaspoons (1 tablespoon) of added carbohydrate or sugar. My Power Eating definition of added carbohydrate and sugar includes both simple sugars and refined starches found in sport beverages. In this new *Power Eating*, I have adjusted the term to be specific: teaspoons of added carbohydrate or sugar. On the 2,000-calorie diet, you should put the added carbohydrate or sugar to work for you immediately after exercise to begin recovery. You need the rest of those calories for robust, nutrient-dense carbohydrate, protein, and high-performance fats. As the amount of calories increases, the amount of added carbohydrate or sugar increases to allow for greater refueling of a more active and larger, more muscular body. The added carbohydrates or sugars are almost completely for exercise nutrition: before, during, and after exercise for recovery. That's when they work for you.

Besides the fact that sugar provides almost no nutrients but plenty of calories, too much of it in your diet can harm your health in various ways, as discussed above. What follows is a more specific list of sugar's detrimental effects, culled from the scientific literature on sugar consumption.

- Decreases levels of the helpful, protective cholesterol, high-density lipoprotein (HDL)
- Increases triglycerides (elevated triglycerides increase your risk of coronary artery disease)

- Causes fluctuations in blood glucose levels—a situation that can be problematic in people with diabetes
- Contributes to the formation of advanced glycation end products (AGEs) in a process in which sugar links to protein (AGEs are implicated in aging, diabetic nerve damage, vascular problems, and impaired cellular function)
- Increases the risk of obesity
- Is directly related to the formation of dental cavities
- Displaces the intake of whole foods in the diet

Source: B.V. Howard and J. Wylie-Rosett, "Sugar and Cardiovascular Disease: A Statement for Healthcare Professionals from the Committee on Nutrition of the Council on Nutrition, Physical Activity, and Metabolism of the American Heart Association," *Circulation* 106, no. 4 (2002): 523-527.

Carbohydrate: How Much, How Often?

Clearly, there are plenty of reasons to fill up on carbohydrate, particularly the whole, unrefined kind. First, though, you have to understand that there is a ceiling on how much carbohydrate your body will stock. Think of a gas tank; it can hold only so many gallons. If you fill it with more than it can hold, it will just overflow. Once your carbohydrate stores fill up in the form of glycogen, the liver turns the overflow into fat, which is then stored under the skin and in other areas of the body.

The amount of muscle glycogen you can store depends on your degree of muscle mass. Just as some gas tanks are larger, so are some people's muscles. The more muscular you are, the more glycogen you can store. To make sure you get the right amount of carbohydrate and not too much, figure your daily carbohydrate intake as follows: To build muscle, consume 4.5 to 7 grams of carbohydrate per kilogram of body weight daily. Divide your body weight in pounds by 2.2 to get your body weight in kilograms; then multiply by a number in the range of 4.5 to 7. If you want to maintain your weight, lose fat, or cut, you can find your customized carbohydrate needs in chapters 15, 18, and 19. While this advice is generally correct for most serious athletes, active females commonly have somewhat different fueling needs than active males. Chapter 7 addresses the latest research on fueling an active female, and chapters 15 through 19 for include plans for female-specific menus.

Once you increase your carbohydrate to the right level, you should start making additional strength gains. Ample amounts of carbohydrate will give you the energy to push harder and longer for better results in your workout.

Bread, Cereal, Rice, and Pasta

Along with many fruits and vegetables, the grain food group contains complex carbohydrate, which you know best as starch. Starch is to a plant what glycogen is to your body, a storage form of glucose that supplies energy to help the plant grow. At the molecular level, starch is actually a chain of dozens of glucose units. The links holding the starch chain together are broken apart by enzymes during digestion, leaving single glucose units that are circulated to the body's cells.

Although primitive humans probably gnawed on whole kernels, today we grind or mill grains to ease their preparation and improve their palatability—hence the term *refined grains.* Milling subdivides the grain into smaller particles. For example, the wheat kernel can be milled to form cracked wheat, fine granular wheat, or even finer whole-wheat flour. Refining processes also remove the germ or seed, as well as the bran, a covering that protects the germ and other inner parts of the grain.

When the endosperm, a starch layer that protects the germ, is separated from a corn kernel, you get such products as grits and cornmeal. Another processing technique is abrasion, in which the bran of rice or barley is removed and the remaining portion is polished. The result is white rice or pearled barley. As parts of the kernel such as the germ or bran are removed, so are the nutrients they contain—fiber, unsaturated fat, protein, iron, and several B-complex vitamins. Some of these are partially replaced in cereal products in a process known as enrichment. However, enriched cereals are not nearly as nutritious as the original grains, so you should minimize your consumption of them. Furthermore, they lack the fiber found in whole grains.

I recommend that most of the starchy grains in your diet be whole grains. First, they are higher in fiber. Second, unlike refined foods, whole grains are less likely to cause insulin resistance, when elevated blood sugar circulates in the blood because body cells respond abnormally to the action of insulin. High intakes of refined foods can lead to insulin resistance, even in active people.

As a strength trainer, you're probably used to eating a lot of oatmeal, rice, and other common grains. For variety, you might experiment with grains that are less well known but are now widely available in supermarkets. For instance, tabbouleh, a Middle Eastern dish, is a delicious cold salad made from bulgur wheat. The Russians traditionally use kasha, or roasted buckwheat groats, to make both warm and cold dishes and stuffings. Barley makes a hearty soup. Quinoa, more of a seed than a grain, is cooked like a grain but is higher in protein, calcium, magnesium, iron, and phosphorus than typical grains. Its nutty flavor adds variety and nutrition to warm and cold dishes. Several new ancient grains are finding their way into our diets from global cultural food patterns and can support a gluten-free diet.

Fruits and Vegetables

You've heard it since grade school: Eat your fruits and vegetables, and you'll be healthy. Somewhere between then and now, you may have become skeptical of that advice. It seems too simplistic. After all, human health and nutrition science must be more complicated than that! But science has put grade school advice to the test and turned up some provocative findings. In a nutshell, the advice you heard as a kid is not only sound, it may also be lifesaving.

Thanks to continuing research, there are now more reasons than ever to eat lots of fruits and vegetables. In addition to their high vitamin, mineral, and fiber content, fruits and vegetables are full of other nutritional treasures such as the following:

- *Antioxidants.* Vitamins and minerals such as vitamin A, beta-carotene, vitamins C and E, and selenium fight disease-causing substances in the body called free radicals. Antioxidants have some real benefits for strength trainers; see chapter 9 for more details.

- *Phytochemicals.* These plant chemicals protect against cancer, heart disease, and other illnesses. They signal your protein and enzyme manufacturing systems to turn the volume up or down on production. These compounds are strategically linked to your body's ability to stay healthy, prevent disease, and slow down aging. Table 3.2 lists some of the important phytochemicals found in various types of carbohydrate.

- *Phytoestrogens.* These are special phytochemicals found in tofu and other soy foods that, in moderation, may protect against some cancers, lower dangerous levels of cholesterol, and promote bone building. Phytoestrogens are listed in table 3.2.

TABLE 3.2　Phytochemicals for Fitness

Phytochemical	Food source	Protective action
Allyl sulfides	Garlic, onions, shallots, leeks, chives	Lower risk of stomach and colon cancers
Sulforaphanes, indoles, isothiocyanates	Broccoli, cabbage, Brussels sprouts, cauliflower, kohlrabi, watercress, turnips, Chinese cabbage	Lower risk of breast, stomach, and lung cancers
Carotenes	Carrots, dried apricots and peaches, cantaloupe (rock melon), green leafy vegetables, sweet potatoes, yams	Lower risk of lung and other cancers
Lycopene, p-coumaric acid, chlorogenic acid	Tomatoes	Lower risk of prostate and stomach cancers
Alpha-linolenic acid, vitamin E	Vegetable oils	Lower risk of inflammation and heart disease
Monoterpenes	Cherries, orange-peel oil, citrus-peel oil, caraway, dill, spearmint, lemongrass	Lower risk of breast, skin, liver, lung, stomach, and pancreatic cancers
Polyphenols	Green tea	Lower risk of skin, lung, and stomach cancers
Phytoestrogens	Soy foods, including tofu, miso, tempeh, soybeans, soy milk, isolated soy protein	Lower risk of breast and prostate cancers; decrease symptoms of menopause

There are lots of reasons for piling more fruits and vegetables onto our plates. First, plant foods provide significant protection against many types of cancer. People who eat greater amounts of fruits and vegetables have about half the risk of getting cancer and less risk of dying of cancer than those who eat lesser amounts. For example, tomatoes may protect against prostate cancer. In a study sponsored by the National Cancer Institute, researchers identified lycopene as the only carotenoid associated with a lower risk of prostate cancer. Cooked tomato products are concentrated sources of lycopene. Thus, tomato sauce, stewed tomatoes, tomato paste, tomato juice, pizza sauce, and spaghetti sauce are rich in lycopene. People who consumed more than 10 servings of these combined foods per week had a significantly decreased risk of developing prostate cancer compared with those who ate fewer than one and a half servings per week.

Here's more proof of the cancer-fighting power of fruits and vegetables: A study of 2,400 Greek women showed that women with the highest intake of fruit (six servings a day) had a 35 percent lower risk of breast cancer compared with women who had the lowest fruit intake (fewer than two servings a day).

The number of fruits and vegetables in your daily diet makes a difference in cardiovascular health, too. Researchers tracked 832 men aged 45 to 65 as part of the famous Framingham Heart Study, which has followed the health of residents of a Boston suburb since 1948. For every increase of three servings of fruits and vegetables that the men ate per day, there was approximately a 20 percent decrease in their risk of stroke. A previous study reported a similar finding among women. Those who ate lots of spinach, carrots, and other vegetables and fruits rich in antioxidants had a 54 percent lower risk of stroke than other women.

There's more: In the United States, men with low vitamin C intakes have a significantly higher risk of cardiovascular disease and death compared with men who eat the highest levels of vitamin C. Risk of heart disease appears to be the lowest in people who eat an average of at least 11 pounds (5 kg) of citrus fruit per year.

Want to better control your blood pressure? Eat more fruit. It's loaded with potassium and magnesium—two minerals that have been credited with possibly lowering blood pressure. Research shows that people who follow the traditional dietary patterns of various ethnic groups tend to have lower blood pressure than those who follow the typical American diet. The reason is that people with these traditional diets eat twice as many servings of fruits and vegetables as people who transition to the average American diet. Other research indicates that high blood pressure can be lowered—without medication—if you eat a diet packed with fruits and vegetables.

Can you get the same health benefits from popping supplements as you can from food? Not exactly. New research has discovered that factors such as antioxidants and phytochemicals work best to fight disease when you get them from food rather than when they are isolated as supplements. In other words, a vitamin and mineral supplement, or any other kind of nutritional supplement, can't match the power of food.

To get the disease-fighting benefits of fruits and vegetables, you should eat a minimum of three servings of vegetables and two servings of fruit every day. One

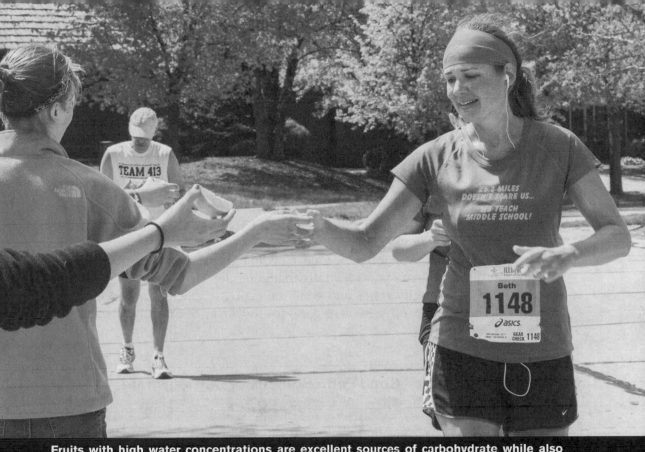

Fruits with high water concentrations are excellent sources of carbohydrate while also being low in calories.

serving of a vegetable is equal to 1/2 cup (91 g) of cooked or chopped raw vegetables; 1 cup (38 g) of raw, leafy vegetables; 1/2 cup (90 g) of cooked legumes; or 3/4 cup (178 ml) of vegetable juice. One serving of a fruit is equal to 1 medium piece of raw fruit, half of a grapefruit, 1 melon wedge, 1/2 cup (62 g) of berries, 1/4 cup (37 g) of dried fruit, or 3/4 cup (180 ml) of fruit juice.

Energy Bars

Energy bars, which are a convenient, ready-to-eat source of carbohydrate, have come a long way since I first ate a PowerBar around 30 years ago. There was no question then that food was a better choice, but it was hard to eat a cheese sandwich and an apple while cycling along the rugged coast of Maine. A PowerBar was desirable because I could wrap it around my handlebars, peel it off, and eat it as I rode. Although still not my favorite source of nutrition, bars have now become specialized to boost energy for activity, add protein for dieting or building muscle, or generally replace a small meal or snack. Most important, they are convenient to have with you when you need them.

For the most part, energy bars come in three varieties: those containing lots of carbohydrate and little fat; those formulated with a more equal combination of carbohydrate, protein, and fat; and those that emphasize protein and often use noncaloric or low-calorie sweeteners for taste.

For strength trainers, eating energy bars is a fast way to replace glycogen stores (which are depleted during heavy exercise) to help your body recover. If you need to add fiber to your diet, look for bars that contain fiber-rich whole foods such as oats, nuts, and fruit, whose carbohydrate content provides a steady release of energy. Some of these often have as much as 5 grams of fiber in them. You'd be wise to check the calorie counts of these products, however. They can contain anywhere from 200 to 400 calories or more per bar. So if you're trying to shed body fat, you could unwittingly sabotage your diet by eating bars as snacks instead of whole foods such as fruits and vegetables.

With some planning you might be able to avoid bars most of the time by having a convenient food source of carbohydrate that you take with you in the morning. Pair it with a rich protein source and you'll be eating whole, natural food rather than an engineered bar. Table 3.3 lists good food sources of carbohydrates.

TABLE 3.3   Good Food Sources of Carbohydrate

Source	Serving size	Carbohydrate (g)	Calories
Fruits			
Apples, raw, with skin	1 medium (3 in. diameter)	25	95
Applesauce, canned, unsweetened, with added ascorbic acid	1/2 cup (122 g)	14	51
Apricots, dried, sulfured, uncooked	1/4 cup (33 g)	20	78
Bananas, raw	1 medium (7-8 in. long)	27	105
Blueberries, frozen, unsweetened	1 cup (155 g)	19	79
Cherries, sweet, raw	1 cup (138 g)	22	87
Cherries, tart, dried, sweetened	1/4 cup (40 g)	32	133
Dates, Deglet Noor	5 dates (36 g)	27	100
Fruit cocktail, (peach, pineapple, pear, grape, and cherry), canned, extra light syrup, solids and liquids	1 cup (246 g)	29	111
Grapefruit (pink, red, and white) raw, all areas	1 large (4.5 in. diameter)	27	106
Grapes, red or green (European type, such as Thompson seedless), raw	1 cup (151 g)	27	104

Source	Serving size	Carbohydrate (g)	Calories
Jackfruit, canned, syrup pack	1/2 cup (89 g)	21	82
Mangos, raw	1 cup (165 g)	25	99
Melons, cantaloupe, raw	1 cup, chopped (160 g)	13	54
Nectarines, raw	1 medium (2.5 in. diameter)	15	62
Oranges, clementine, raw	1 piece (74 g)	9	35
Oranges, navel, raw	1 medium (3 in. diameter)	18	69
Peaches, canned, extra light syrup, solids and liquids	1 cup (247 g)	27	104
Pears, canned, extra light syrup pack, solids and liquids	1 cup (247 g)	30	116
Raisins, seedless	1/4 cup (36 g)	29	108
Raspberries, frozen, unsweetened	1 cup (140 g)	17	73
Strawberries, raw	1 cup (152 g)	12	49
Vegetables			
Beans, snap, green, frozen, cooked, boiled, drained without salt	1 cup (135 g)	9	38
Carrots, raw	1 large (7-8.5 in. long)	7	30
Cauliflower, raw	1 cup, chopped (107 g)	5	27
Corn, sweet, yellow, frozen, kernels cut off cob, boiled, drained, without salt	1/2 cup (83 g)	16	67
Edamame, frozen, prepared	1 cup (155 g)	14	188
Eggplant, cooked, boiled, drained, without salt	1 cup, chopped (99 g)	9	35
Peas, green, frozen, cooked, boiled, drained, without salt	1/2 cup (80 g)	11	62
Potatoes, Russet, flesh and skin, baked	1 medium (2-3 in. diameter)	37	168
Potatoes, sweet potato, cooked, baked in skin, flesh, without salt	1 cup (200 g)	41	180
Pumpkin, canned, without salt	1/2 cup (123 g)	10	42
Squash, summer, zucchini, includes skin, raw	1 medium (196 g)	6	33

> continued

TABLE 3.3 > *continued*

Source	Serving size	Carbohydrate (g)	Calories
Vegetables *(continued)*			
Squash, winter, acorn, cooked, baked, without salt	1/2 cup (103 g)	15	57
Squash, winter, butternut, cooked, baked, without salt	1/2 cup (103 g)	11	41
Squash, winter, spaghetti, cooked, boiled, drained, or baked, without salt	1 cup (155 g)	10	42
Breads and crackers			
Bagels, plain, enriched, with calcium propionate (includes onion, poppy, sesame)	1 medium (3.5-4 in. diameter)	55	277
Bread, naan, whole wheat, commercially prepared, refrigerated	1 piece (106 g)	49	303
Bread, pita, whole-wheat	1 large (6.5 in. or 16 cm diameter)	36	168
Bread, wheat	2 slices (58 g)	28	159
Crackers, matzo, plain	1 sheet (26 g)	23	11
Crackers, whole-wheat, TRISCUITS	6 crackers (28 g)	19	120
English muffins, whole-wheat	1 whole (66 g)	27	134
Pancakes, whole-wheat, dry mix, incomplete, prepared	2 pancakes (4 in. diameter)	26	184
Rolls, dinner, whole-wheat	1 med (36 g)	18	96
Tortillas, ready-to-bake or fry, flour, refrigerated	1 tortilla (10 in. diameter)	36	220
Cereals			
Cereals ready-to-eat, GENERAL MILLS, Corn CHEX	1 cup (31 g)	26	115
Cereals ready-to-eat, GENERAL MILLS, Multi-Grain CHEERIOS	1 cup (29 g)	24	107
Cereals ready-to-eat, GENERAL MILLS, Rice CHEX	1 cup (27 g)	23	101
Cereals ready-to-eat, KASHI, 7 Whole Grain Puffs	1 cup (19 g)	15	64
Cereals ready-to-eat, POST, Raisin Bran Cereal	1/2 cup (31 g)	23	96
Cereals ready-to-eat, POST, Grape-Nuts Cereal	1/4 cup (29 g)	23	105

Source	Serving size	Carbohydrate (g)	Calories
Cereals ready-to-eat, POST, Shredded Wheat, original spoon-size	1/2 cup (25 g)	20	86
Cereals ready-to-eat, QUAKER, QUAKER OAT LIFE, plain	1/2 cup (21 g)	16	79
Cereals, CREAM OF WHEAT, instant, prepared with water, without salt	1/2 cup (121 g)	16	75
Granola, homemade	1/4 cup (31 g)	16	149
Oatmeal, instant oats, fortified, plain, prepared with water	1/2 cup, dry	29	170
Oatmeal, QUAKER, Instant Oatmeal, Cinnamon-Spice, dry	1 packet (43 g)	32	159
Oatmeal, steel cut oats, uncooked	1/2 cup (44 g)	29	170
Cereals ready-to-eat, rice, puffed, fortified	1 cup (14 g)	13	56
Sport drinks and bars			
6% glucose–electrolyte solution, Gatorade	8 oz (240 ml)	14	50
High-carbohydrate replacer, Vitargo	12 oz (360 ml)	35	140
Meal replacer	11 oz (325 ml)	59	360
KIND, FRUIT & NUT BAR	1 bar (40 g)	23	190
LARABAR FRUIT & NUT BAR CHERRY PIE, UNPREPARED	1 bar (48 g)	30	200
LUNA, WHOLE NUTRITION BAR, NUTZ OVER CHOCOLATE	1 bar (48 g)	24	200
POWERBAR, PERFORMANCE ENERGY BAR, CHOCOLATE	1 bar (65 g)	45	240
Snacks, CLIF BAR, mixed flavors	1 bar (68 g)	45	235
Snacks, granola bar, QUAKER, chewy, 90 Calorie Bar	1 bar (24 g)	19	90
Snacks, granola bars, hard, oats and honey, like NATURE VALLEY	1 bar (21 g)	15	100

> continued

TABLE 3.3 > *continued*

Source	Serving size	Carbohydrate (g)	Calories
Sport drinks and bars *(continued)*			
Snacks, granola bars, hard, plain	1 bar (25 g)	16	118
Snacks, granola bars, soft, uncoated, plain	1 bar (28 g)	19	124
Grains			
Barley, pearled, cooked	1 cup (157 g)	44	193
Couscous, cooked	1 cup (157 g)	36	176
Pasta, cooked, enriched, without added salt	1 cup (120 g)	37	190
Pasta, whole-wheat, cooked	1 cup (117 g)	35	174
Quinoa, cooked	1 cup (185 g)	39	222
Rice noodles, cooked	1 cup (176 g)	42	190
Rice, brown, medium-grain, cooked	1 cup (195 g)	46	218
Rice, white, medium-grain, enriched, cooked	1 cup (186 g)	53	242
Rice, wild rice, cooked	1 cup (164 g)	35	166
Pasta, gluten-free, brown rice flour, cooked, TINKYADA	1 cup (155 g)	49	211
Pasta, gluten-free, corn and rice flour, cooked	1 cup (141 g)	54	252
Pasta, gluten-free, corn flour and quinoa flour, cooked, ANCIENT HARVEST	1 cup (132 g)	41	201
Pasta, gluten-free, corn, cooked	1 cup (140 g)	39	176
ANCIENT HARVEST, BEAN & QUINOA ELBOWS PASTA, UPC: 089125220302	100 g	63	339
PROTEIN ROTINI PASTA, WHEAT, FAVA BEAN, CHICKPEA & LENTIL, UPC: 708820040281	1 cup (75 g)	51	267
LENTIL PENNE BEAN PASTA, UPC: 888683106727	1 cup (83 g)	53	288

Source	Serving size	Carbohydrate (g)	Calories
Legumes			
Beans, baked, canned, plain or vegetarian	1 cup (254 g)	54	239
Beans, black, mature seeds, canned, low sodium	1 cup (240 g)	40	218
Beans, kidney, red, mature seeds, canned, drained solids, rinsed in tap water	1 cup (158 g)	33	191
Beans, navy, mature seeds, canned	1 cup (262 g)	54	296
Beans, pinto, mature seeds, cooked, boiled, without salt	1 cup (171 g)	45	245
Beans, refried beans, canned, vegetarian	1 cup (242 g)	33	201
Chickpeas (garbanzo beans, Bengal gram), mature seeds, cooked, boiled, without salt	1 cup (164 g)	45	269
Lentils, mature seeds, cooked, boiled, without salt	1 cup (198 g)	40	230
Lima beans, immature seeds, frozen, baby, cooked, boiled, drained, without salt	1 cup (180 g)	35	189

Source: United States Department of Agriculture.

Carbohydrate Before and During Your Workout

Preworkout carbohydrate: Is it a good idea? It depends. If you're in a mass-building phase and want to push to the max, fuel yourself with carbohydrate before and during your workout. The best timing recommendations for eating before exercise is to eat a small meal of carbohydrate and protein one and a half to two hours before working out (for building). This meal should contain about 40 to 50 grams of carbohydrate (200 calories) and 20 to 30 grams of protein (80 calories).

If you are trying to taper or cut, you might minimize the amount of carbohydrate you take in prior to a moderate-intensity workout, because you are training to burn fat. I suggest cutting your carbohydrate–protein meal in half. Thus, your meal would contain about 25 grams of carbohydrate and 20 grams of protein. On the other hand, if you are training at a high or heavy intensity, don't decrease your carbohydrate fueling. The only way you can maintain high-intensity training is by having carbohydrate fuel available to burn. Without carbohydrate on board you may feel like you're working out at a high level, but if you measured your actual work output, it would look more like a lower-intensity level.

And, of course, you should make sure you are always well hydrated. Drink 2 cups (480 ml) of fluid within 2 hours of working out and another cup (240 ml) 15 minutes before exercise. Following this pattern will ensure that you gain the greatest energy advantage from your preexercise meal without feeling full while you exercise. If you want a little extra boost, try drinking a liquid carbohydrate beverage just before your workout. In a study of strength trainers, one group consumed a carbohydrate drink just before training and between exercise sets. Another group was given a placebo. For exercise, both groups did leg extensions at about 80 percent of their strength capacity, performing repeated sets of 10 repetitions with rest between sets. The researchers found that the carbohydrate-fed group outlasted the placebo group, performing many more sets and repetitions.

Another study turned up a similar finding. Exercisers drank either a placebo or a 10 percent carbohydrate beverage immediately before starting to exercise as well as before the 5th, 10th, and 15th sets of a strength-training workout. They performed repeated sets of 10 repetitions, with three minutes of rest between sets. When fueled by the carbohydrate drink (1 g per kg of body weight), they could do more total repetitions (149 versus 129) and more total sets (17.1 vs. 14.4) than when they drank the placebo. All this goes to show that carbohydrate clearly gives you an energy edge when consumed before and during a hard workout lasting longer than one hour. The harder you can work out, the more total calories you burn and the more you can stimulate your muscles to grow.

If you sip a carbohydrate drink over the course of a long workout, be aware that you can take in too many calories. When counseling clients, I recommend that they drink their first premeasured carbohydrate-fueling beverage 20 to 60 minutes before training. Then during successive hours of training, they should down their premeasured carbohydrate sport drink all at once at the beginning of each hour, and then go with water for the rest of the hour, continuing this pattern for each hour of training. That way, they don't consume too many calories from an unlimited amount of carbohydrate drink.

Get Your Workout Carbohydrate Count

The real key is to figure out how many grams of carbohydrate you need daily, from the menus in chapters 15 through 19. Then determine the carbohydrate you need for fueling exercise and include your workout carbohydrate into your total daily carbohydrate calculations. I like the idea of putting your fast carbohydrate, such as energy bars, to work for you around your training. This is a good diet planning strategy and leaves room for your more water-filled, fiber-rich vegetables and fruits to fill up your meals and snacks, especially if you are trying to taper or cut.

Consider your goals—mass building, performance enhancement, or fat burning—and listen to your body for signs of fatigue. Adjust your carbohydrate intake accordingly, depending on your goals and energy level. These are some factors that I consider, and simple formulas that you can use to get an idea of where to begin to count your workout carbohydrate. Start by figuring out your calorie burn during exercise. If you use an exercise tracker, that may give you your personalized data. This is a very general formula that can be used for any sport or exercise (kcal = calories):

0.1 kcal/kilogram of body weight/minute

OR

0.22 kcal/pound of body weight/minute

Use the appropriate equation to find a rough approximation of the number of calories you burn per minute of exercise. Then multiply that value by the number of minutes that you exercise. So if you exercise for one hour (60 minutes), use the following equation:

kcal × 60 minutes = kcal per hour

Of the total calories you burn, the proportion that comes from carbohydrate is based on the intensity of your exercise: The higher the intensity the more carbohydrate (and less fat) you burn. You can use general factors to account for exercise intensity.

- Moderate intensity: 40 percent carbohydrate fueled. Therefore, kcal/hour × 0.4 = carbohydrate calories used during moderate-intensity exercise.
- High intensity: 70 percent carbohydrate fueled. Therefore, kcal/hour × 0.7 = carbohydrate calories used during high-intensity exercise.
- Maximum intensity (this can be held for only a few minutes): 95 percent carbohydrate fueled. Therefore, kcal/hour × 0.95 = carbohydrate calories used during maximum-intensity exercise.

Now you need to turn these calories into grams of carbohydrate. Since 1 gram of carbohydrate contains 4 calories, divide your carbohydrate calories used by 4.

Carbohydrate kcal used/4 = grams of carbohydrate used per hour

You can go a little further to personalize your calculations. Here are all the different occasions where I shave a little more off of my carbohydrate recommendations around exercise.

- Females burn a little less carbohydrate than males, especially during moderate intensities of exercise.
- People with a smaller body size, and therefore less muscle mass, sometimes require fewer total calories than what is determined from the research, most of which is done on 154 pound (70 kg) or heavier males.
- Less well-trained or nonelite exercisers may burn fewer carbohydrate calories during exercise because they may not reach the higher levels of workout intensity for as long a duration as more highly trained, elite athletes.

Go for Carbohydrate

As you plan to include carbohydrate in your diet, keep in mind these important principles:

- Choose the right source of carbohydrate (unrefined, whole foods) to get the best elevations of insulin for muscle building.
- Combine carbohydrate with protein and fat, and eat multiple meals featuring this combination throughout the day.
- Use simple and refined sugars and starches such as honey, sport drinks, and other foods that quickly empty from your stomach in a targeted way, usually just before, during, and after a workout to accelerate stomach emptying and the recovery process.

Giving careful thought to what you eat—and making sure you get plenty of carbohydrate—will provide a solid foundation for optimizing both your performance and your health.

What type of carbohydrate should you consume during cross-training exercise? The answer is a carbohydrate that digests quickly, absorbs into your bloodstream rapidly, and reaches your muscle cells fast. This translates into easily digestible carbohydrate sources such as a sport drinks, or even bagels or white potatoes while you are on your bike. Rapidly digesting carbohydrate sources cause an insulin surge that reverses the catabolic state associated with training. This type of carbohydrate also helps the body quickly enter an anabolic state by carrying amino acids into muscle cells.

Plenty of research has been conducted into the effect of consuming high-glycemic carbohydrate sources around exercise, but the research often conflicts, reinforcing the tale of glycemic index mythology that I discussed above. Case in point: When eight untrained healthy men underwent three experimental conditions (consuming low-glycemic carbohydrate sources, high-glycemic carbohydrate sources, or a placebo), it didn't matter what type of carbohydrate sources were ingested. This indicates that what matters is that you consume carbohydrate to fuel your workout, and not the glycemic rating.

Other research does indicate that consuming high-glycemic carbohydrate foods increases the resynthesis of glycogen in the muscle cells, which just means that they coincidentally chose foods that actually do digest rapidly. Based on current findings, I recommend that you use your own personal experience and examine your own practical issues, such as stomach comfort and sense of energy, to decide which type of carbohydrate works best for you.

Remember that this is a starting point. You may find that when applied to your body and your personal training program, you need a little more or a little less carbohydrate. This is where the art of sport nutrition counseling becomes as important as the science.

Recovery Nutrition

After working out, you want your muscles to recover. Recovery is essentially the process of replenishing muscle glycogen. The better your recovery, the harder you'll be able to train during your next workout. The current research on nutrient timing finds that the critical factor is the presence of the nutrients and energy you need when your body starts to seek them out for recovery. The timing of when you eat the nutrients and fuel is not really the pivotal point. However, most people who have training goals like to have an eating plan as well as a training plan. So here is a very practical suggestion for planning your recovery nutrition strategy.

Immediately After Your Workout

Your muscles are most receptive to producing new glycogen within the first few hours after your workout. That's when blood flow to muscles is much greater, a condition that makes muscle cells practically sop up glucose like a sponge. Muscle cells are also more sensitive to the effects of insulin during this time, and insulin promotes glycogen synthesis. You should therefore take in some carbohydrate, along with protein, after your workout. (Remember that protein helps jump-start the manufacture of glycogen.) The question is this: What's the best type of carbohydrate for refueling? Answer: Carbohydrate that is easiest for you to consume and quickest to empty from your stomach.

If you are in a building phase, I suggest that you consume 1.0 to 1.2 grams of carbohydrate per kilogram of body weight as soon as possible after exercise. If you are in a tapering phase, consume 0.5 to 1 gram of carbohydrate per kilogram of body weight as soon as possible after exercise if you are a man; consume less (on the lower end of the range) if you are a woman or have a smaller body size. Your protein serving can be about 0.5 gram per kilogram of body weight.

Think of it this way: Have a 3:1 ratio of carbohydrate to protein as soon as possible after exercise. Protein is the big key to building muscle after exercise; carbohydrate is more about refueling. The more you are trying to enhance performance for your next bout of exercise, the more you'll depend on carbohydrate. If, however, weight and fat loss are the goals of your current training, then you will depend less on carbohydrate, and use closer to a 2:1 ratio in your postexercise meal.

The following recipe is for a smoothie that contains the proper ratios of carbohydrate, protein, and fat for refueling.

Honey, particularly in the form of a carbohydrate gel, is also a good postworkout choice. A research study published in the *Journal of the International Society of Sports Nutrition* in 2007 found that combining honey with a whey protein supplement may boost postworkout recovery and help prevent drops in blood sugar after exercise. In this particular study, honey powder performed as well as maltodextrin—a starch that has been the standard among recovery carbohydrate sources.

Another supplement carbohydrate source is a patented amylopectin (starch) fraction called Vitargo, a unique complex carbohydrate ingredient. It's derived and fractionated from any source of food starch, such as barley, corn, or potatoes, and contains no sugar. Fractionation separates a naturally occurring unique starch

Kleiner's Muscle Formula PLUS

21 g isolated whey protein

1 cup frozen unsweetened strawberries

1 medium banana

1 cup (240 ml) nonfat cow's milk or vanilla soy milk fortified with calcium and vitamins A and D

1 cup (240 ml) orange juice fortified with calcium and vitamin C

Blend for 60 seconds until smooth.

One serving contains:

Nutrients	Food group servings
436 calories	4 fruit servings
86 g carbohydrate	3 very lean protein servings
27-29 g protein	1 nonfat milk serving
0 g fat	3 tsp added carbohydrate or sugar (from soy
8 g dietary fiber	milk)

molecule from the other common starch molecules. Unlike other types of carbohydrate added to drinks and powders, such as maltodextrin, this fractionated starch is emptied from the stomach, enters the small intestine, and arrives in the bloodstream twice as fast as does maltodextrin or multitransport carbohydrate, which is known to be the next fastest carbohydrate supplement. Glycogen is replenished in muscle cells within two hours—again nearly twice as fast as any other rapid sport drink, and performance studies have shown up to a 23 percent higher work output two hours after exhaustive exercise. Therefore, recovery is very rapid. Vitargo is very easy on the gut, and can be used before, during, and after both resistance and endurance exercise.

Every Two Hours After Your Workout

Continue to take in carbohydrate every two hours after your workout until you have consumed at least 100 grams within 4 hours after exercise and a total of 600 grams within 24 hours after your workout. That equates to roughly 40 to 60 grams of carbohydrate an hour during the 24-hour recovery period. (Many women and smaller athletes may not need this much. Follow the menu plans for customized postworkout meals.)

A word of caution: There is a drawback to consuming simple and refined carbohydrate foods at times other than around exercise. They may produce an undesirable surge of blood sugar without any other healthful nutrients of food factors attached, yet stimulating a big reward and sense of elation in your brain. When this happens, you might love the taste from the food and think you feel great, but you are left having spent a calorie wad without any supporting nutrition to go with it. Repeated again and again this habit can lead to cravings for very sweet foods to satisfy your brain's nature to seek rewards. Whole foods, especially when consumed as part of a mixed diet of macronutrients, on the other hand, provide a more constant release of energy and so are unlikely to lead to depletion and cravings. By mixing and matching whole foods in your diet, you can keep your blood sugar levels stable from meal to meal. The watchword here is *moderation*. These fast-acting products such as sport drinks are useful when you train hard, or for long periods of time, and only around exercise. They are not beverages to choose and drink all day long.

Throughout the Week

So what kind of carbohydrate should you eat all day long and throughout the week? Because the goal of Power Eating is to help you increase muscle and reduce body fat, the type of carbohydrate you eat, the timing of your eating, and the carbohydrate combination are all very important. All forms of whole-food carbohydrate are important: fruits, vegetables, beans and legumes, and starchy vegetables such as potatoes, yams, and winter squash. But one type of carbohydrate shines: whole grains.

Whole grains, first of all, are best known for their fiber content, as discussed earlier. Fiber increases fullness, reduces transit time through the gut, and helps in blood sugar management. But there's more to whole grains than fiber, according to recent scientific research. Whole grains

- have strong antioxidant and anticancer properties;
- are excellent sources of minerals, trace elements, vitamins, and phytochemicals;
- are high in B vitamins and thus help enhance the nervous system;
- supply prebiotics, which are food factors that feed probiotics (healthy bacteria) in the gut and thus are integral to the health of the gastrointestinal system;
- help reduce abdominal fat, body weight, and body fat; and
- decrease the risk of developing metabolic syndrome, especially in the teen years.

Clearly, whole grains are a super-carbohydrate!

Should You Practice Carbohydrate Loading?

Endurance athletes practice a type of nutritional jump start known as carbohydrate loading. Basically, it involves increasing the amount of glycogen stored in the muscles just before an endurance competition. With more glycogen available, the athlete can run, cycle, or swim longer before fatigue sets in and thus gain a competitive edge. When done properly, carbohydrate loading works wonders for endurance athletes.

The Gluten Issue

Today, no discussion of whole wheat and whole grains in the diet can sidestep the topic of gluten, a protein component of wheat, rye, and barley. Some people are sensitive to gluten and may have either a gluten intolerance or celiac disease, which is inherited. For those who have an inherited tendency to develop celiac disease, eating foods that contain gluten damages the lining of the small intestine, which leads to nutritional deficiencies and possibly other diseases. Celiac disease, which may affect 1 percent of the population, is an immune system response to gluten that causes severe abdominal pain, bloating, and appetite loss. A lifelong illness, it begins at birth, although the symptoms may not appear for years. If you have celiac disease, which is diagnosed through an endoscopic biopsy and a special blood test, you must avoid all gluten-containing foods.

People with a self-reported intolerance to gluten make up approximately 10 percent of the population. Whereas people with celiac disease can take months to recover from exposure to gluten, those with an intolerance can recover quickly, within a few days. Symptoms of a gluten intolerance include upset stomach, bloating, rash, heartburn, nausea, headaches, and other less specific symptoms.

If you think you have an intolerance to gluten, include some gluten-containing foods in your diet for several weeks; then follow that with a gluten-free diet. Carefully record your responses. Then add gluten-containing foods back into your diet and document what happens. You must be very strict to get a clear picture of what your body is actually responding to. If you suspect celiac disease, do not do this on your own; see your physician.

You might find that some gluten-containing foods bother you but others do not. In this case, the gluten may be a coincidental factor in the foods but not the source of your discomfort. Research has shown that carbohydrate classified as fermentable oligo-, di-, monosaccharides and polyols, otherwise known as FODMAPs, may be the culprit for you, and not gluten. A very simple list of foods are considered to be FODMAPs. If you think you are sensitive to these kinds of foods, I recommend that you talk to a registered dietitian to help you create a healthy diet plan.

These types of carbohydrate-rich foods are FODMAPs:

- *Fructose:* Fruits, honey, high-fructose corn syrup, and agave syrup
- *Lactose:* Dairy
- *Fructans:* Wheat, onions, garlic
- *Galactans:* Legumes, such as beans, lentils, and soybeans
- *Polyols:* Sugar alcohols and fruits that have pits or seeds, such as apples, avocados, cherries, figs, peaches, or plums

Be very careful about eliminating such important foods from your diet unnecessarily. Although 10 percent of the population may be self-reported gluten sensitive, that means that 90 percent is not; however, we are all being targeted by Madison Avenue to buy gluten-free foods, and now they've got FODMAPs to add on top of that. Highly processed gluten-free foods can still be high in sugar and low in nutrition just like other processed foods. You can still eat whole grains even if you must eliminate gluten.

Grains With Gluten

Wheat, including varieties such as durum and semolina

Spelt

Barley

Rye

Triticale

Kamut

Farro

Sorghum

Bulgur

Gluten-Free Grains

Amaranth

Corn

Oats*

Millet

Montina (Indian rice grass)

Rice

Wild rice

Buckwheat

Teff

Quinoa

*Oats are inherently gluten free but are frequently contaminated with wheat during growing or processing.

Among strength athletes, bodybuilders have experimented the most with carbohydrate loading. Their goal is not endurance but bigger muscles. In general, about seven days before the contest, the bodybuilder cuts way back on carbohydrate. This is the depletion stage. Then, a few days before the contest, the bodybuilder starts increasing carbohydrate intake. This is the loading stage. The depletion stage theoretically prepares the muscles to hold more glycogen than before the depletion. So when the athlete increases carbohydrate consumption just before competition, the muscles hold more glycogen and supposedly look fuller.

But does this actually happen? Not really, says one study. Researchers put nine men, all bodybuilders, on a carbohydrate-loading diet. The diet involved three days of heavy weight training (designed to deplete muscle glycogen) and a low-carbohydrate diet (10 percent of the calories were from carbohydrate, 57 percent from fat, and 33 percent from protein). This was followed by three days of lighter weight training (to minimize glycogen loss) and a diet of 80 percent carbohydrate, 5 percent fat, and 15 percent protein. A control group followed the same strength-training program but followed a standard diet. At the end of the study, the researchers measured the muscle girth of all the participants. The results? Carbohydrate loading did not increase muscle girth in any of the bodybuilders.

Data in the sport nutrition literature allow us to conclude that strength athletes derive no real benefit from carbohydrate loading. Your diet should contain ample carbohydrate on a daily basis, but this is not the same as carbohydrate loading. Keep in mind, too, that carbohydrate depletion can actually result in the loss of hard-earned muscle. And since you lose intercellular water when you deplete carbohydrate, your muscle cells shrink. Carbohydrate in the diet helps to volumize your muscle cells and promote muscle protein synthesis. So stick with carbohydrate all the way to contest day.

4

Managing Fat

After a couple of hours of intense exercise, your glycogen supply can dwindle to nothing. But not so with your fat stores—another energy source for muscles. Compared with the limited but ready-to-use glycogen stores, fat stores are practically unlimited. In fact, it's been estimated that the average adult man carries enough fat (about 1 gal, or 4 L) to ride a bike from Chicago to Los Angeles, a distance of roughly 2,000 miles (3,219 km).

If fat stores are nearly inexhaustible, why worry about carbohydrate intake and glycogen replenishment? And why not supplement your diet with fat as an extra source of energy? True, there is a large enough tank of fat on your body to fuel plenty of exercise. (That's one reason there's no need to supplement with extra fat.) But the problem is that fat can be broken down only as long as oxygen is available. Oxygen must be present for your body to burn fat for energy but not to burn glycogen. In the initial stages of exercise, oxygen is not yet available. It can take 20 to 40 minutes of exercise before fat is maximally available to the muscles as fuel. The glucose in your blood and glycogen in your muscles are pressed into service first.

That's not to say that fat is hard to burn. It isn't. But how efficiently your body burns fat depends on your level of conditioning and your diet. One of the advantages of strength training and aerobic exercise is that your body improves its ability to burn fat as fuel in two major ways.

First, exercise (particularly aerobic exercise) enhances the development of capillaries that lead to muscle cells, thus improving blood flow where it's needed. In addition, exercise increases myoglobin, a protein that transports oxygen from the blood into muscle cells. With better blood flow and more oxygen in the muscles, the body becomes more efficient at burning fat, which is why you should not neglect the aerobic portion of your training.

Second, exercise stimulates the activity of hormone-sensitive lipase, an enzyme that promotes the breakdown of fat for energy. The more fat you can break down and burn, the more defined you will look.

Fat is definitely an exercise fuel, but it is a second-string source of energy for strength trainers. During strength training, your body still prefers to burn carbohydrate for energy, either from glucose in the blood or glycogen in the muscles. Fat is certainly one of the more controversial topics in nutrition. It is crucial in your diet, but it also has a bad reputation. Let's try to clear up the confusion once and for all.

Fat Facts

There are three major types of fatty material in the body: triglycerides, cholesterol, and phospholipids. Triglycerides, true fats, are stored in fat tissue and in muscle. A small percentage of fatty material is found in the blood, circulating as free fatty acids, which have been chemically released from the triglycerides. Of the three types of fatty material, triglycerides are the most involved in energy production. Research with bodybuilders has found that triglycerides, including the fat found in muscle, serve as a significant energy source during intense strength training. Not only will strength training help you build muscle but also will help you burn body fat.

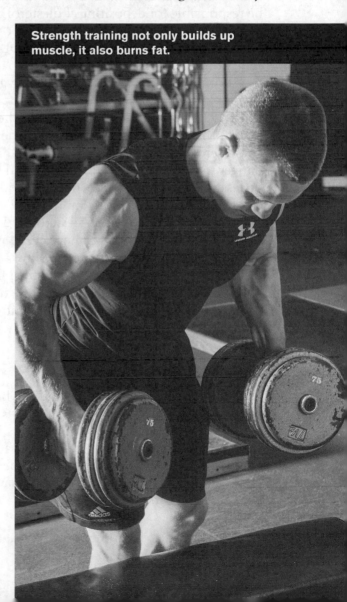

Strength training not only builds up muscle, it also burns fat.

Cholesterol is a waxy, light-colored solid that comes in two forms. You might call the first kind "the cholesterol in blood," and the second, "the cholesterol in food." Required for good health, blood cholesterol is a constituent of cell membranes and is involved in the formation of hormones, vitamin D, and bile (a substance necessary for the digestion of fat). Because your body can make cholesterol from fat, carbohydrate, or protein, you don't need to supply any cholesterol from food.

When you eat a food that contains cholesterol, that cholesterol is broken into smaller components that are used to make various fats, proteins, and other substances that your body requires. The cholesterol you eat doesn't become the cholesterol in your blood. Although it is important to reduce your intake of high-cholesterol foods, it is even more important to lower your intake of saturated fat (the kind found mostly in animal foods). That's because the liver manufactures blood cholesterol from saturated fat. The more saturated fat you eat, the more cholesterol your liver makes.

If your liver produces large amounts of cholesterol, the excess circulating in the bloodstream can collect on the inner walls of the arteries. This accumulation is called plaque. Trouble starts when plaque builds up in an artery, narrowing the passageway and choking blood flow. A heart attack can occur when blood flow to the heart muscle is cut off for a long period of time and part of the heart muscle begins to die. High blood cholesterol is therefore a major risk factor for heart disease, but it is one that in many cases can be controlled with exercise and a healthy diet.

Cholesterol may be present in blood as a constituent of low-density lipoprotein (LDL) or of high-density lipoprotein (HDL). LDL and HDL affect your risk of heart disease differently. LDL contains the greater amount of cholesterol and may be responsible for depositing cholesterol on the artery walls. LDL is known as bad cholesterol; the lower your blood value of LDL, the better.

HDL contains less cholesterol than LDL. Its job is to remove cholesterol from the cells in the artery wall and transport it back to the liver for reprocessing or excretion from the body as waste. HDL is the good cholesterol; the higher the amount in your blood, the better.

The science is far more complex and the details about oxidized fractions of LDL may further explain the development of heart disease, but suffice it to say that a total cholesterol reading of greater than 200 milligrams per deciliter of blood may be a danger sign. Generally, your HDL should be greater than 35 and your LDL should be less than 130. High levels of triglycerides in your blood can reflect an excess of alcohol or saturated fat in your diet and can increase your risk of heart disease. It is advisable to have your cholesterol and triglycerides checked annually. In time, scientists and physicians will have even better laboratory tools to predict your risk and protect your health. Table 4.1 shows what your cholesterol numbers mean.

The third type of fatty material, phospholipids, is involved in the regulation of blood clotting. Along with cholesterol, an important role of phospholipids is to form part of the structure of all cell membranes; they are critical in the membranes of brain cells and nervous system cells.

Fat in Foods

As an exerciser, strength trainer, or bodybuilder concerned with your appearance, you may be confused by mixed messages concerning dietary fat. What is the real story? The big thing to know about fats is that they can modulate the way cells work, in ways that are good for you and in ways that are bad for you. Whether it's good or bad depends on the specific type of fat, and also the ratio of the different kinds of fats in your diet. The thing to pay attention to is that these influences on the way cells work can be profound.

TABLE 4.1 Cholesterol Numbers

Total cholesterol	
<200 mg/dl	Desirable
200-239 mg/dl	Borderline high
≥240 mg/dl	High
LDL cholesterol	
<100 mg/dl	Optimal
100-129 mg/dl	Near optimal/above optimal
130-159 mg/dl	Borderline high
160-189 mg/dl	High
≥190 mg/dl	Very high
HDL cholesterol	
<40 mg/dl	Low: a major risk factor for heart disease
40-59 mg/dl	The higher, the better
≥60 mg/dl	Considered protective against heart disease
Triglycerides	
<150 mg/dl	Desirable
150-199 mg/dl	Borderline high
200-499 mg/dl	High
≥500 mg/dl	Very high

Source: National Heart, Lung, and Blood Institute, "Third Report of the National Cholesterol Education Program (NCEP) Expert Panel on Detection, Evaluation, and Treatment of High Blood Cholesterol in Adults (Adult Treatment Panel III) Executive Summary." NIH Publication No. 01-3670, May 2001, http://www.nhlbi.nih.gov/guidelines/cholesterol/atp3xsum.pdf.

The latest word is that fat is actually good for you and good for weight control, as long as you eat the right kinds. Sure, too much fat, just like too much carbohydrate or protein, can turn into body fat if you eat too many calories. But the right kinds of fat actually help you lose body fat and keep you healthy in body and mind. You'll need help figuring out how much fat and what kind of fat to eat to stay healthy. Here's a closer look.

Fatty acids from food, the tiny building blocks of fat, are classified into three groups according to their hydrogen content: saturated, polyunsaturated, and monounsaturated. Saturated fatty acids are usually solid at room temperature and, with the exception of tropical oils, come from animal sources. Beef fat and butter fat are high in saturated fatty acids. Butter fat is found in milk, cheese, cream, ice cream, and other products made from milk or cream. Low-fat or skim milk products are much lower in saturated fat. Tropical oils high in saturated fat include coconut oil, palm kernel oil, and palm oil and also the cocoa fat found in chocolate. They are generally found in commercial baked goods and other processed foods.

Polyunsaturated and monounsaturated fats are usually liquid at room temperature and come from nuts, vegetables, and seeds. Polyunsaturated fats such as vegetable shortening and margarines are solid because they have been hydrogenated—a process that changes the chemical makeup of the fat to harden it. The resulting fat is composed of substances known as trans-fatty acids or trans fat, which many studies have shown to raise blood cholesterol. Trans-fatty acids are more harmful than saturated fats when it comes to your heart; no level of trans fat is safe, and it should be avoided altogether. Fortunately, food manufacturers are now required to label the existence of trans fat on their products if their packaged foods enter interstate commerce in the United States. Look at the Nutrition Facts label to see how many grams of trans fat are in your food. Be aware, though, that companies are allowed to label their trans fat content as zero if one single serving of the food contains one-half gram of trans fat or less. That means that there still could be some trans fat in a single serving, and if you eat more than one serving, you are consuming an appreciable amount of trans fat. Remember, no level of trans fat is safe.

Monounsaturated fatty acids are found in large amounts in olive oil, canola oil, peanut oil, and other nut oils. Monounsaturated fats appear to have a protective effect on blood cholesterol levels. They help lower the bad cholesterol (LDL) and maintain the higher levels of good cholesterol (HDL).

Essential Fats

Of all dietary fat, certain types of polyunsaturated fat are considered essential. Two of these are linoleic acid and alpha-linolenic acid (ALA). The chemical structure of linoleic acid is referred to as an omega-6 fat, and the chemical structure of alpha-linolenic acid is an omega-3 fat. Although these fats are essential, they are not needed in very large amounts. Your body can't make them; you have to get them from food. They are required for normal growth, the maintenance of cell membranes, and healthy arteries and nerves. As well, essential fats keep your skin smooth and lubricated and protect your joints. They also assist in the breakdown and metabolism of cholesterol. Vegetable fats such as corn, soybean, safflower, and walnut oils are all high in essential fats, as are nuts and seeds. The total amount required for good health is 6 to 10 percent of total fat intake, or a total of 5 to 10 grams a day.

In addition to alpha-linolenic acid, two other omega-3 fats are considered essential and are found primarily in fish and shellfish: eicosapentaenoic acid (EPA) and docosahexaenoic acid (DHA). EPA and DHA are found predominantly in marine oils, whereas ALA is found in mostly all plant foods. All three are important and should not be substituted for one another. They are not interchangeable in amounts that will support health and performance, and they cannot be manufactured by the body in amounts that will support health.

Unfortunately, most people's intake of omega-3 fat is pitifully low. One reason is that we are eating more omega-6 fat, displacing omega-3 fat and creating an unhealthy imbalance. Sources of omega-6 fat include all the types of oils used in commercial cooking, baking, and food processing, including safflower, sunflower, soybean, corn, and cottonseed oils. Nutrition experts now recommend that we eat omega-6 fat and omega-3 fat in a healthier ratio, increasing our intake of omega-3 oils and decreasing our intake of omega-6 oils. You should substitute olive oil and canola oil, which are lower in omega-6 fat and higher in monounsaturated fat, for the other oils in your diet. Then increase the amount of fish you eat to increase your omega-3 intake. Some have suggested a 1:1 or 2:1 ratio of omega-6 fat to omega-3 fat; others advocate a 4:1 ratio. These ratios have been associated with lower incidences of heart disease and cancer in populations in which the consumption of omega-3 fat is traditionally higher.

Evidence is emerging that when this ratio is out of whack—when there is a high intake of omega-6 fat and a low intake of omega-3 fat—the fatty acid metabolism is altered in the body. The brain releases hormones and neurotransmitters (brain chemicals involved in sending messages) that tell the body to hold on to fat and not to burn it. It appears, then, that by raising levels of omega-3 fat in your diet, you create a better fat-burning effect. You really do need to eat the right kind of fat to feed your brain and burn body fat.

Omega-3 fatty acids, in particular, have far-reaching benefits for health and the management of chronic disease. Current research shows that they lower blood levels of triglycerides and a heart-damaging form of cholesterol called very low-density lipoprotein (VLDL). In addition, omega-3 fat lowers blood pressure in people with high blood pressure and may reduce the risk of sudden cardiac death. Omega-3 fat is also required for the development of the retina and neurological tissues. A lack of omega-3 fat in the diets of pregnant women may adversely affect the eyesight and even brain development of newborns.

Omega-3 Supplementation

The data are really quite clear about how important the marine oils DHA and EPA are in the treatment of diseases of chronic inflammation. For instance, research has shown that periodontal disease, a chronic inflammatory disease, responds well to DHA treatment. A significant association has been established between periodontal disease and an increased risk for cardiovascular disease, diabetes, hypertension, cancer, low birth weight, and even miscarriage; the physiological connection is chronic systemic inflammation.

It is a good idea to supplement your diet with fish oil. Enough research justifies its use; however, you need to choose wisely. The product you choose should be a good source of EPA and DHA, with at least 1,000 milligrams combined of DHA and EPA.

DHA is important for healthy brain function, eyes, and the entire central nervous system. DHA is strongly associated with mood; low levels are associated with depression, loss of mental focus, and loss of memory.

DHA and EPA supplementation is recommended for both the treatment and prevention of virtually all of the chronic diseases. The recommended dose for supplementation or through diet is 1,000 milligrams per day of a combination of DHA and EPA. Under certain circumstances DHA or EPA are recommended alone,

Omega-3 Fatty Acids and Brain Health

Treatment of depression, anxiety, and stress with omega-3 fatty acids is garnering a lot of attention in medical circles. About 60 percent of the brain is composed of fat, and the primary fat in the brain is omega-3 fat. When omega-3 fat is in short supply in the diet, other fat gets involved in brain building, and as a result, the health of brain cells is impaired. The membrane of each brain cell, for example, becomes rigid, and it takes longer for electrical impulses to travel from one cell to another. This means that messages are not being carried rapidly from brain cell to brain cell. Consequently, you don't think clearly, and your memory may become foggy. Depression and anxiety can also set in. Increasing levels of omega-3 fat in the diet has been shown to alleviate these problems.

There is an important ratio of omega-6 to omega-3 fats in the diet that also helps to limit inflammatory processes. In recent years, scientists have discovered that the development of many diseases is influenced by chronic inflammation in the body. Inflammation is an essential part of the body's healing process, brought on when the immune system tries to battle disease-causing germs and repair injured tissue. When that battle is over, the army of inflammation-triggering substances is supposed to withdraw, but in many cases it does not. Chronic inflammation is the result, and it has been implicated in heart disease, diabetes, arthritis, multiple sclerosis, cancer, and even Alzheimer's disease. Omega-3 fat appears to halt chronic inflammation. Omega-6 fat is pro-inflammatory, whereas omega-3 fat is anti-inflammatory. However, omega-6 fat is far more abundant in our food supply. So it takes planning and effort and good choices to create a healthy ratio of omega-6 to omega-3 fat. Although the average American diet reflects a ratio of 20:1, a more ideal ratio is 2:1 to 4:1.

The fat cells in your body create their own inflammatory processes—which is yet another reason to stay lean. In fact, overweight people show symptoms of chronic, low-grade inflammation, perhaps indicating early atherosclerosis, according to research. A study conducted by researchers at the Free University in Amsterdam and scientists at the National Institute on Aging in Bethesda, Maryland, found overweight people to be far more likely than lean ones to have excess concentrations of C-reactive protein (CRP) in their blood—a marker of inflammation. In fact, it is possible that chronic systemic inflammation precedes overweight and obesity due to poor lifestyle choices. As mentioned above, fat tissue is not benign. It is considered to be its own endocrine organ, pumping out hormones that create inflammatory markers that help sustain and create more fat tissue and keep inflammation chugging along. These compounds also contribute to increased risk of all the chronic diseases noted above. So if you are overweight, losing weight is the first step toward protecting your health.

but in general the combination works quite well. If you have a larger body, do a lot of physical activity where you become sore or get banged up, or have chronic inflammation, you can safely consume 2,000 milligrams daily. Always tell your physician or health care provider before taking supplements if you also take prescription medications or need any kind of medical intervention or surgery. You

Enhance Healing Ability

Some interesting laboratory data have shown that DHA and EPA supplementation enhances wound healing. Athletes become injured fairly regularly, so having adequate levels of these fats is important for healing.

---

should be able to find high-quality supplements that combine DHA and EPA in online and retail stores.

To consume this much DHA plus EPA daily, you should consume five fish meals per week from predominantly fatty fish. Serving sizes should be 4 to 6 ounces (120 to 180 g). The best fish sources of omega-3 fatty acids are wild salmon, mackerel, black cod, cod, halibut, rainbow trout, shellfish, sardines, herring, and tuna. (See table 4.2 for nutritional information on seafood.)

Omega-3 fat is also found in green leafy vegetables, nuts, canola oil, tofu, and flaxseed. However, it is not the same omega-3 fat as that found in fish oil. It is ALA, the third kind of omega-3 fat besides EPA and DHA. ALA has its own important anti-inflammatory pathway, but, in limited amounts, it can be converted to EPA and DHA in the body. On the best of days, when you eat flax or get ALA from any of the other sources, only 5 percent of it is changed into EPA and DHA. Furthermore, you must be well nourished and very healthy to get that 5 percent exchange rate. Most people don't have the capability to fully reach 5 percent. Although fat from flaxseed and sources of ALA other than fish has important benefits, it is not a good substitute for EPA and DHA.

If you are on the road and can't get fish, I recommend that you supplement your diet with fish oil. For non-fish eaters or vegetarians, other fortified foods contain vegan sources of DHA and EPA, primarily milk and eggs (make sure they are labeled as fortified with these oils). If you cannot consume enough of these foods in your regular diet, I highly recommend supplementation from a fish or vegan algae-based product. With either form of supplement, read the Supplement Facts label to determine how much DHA and EPA are in the daily recommended dose of that product. Very often, a product's own recommended dosage is much lower, so it there are more doses per bottle, making the product seem less expensive. However, you need to take the number of capsules that will bring the total milligrams up to my recommended dosage of 1,000 milligrams of DHA plus EPA daily.

One of the most exciting areas of research with omega-3 fat for physique athletes is the animal research looking at the influence of omega-3 fat on fat burning. Research with mice has shown that omega-3 fat reduces both fat cell numbers and fat cell size. Epidemiological data on humans show that following a Mediterranean-style diet (which includes regular fish meals and plenty of high-performance fat) leads to better total body weight control and better abdominal fat control.

Olive Oil

Olive oil is one of the "good fats." Please understand, however, that there is a difference between extra-virgin olive oil and olive oil. Extra-virgin olive oil comes

TABLE 4.2 A Guide to Nutritional Values for Alaska Seafood

Wild Alaska seafood nutrition: More reasons to feel good about eating wild Alaska seafood!

	Calories	Protein (g)	Fat (g)	Saturated Fat (g)	Sodium (mg)	Cholesterol (mg)	Omega-3s (mg) (EPA + DHA)	Vitamin D [IU (mcg)]
Alaska whitefish								
Halibut	100	20	2	–	70	51	201	200 (5.0)
Cod	70	15	0	–	156	40	141	16 (0.4)
Pollock	70	16	0	–	142	63	285	44 (1.1)
Rockfish	90	19	2	–	76	52	300	156 (3.9)
Sole	70	13	2	–	90	51	257	120 (3.0)
Black cod (Sablefish)	210	15	17	–	62	54	1543	N/A

Surimi seafood: Nutritional values for Alaska Surimi seafood vary depending on brand and product form; please check the package label for specifics.

	Calories	Protein (g)	Fat (g)	Saturated Fat (g)	Sodium (mg)	Cholesterol (mg)	Omega-3s (mg) (EPA + DHA)	Vitamin D [IU (mcg)]
Alaska shellfish								
King crab	70	16	1	0.1	911	45	351	N/A
Snow crab	100	20	1	0.16	572	60	405	N/A
Dungeness crab	90	19	1	0.1	321	65	501	N/A
Scallops*	90	17	1	0.2	567	35	149	80 (2)
Shrimp*	80	20	0	0.4	94	160	260	N/A
Alaska salmon								
King	200	22	11	3	51	70	1476	N/A
Sockeye	130	23	5	1	78	50	730	570 (14)
Coho	120	20	4	1	49	50	900	383 (10)
Keta	130	22	4	1	54	80	683	N/A
Pink	130	21	4	1	76	50	524	444 (11)
Alaska canned salmon (traditional)**								
Sockeye (red)	140	20	6	1	350	70	1,077	715 (18)
Pink	120	20	4	1	320	70	916	493 (12)
Keta	120	18	5	1	330	35	1,099	328 (8)

Serving size: 3.0 oz./85g cooked portions.

N/A means data not available.

*Values are for mixed species.

**Traditional values include skin and bones.

Source: USDA National Nutrient Database for Standard Reference, Release #28. Used with permission of Alaska Seafood Marketing Institute.

from the first pressing of a single variety of olive or fruit, not a blend. That gives it a distinct taste, smell, and color. What is not so well known about extra-virgin olive oil is that it uniquely contains an anti-inflammatory phenolic compound called oleocanthal, which is almost identical to the nonsteroidal anti-inflammatory drug ibuprofen. This makes extra-virgin olive oil an excellent anti-inflammatory food. Although olive oil in general is a good anti-inflammatory food, extra-virgin olive oil is significantly better. Use it whenever possible. You'll know when you've got a potent variety when you get that peppery catch, or finish, in the back of your throat when you drink it plain. That's the oleocanthal, and that's the good stuff!

Fat and Your Gut

When you have an upset stomach or uncomfortable intestines, it's tough to train hard day after day, and certainly you will not perform at your best. One solution is to populate your diet with good fat, such as olive oil and omega-3 fat. Remember, these fats exert an anti-inflammatory effect that is healing to your gastrointestinal tract. By contrast, an excess of omega-6 fat promotes inflammation everywhere, including in the gut, which is why you want to steer clear of fried foods, packaged snack foods, foods high in saturated fat, and fast foods. By substituting good fat—or what I like to call high-performance fat—you'll notice a quick improvement in how you feel.

Seeds, another high-performance source of fat, are also helpful in promoting gut health because of their fibrous structure. Lignin, a type of fiber found in plant foods, is present in large amounts in flaxseed. While probiotic bacterial cultures help to promote health in your intestines, lignin keeps the bacterial cultures well fed. For this reason, lignin is called a prebiotic. Including 1 to 2 tablespoons of ground flaxseed in your diet every day is a wonderful way to ingest healthy fibers as well as the strong anti-inflammatory omega-3 fat, ALA. Flaxseed must be ground; our teeth cannot grind the seeds well enough for digestion. If the seeds are not preground, as in flaxseed meal, they will exit the body whole without bestowing any of their benefits.

Essential Fat Needs

If you slash fat to miniscule levels or cut it out altogether, you risk developing an essential fat deficiency. This is not a widespread problem, because Americans get their fill of fat. Even so, I have seen many athletes, bodybuilders in particular, go to extremes in cutting fat. When this happens, the body has trouble absorbing the fat-soluble vitamins A, D, E, and K. Furthermore, the health of cell membranes is jeopardized because low-fat diets are low in vitamin E. Vitamin E is an antioxidant that prevents disease-causing free radicals from puncturing cell membranes, and it also helps in the muscle repair process that takes place after exercise. Men who go on low-fat diets put their bodies in hormonal jeopardy, because fat is required to make the male hormone testosterone. Women who slash their fat feel terrible in general, and even start to crave processed carbohydrate.

You can also go overboard on fat. Too much dietary fat often causes weight gain and gradually leads to obesity and related health problems. While this may not be due to the fat per se, because fat is so dense in calories, most people who don't plan their food and energy intake end up eating an excess of calories when they eat a diet heavily balanced toward fat. Excessive saturated fat in the diet can also elevate cholesterol, particularly the dangerous type (LDL). On the other hand, polyunsaturated and monounsaturated fats have been shown to cut cholesterol levels. However, polyunsaturated fat may also lower the protective type of cholesterol (HDL). Very high intakes of polyunsaturated fat have been linked to higher risks of cancer.

So where's the happy medium between too much fat and too little? According to the American Heart Association, for the purposes of prevention, they recommend a diet very similar to what I recommend in *The New Power Eating*: a plant-based diet that is rich in vegetables, fruits, and whole grains; includes low-fat dairy products, fish, poultry, legumes, high-performance fats, and oils, nuts, and seeds; and limits intake of sodium, sweets, sugar sweetened beverages, and red meats. By following this kind of dietary structure, your total fat intake and the types of fats that you eat will be well balanced. You don't need to be counting fat grams and calories. A diet that contains this variety is considered beneficial for managing depression, anxiety, and stress. Of course, the American Heart Association also includes targeted exercise recommendations to encourage the average person to become more active.

Although these AHA guidelines serve a general purpose for the kind of healthy diet that can be helpful for anyone, this is not an athlete-specific diet plan. In the same vein, the DRIs are not written for very active individuals. But like the AHA diet plan, they give us a place to start. To be more specific, here are some recommendations. I will follow them up with more specific, Power Eating fat recommendations.

DRIs for Essential Fats

Linoleic acid: 12 grams daily for women; 17 grams daily for men

Alpha-linolenic acid: 1.1 grams daily for women; 1.6 grams daily for men

EPA and DHA combined: 2 grams daily, based on a 2,000-calorie diet (This is a United Kingdom recommendation because there is no EPA and DHA DRI for the United States. For clarity on the safety of this dose, a study published in 2016 noted no safety concerns with levels of EPA + DHA from 5.0 to 6.9 grams per day—levels at least 20 times higher than the FAO minimum recommended intake of 250 milligrams/day.)

Fat Recommendations for Active People

If you're an exerciser, bodybuilder, or strength trainer trying to stay lean, you should control your total fat intake to control your total calorie intake. For reasons around both physical training, health and emotional well-being, I like my clients to hover around 25 to 35 percent, of their total calories from fats, depending on their total calorie intake and specific training goals at the time. There are reasons that you might alter this percentage, and we will discuss those below.

There are many strategies for accomplishing this fat intake level. One less-structured way is to follow the AHA guidelines for food choices. If the majority of your food choices are plant-rich from a variety of vegetables, fruits, whole grains, beans, nuts, and seeds, and you add in animal protein-rich foods from fish, meat, and dairy to round out your diet, your total fat intake is most likely to be in a well-controlled zone of about 25 to 35 percent of calories each day. I want to emphasize the word "variety." If you neglect variety and choose a majority of high fat plant foods, like avocados, oils, nut butters, and seeds, you will have created a high-fat diet. Or, if you include dairy but avoid meats, and eat a high volume of cheese, you are also creating a high-fat diet. So the label that you put on your diet doesn't protect you from less healthy choices. You have to ensure the variety in your diet, which promotes health and performance.

Your diet should contain much more unsaturated than saturated fat: 5 percent saturated, 10 to 15 percent monounsaturated, and 7 to 10 percent polyunsaturated.

A much more structured way to monitor your fat intake is by counting the grams of fat in your diet each day. To be honest, counting calories and macronutrient grams daily is probably my least favorite way to live life. I prefer that you plan a food template, perhaps monthly, of what you will include in your diet each day using food groups, with the knowledge of the macronutrient content of the foods in those groups. Then you can choose from within those groups as they fall in your plan each day, without constantly counting, and know that you are on your plan. This gives you so much more freedom to choose as life presents itself in your day, rather than structuring and restricting your life around your food plan. And you can be more comfortable with your diet at the same time. In all the menu chapters in *The New Power Eating*, you will see how I use a food group template down the left column of the page to fill in a daily menu of food choices.

You can calculate your own daily fat intake by using the following formulas:

Total Fat

Total calories × 30% = daily calories from fat / 9 = g total fat

Example: 2,000 calories × 0.3 = 600 / 9 = 67 g total fat

Saturated Fatty Acids (SFA)

Total calories × 5% = daily calories from SFA / 9 = g SFA

Example: 2,000 calories × 0.05 = 100 / 9 = 11 g SFA

Following the Power Eating plan, first determine your protein and carbohydrate needs. All of your leftover calories are fat calories—most of which should be monounsaturated and polyunsaturated fats. Be sure to read food labels for the fat content per serving of the foods you buy in the supermarket. The grams of fat are listed on any food package that provides a nutrition label.

Fat Substitutes and Fat Replacers

Many low-fat foods replace the fat with starch, fiber, protein, and other forms of fat. But why even bother with fat substitutes and fat replacers when you need the right kinds of fat in your diet? Go ahead and continue to enjoy healthy fat in foods such as extra-virgin olive oil, nuts, avocados, and nut and seed oils. Your body needs and deserves them.

What's more, we don't yet know what effect artificial fat has on health. Some nutritionists and other health advocates are concerned that consumers may get so carried away with eating fat-free foods that they won't obtain enough of the healthy fat their bodies truly need.

Reducing Less-Healthy Fat in Your Diet

Trans fat, saturated fat, and to a lesser extent, cholesterol (especially if you have a genetic tendency toward high blood cholesterol) in your diet can lead to high cholesterol in your blood, which in turn clogs blood vessels, contributing to heart disease and stroke. You should be vigilant about reducing these fats in your diet.

As we discussed in chapter 3, simple and refined sugars and starches are also a big part of the problem, raising levels and likely causing oxidation of blood cholesterol, dramatically increasing the risk of clogged blood vessels. These ingredients cannot be left out of the discussion. Read labels to understand the hidden and added sugars in your food, and focus on whole grains and whole starchy vegetables rather than refined flours and processed starches.

The major sources of saturated fat are meats and whole-milk dairy products. However, fat from animals is not necessarily bad in and of itself. The real problem with animal fat may be the industrial farming methods used to raise animals. Caged animals fed corn develop very different, and harmful, fat composition compared to wild animals that eat grasses. Meat and dairy from wild animals may not have unhealthy levels of fat, and in fact may have healthy fatty acid profiles. In addition, most farming chemicals such as pesticides and herbicides are fat soluble. So when you eat foods that have fat in them on a regular basis, it's wise to choose organic. However, because research is ongoing on this topic, you should limit your consumption of animal-based saturated fats in general. When no nutrition information is available for a particular food, remember these helpful hints about the sources of saturated fat, trans fat, and cholesterol in foods.

- Choose lean cuts of select meat such as round, sirloin, and flank, and eat portions that are no larger than the palm of your hand. Chicken, turkey, and fish are always leaner meat choices. To give an example, a 3-ounce (90 g) portion of beef has at least 2 grams of saturated fat; skinless chicken has 0.5 gram of saturated fat. Chicken breast with skin is equal to beef, at about 2 grams of saturated fat.

- When preparing and eating meat, make sure to trim all visible fat and skin. Use cooking racks when baking, broiling, grilling, steaming, or microwaving the meat to avoid melting the fat back into the meat.

- When eating lunch meat, select low-fat chicken or turkey breast rather than high-fat bologna or salami. Know that any lunch meat has additives for flavoring, even if it just says "broth" on the label.

- Dairy foods are very important in your diet, including for weight control. To cut the fat in dairy foods, choose low-fat products rather than whole-milk products and include them in your diet two or three times each day.

- Cholesterol is found only in animal products, and egg yolk is a concentrated source. There has never been a research study showing that egg yolks raise cholesterol levels, and in fact there are several that have shown that an egg yolk a day does not raise blood cholesterol levels in healthy individuals. I have always known this and I never recommended eliminating eggs from the diet, but it was a poorly substantiated public health recommendation that took on a life of its own. There are several reasons to add egg yolks back to your diet, including that yolks are a primary source of phospholipids and the B vitamin choline in our diet. Phospholipids are important for cell membrane health and may have a positive impact on blood cholesterol and inflammation. Choline is half of the neurotransmitter acetylcholine, the most abundant neurotransmitter in the body. Acetylcholine is at work all the time, every time we think or move. After Americans started dumping egg yolks down the drain, nutrition scientists discovered that our diets had become deficient in choline. Alarm bells went off in the nutrition world, and today you should be hard pressed to find a nutrition specialist who recommends eliminating egg yolks for everyone.

- If you know that you have a difficult time controlling your blood cholesterol or you are a type 2 diabetic, consider substituting two egg whites for one yolk, and limit your intake to one egg yolk per day. If you are vegetarian or vegan and do not eat egg yolks, or you are allergic to egg yolks, you can get choline from whole soy foods and milk that contain their fat fraction. Choline is found in the compound lecithin, which occurs in soy. However, most people do not eat enough soy to get their daily need. Consider a daily choline supplement, usually found in one-a-day type vitamin supplements. You can find more information on choline in chapter 9.

- Processed and prepared foods, especially snack foods, can be concentrated sources of fat. Hydrogenated vegetable fat contains trans-fatty acids that promote heart disease, so pay the most attention to the types and total amounts of fat in the food you eat. Read labels carefully, even if the packaging says that the product is light, to determine whether products really are low in fat. Be aware, also, that legally any product that has 0.5 gram of trans fat or less can be labeled trans fat free. So you probably are eating plenty of trans fats if you are eating a lot of packaged baked goods that say 0 trans fats per serving. Each serving may have up to 0.5 gram of trans fat.

All of the accumulated sport nutrition information tells us that the right kinds of dietary fat have profound effects on weight management, mood, and overall health. If we cut out all the fat in our diets, we eliminate not only the unhealthy saturated fat but also the very healthy unsaturated fat. In today's world, the effective message is that the wrong fat can hurt, and the right fat can help. As long as you balance your calories, a diet high in lean protein, good carbohydrate, and good fat will leave little room for unhealthy foods to creep in. Keep your sight on all the good foods you need to eat every day and then the bad foods won't get you down.

Sport Nutrition Fact Versus Fiction: Is Chocolate Healthy or Harmful?

Answer: Healthy! Chocolate is a healthy choice in prudent amounts. First, when you're feeling low or run-down, a bit of chocolate not only pampers you but also works with your brain chemistry to lift your mood and make you feel better. The combination of sugar and fat in chocolate elevates two key neurotransmitters, serotonin and endorphins. Low levels of these brain chemicals are linked with depression and anxiety. By raising them, you feel calmer, more relaxed, and happier. Not bad for a few hundred calories!

Second, eating chocolate may actually make you healthier. This finding originated with the research on dietary saturated fat and its association with an increased risk of developing heart disease. Over a decade ago, the discovery that stearic acid, the predominant saturated fat in chocolate, actually has a neutral effect on blood cholesterol levels exonerated chocolate, removing it from the list of foods that are bad for your heart. Even feeding subjects one whole chocolate bar a day didn't change their levels of blood cholesterol.

What's more, scientists have discovered that chocolate is full of antioxidants, including flavonols and flavonoids. These compounds appear to have cardioprotective effects, including antioxidant properties, the ability to reduce the stickiness of blood cells, and the ability to help the lining of blood vessels remain dilated, allowing blood to pass more freely and keeping blood pressure at normal levels.

The richest source of flavonols is natural, non-Dutched (no alkali) cocoa powder. It is also the healthiest source because it is devoid of sugar and very low in fat and calories. Next on the list are baking chocolate and dark chocolate. Dark chocolate has twice the amount of flavonols as milk chocolate.

Curious about the antioxidant content of cocoa compared with wine and tea, Dr. Chang Yong Lee of Cornell University tested the antioxidant content of the following beverages: 1 cup (240 ml) of hot water containing 2 tablespoons of pure cocoa powder, 1 cup (240 ml) of water containing a standard-size bag of green tea, 1 cup (240 ml) of black tea, and a 5-ounce (150 ml) glass of California merlot (red wine). On a per-serving basis, the antioxidant concentration in cocoa was the highest. Its concentration was almost two times stronger than the concentration in red wine, two to three times stronger than in green tea, and four to five times stronger than in black tea. Dr. Lee also found that hot cocoa triggers the release of more antioxidants than cold cocoa.

Dr. Mary Engler and colleagues of the University of California at San Francisco investigated the effects of a flavonoid-rich dark chocolate on endothelial function (the function of the cells lining blood vessels), oxidative stress, blood lipids, and blood pressure in 21 healthy adults. The subjects were assigned to eat either a daily high-flavonoid or low-flavonoid dark chocolate bar for two weeks. There were no obvious differences between the two bars. The subjects were instructed to keep their diets the same as usual, except to eliminate all other foods and beverages high in flavonoids, alcohol, vitamin supplements, and nonsteroidal anti-inflammatory drugs. The results showed that endothelial function improved with the consumption of the high-flavonoid chocolate bars. Blood vessels were more dilated and blood flow was freer. Other biochemical measures indicated a strong association with the intake of flavonoids. No differences in oxidative stress or lipid profiles were seen between the two groups.

Deciding which side of the line chocolate falls on goes back to two major tenets of nutrition: variety and moderation. To be sure, chocolate bars, whether they contain dark or milk chocolate, are high in calories, sugar, and fat. The nature of dark chocolate is that it contains more cacao and less sugar. An ounce of 85 percent cacao dark chocolate will automatically have more flavonols and less sugar compared to a 45 percent milk chocolate. When searching for sources of antioxidants in your diet, remember that fruits, vegetables, fish, nuts, seeds, and tea are rich sources of many important nutrients and antioxidants. Flavonol-rich cocoa is available in candy bars, cocoa powder, and even desserts. On a regular basis it is probably best to get your flavonols from a cup of cocoa that is lighter in fat and calories. Then, when you can really enjoy it, savor your piece of dark chocolate as you would a glass of fine wine.

5

Burning Fat

Why do you want to lose body fat? To compete in a lower weight class? Get ready for a bodybuilding or bikini contest? Improve your performance? Be healthier? Look better in your clothes? All are admirable goals for fat loss, and there are umpteen ways to reach them. Two of the most widely used and unhealthy methods are crash dieting and fad dieting.

These strategies come out of the diet world, not the world of sport nutrition science. The diet world is fueled by Madison Avenue and has only financial gain as a goal. Clearly all their advice has not helped to decrease the incidence of overweight and obesity in our world. Why would an athlete with performance goals follow advice aimed at a sedentary, obese target market? Because the diet-aid marketers are weaseling their way into our world of sport nutrition with a marketing megaphone and millions of advertising dollars. Their methods are not evidence-based strategies that will help you, and they most likely will harm your performance. Here's why.

Crash dieting involves a drastic reduction in calories, usually to about 800 calories or fewer a day, and results in equally drastic consequences, such as the following:

- *Muscle and fluid losses along with fat loss.* If you lost 20 pounds (9 kg) in 20 days, depending on your starting weight the first 6 to 10 pounds (2.7-4.5 kg) would be fluid; the rest would be fat and muscle. You are not gaining anything by dropping a lot of weight in a short period of time.

- *Loss of aerobic power.* Your body's capacity to take in and process oxygen, or $\dot{V}O_2$max, will decline significantly. As a result, less oxygen will be available to help your muscle cells combust fat for fuel.

- *Loss of strength.* This is a major handicap if you need strength and power for competition or to get through a workout without fizzling out.

- *Metabolic slowdown.* Crash dieting slows your metabolic rate to a crawl. Your metabolic rate is the speed at which your body processes food into energy and bodily structures. It is made up of two interrelated factors: basal metabolic rate (BMR) and resting metabolic rate (RMR). Your BMR represents the energy it takes just to exist; it is the energy required to keep your heart beating, your lungs breathing, and your other vital internal functions going strong. Basal metabolic needs must be met. If you're a woman, for example, you expend as many as 1,200 to 1,400 calories a day just fueling the basic work of your body's cells. Imagine the harm you are doing to your life processes by subsisting on a diet of 800 calories a day!

RMR includes your BMR plus additional energy expenditures required for the light activities of waking up, getting dressed, sitting up, and walking around. Your RMR accounts for about 60 percent of the energy you expend daily. The higher this rate is, the more efficient your body is at burning fat.

Specifically, it is your RMR that slows down when you restrict calories. In a one-year study of overweight men, those who cut calories to lose weight (as opposed to those who exercised) experienced a significant drop in their RMR. One reason was that they lost muscle tissue, and RMR is closely linked to how much muscle you have. The moral of the story is that following restrictive diets for an extended period will decelerate your RMR, and you can kiss the muscle you worked so hard to build goodbye.

Crash dieting is a losing proposition all the way around. There is nothing to be gained—except more weight! About 95 to 99 percent of all people who go on such diets regain their weight plus interest within a year.

Fad diets—eating plans that eliminate certain foods and emphasize others without any scientific evidence to support their claims—are just as bad as crash diets. A major problem with fad diets is that they are nutritionally unbalanced, and you could be missing out on some of the key nutrients you need for good health. An analysis of 11 popular diets revealed deficiencies in one or more essential nutrients, several of the B-complex vitamins, calcium, iron, and zinc. One diet derived 70 percent of its calories from fat. Such dangerously high levels of fat can lead to heart disease if you are not a serious exerciser. Even then you must understand your own health before following any extreme diet strategy.

But there are other problems, too. Take the mostly protein diet (with hardly any carbohydrate), one of the most popular fad diets among strength trainers. And no wonder it's popular! At first, it works great. You get on the scale, see a huge weight loss, and feel wonderful—until you go off the diet. Then the weight comes back as fast as it left. That is because mostly protein diets are initially dehydrating; they flush water right out of your system to help the body get rid of excess nitrogen. Also, since every molecule of muscle glycogen (stored carbohydrate) gathers three molecules of water around it in the muscle cell, when you deplete your carbohydrate stores you dehydrate your muscle cells. Dehydration is dangerous, too, potentially causing fatigue, lack of coordination, heat illnesses such as heat stress and heatstroke, and in extreme cases (a loss of 6-10 percent or more of body fluid),

Should You Try a Keto Diet?

Many athletes are trying ketogenic diets for performance, endurance, and weight loss. Recent research defines a ketogenic diet as a high-fat diet with less than 50 grams of carbohydrate per day. The diet brings your body into nutritional ketosis, in which it primarily relies on ketones and fatty acids for energy, as an alternative to glucose. To see if they're in nutritional ketosis (called "fat-adapted" or "keto-adapted"), athletes use urine strips or handheld breath analyzers to measure ketone levels. If they are, this means their bodies are oxidizing dietary and stored fat instead of glucose for energy.

But how well does the keto approach work? Let's take a look at some research. In a 1981 study, eight untrained, obese females ages 25 to 33 were studied before, at 1 week and after 6 weeks, while following one of two 830-calorie diets: a high-carbohydrate diet (35 percent protein, 29 percent fat, and 36 percent carbohydrate) and a carbohydrate-restricted, keto-type diet (35 percent protein, 64 percent fat, 1 percent carbohydrate). Basically, there were no differences in weight loss or body composition after 6 weeks. As observed in cycling exercises, endurance dropped by 50 percent on the keto diet. The drop in endurance correlated with depletion of the subjects' muscle glycogen.

Danish researchers placed 10 untrained young men on a carbohydrate-rich diet (65 percent carbohydrate), and 10 untrained men on a high-fat diet (62 percent fat). The men performed endurance training three to four times a week for 7 weeks. For the eighth week of training, both groups followed the carbohydrate-rich diet. After 8 weeks, endurance remained unchanged in the high-carbohydrate group but increased in the high-fat group, though it was still less than in the carbohydrate group. Various other metabolic measures were observed, one being that muscle glycogen broke down at the same rate in both groups. They also found that the respiratory exchange ratio (RER) decreased in the high-fat group only (during the 7 weeks). The RER is the ratio of carbon dioxide (CO_2) produced to the amount of oxygen (O_2) consumed and serves as a guide to the nutrient mixture being catabolized for energy. As the RER increases, so does the percentage of calories derived from carbohydrate, so increased exercise intensity utilizes a smaller proportion of energy from fat. Overall, performance increased 56 percent in the high-carbohydrate group. Performance was significantly lower in the high-fat group, even after switching over to the high-carbohydrate diet at week 8. The researchers concluded that a high-fat diet was detrimental to improvement in endurance.

In a similar study reported in 2006, eight well-trained cyclists completed two trials, ingesting either a high-carbohydrate diet (68% carbohydrate) or a keto diet (68% fat) for 6 days, followed by 1 day of carbohydrate loading. They performed a 100-km time trial on day 1 and a 1-hour cycle at 70 percent of peak oxygen consumption on days 3, 5, and 7, during which resting heart rate variability (HRV) and resting and exercising RER were measured. On day 8, subjects completed a 100-km performance time trial with sprints. In the keto group, performance diminished during the time trials and the sprints even after carbohydrate was replenished.

Certainly, keto diets can work for weight loss, but if you're an athlete in competition or training, proceed with caution. In terms of health, studies have found that keto diets are related to increased inflammation, insulin resistance, poor immunity, harmful changes in the gut biome, fatigue, suppressed thyroid function (which can hinder metabolism), and cognitive problems in the brain. In terms of sport, a keto diet does not give you enough fuel for a winning performance, and you might be setting yourself up for failure.

death. Even with a mere 3 percent drop in body weight as fluid, your performance will diminish. That is the equivalent of 4.5 pounds (2.0 kg) of water loss in a 150-pound (68 kg) person.

It's not the high protein that's the problem, and we'll talk about why a higher-protein diet will help you lose more weight and maintain more muscle while reducing fat. The problem is when protein (or in some cases, protein and fat) becomes virtually the only macronutrient that you are eating. As an athlete under most training scenarios, your training will suffer without any carbohydrate. But we will get to this discussion in a more personalized plan below.

Enough said about what doesn't work. There are antifat exercise and diet strategies that do work—namely a fat-burning training program and an individualized, nutritionally balanced eating plan that emphasizes a balanced combination of carbohydrate, protein, and the right kinds of fat. Before beginning, though, you should set some physique goals.

Go for Your Goal

Whether you realize it or not, you already know what your goal is. Just ask yourself: At what weight, or body-fat percentage, do I look, feel, or perform the best? The answer to that question is your goal.

The first step is to figure out how close to the mark you are. There are lots of ways to figure this out, including height and weight charts, body mass index (BMI) calculations, and bathroom scales. But the problem with most of these is that they are not very accurate for people who strength train. None of these methods takes into account the amount of muscle you have on your body; they might even indicate that you are overweight!

Bathroom scales tempt you to step on them every morning. That can be a downer, because your weight goes up and down daily as a result of normal fluid fluctuations. This is especially obvious in women during reproductive years. It can be easy to get obsessed with the numbers you see on the scale, especially because when you begin a program to lose fat by following the proper diet, exercising, and drinking enough water, you may often gain weight before you lose it. Here's why: For every molecule of glycogen stored in your muscles, you store an additional three molecules of water inside your muscles, which lie there ready to assist in metabolism. When you step on the scale, you may see a gain that is the result of water weight.

Here's what I say to all my clients about the scale: The numbers on a scale only represent the relationship of the mass of your body to gravity. Those numbers have nothing to do with what's going on inside your body relative to fat mass, lean body mass, or hydration.

A better measurement technique is body-composition testing, which determines how much of your weight is muscle and how much is fat. Several methods are in use. One is underwater weighing, considered the gold standard and very accurate if done properly with the right equipment. But it is not convenient (I certainly don't have a water tank in my office), and it can be rather expensive. There are even more expensive options, such as DEXA (dual energy X-ray absorptiometry) testing, which is typically used for bone mineral density testing (BMD) but offers another high-quality measure for body composition. Unless you are seeking research quality data, this is unnecessary.

Another method that is rapidly improving in reliability and validity is bioelectrical impedance analysis (BIA), which involves passing a painless electrical current through the body by means of electrodes placed on the hands and feet. Fat tissue won't conduct the current, but fat-free tissue (namely, water found in muscle) will. Thus, the faster the current passes through the body, the less body fat there is. Readings obtained from the test are plugged into formulas adjusted for height, gender, and age to calculate body-fat and fat-free mass percentages.

You can now purchase bathroom scales on which you can weigh yourself while measuring your body composition with BIA at the same time. These scales are not necessarily accurate, but as long as you follow the weigh-in instructions, you can see trends in your body-composition changes. You should be well hydrated, because if you are dehydrated even a little, as most people are, you won't get an accurate reading. Also, don't eat within four hours of weighing, and don't drink any alcohol or exercise intensely within 12 hours of weighing (this directive alone can make BIA difficult for regular exercisers). When instructions are followed, these scales are fairly reliable in showing whether your body-fat percentage is increasing or decreasing. If you want to keep tabs on your body composition, it is a good idea to check it only once every few weeks because it takes time for this change to occur.

The most reliable BIA available today is a multiple frequency BIA, especially when used to measure body composition of individuals with a normal to overweight body mass index (BMI). This covers athletes quite well. Athletes are usually at a normal BMI, though high levels of lean body mass can disrupt the BMI calculation and land a lean athlete in the overweight BMI category. While BIA is not a gold standard, it can be valuable for long-term monitoring.

Another accurate method of checking body composition is the skinfold technique, which measures fat just under the skin and uses those measurements to calculate body composition, including body-fat percentage. One of the keys to getting accurate and reliable measurements with the skinfold method is to use the same technician, time after time, month after month. That way, you don't get as much variability in the measurements, which are very technique sensitive.

I use another strategy with strength trainers and athletes, one that can be a real motivator as they progress toward their goals. I have them take circumference measurements (with a cloth tape measure) of selected widths on the upper arm, chest, waist, hips, thighs, and calves. You should take these measurements every four to six weeks to see the evidence of the positive changes that strength training, combined with the right diet, makes in your body. Because it is the easiest method, it can also be the most motivating!

Your Optimal Body-Fat Percentage

Exactly what is optimal in terms of body fat? Healthy ranges of body fat are 20 to 25 percent for women and 15 to 20 percent for men. But if you are a strength trainer or bodybuilder, it is desirable to have even lower percentages: 10 to 18 percent for women and 5 to 15 percent for men.

Low Energy Availability and the Female Athlete Triad

Many elite female athletes have less than 10 percent body fat. Female competitive runners, for example, may have as little as 5 or 6 percent body fat, according to some studies. A low percentage of body fat may be perfectly normal and desirable for some female athletes because it enhances sport performance and they are genetically programmed naturally to be very lean. As long as you don't consciously restrict calories while training for a sport, there is nothing unhealthy about having a naturally lean figure. However, calorie restriction combined with overexercising depletes body-fat stores to unhealthy levels, which elevates the risk of a syndrome known as the female athlete triad. The triad refers to three interrelated health problems seen in women: disrupted eating habits, menstrual irregularities, and weak bones. If you have the female athlete triad, you may suffer from an eating disorder such as anorexia or bulimia, or you may have reduced energy because your food intake is too low for your exercise level. Also, your menstrual periods have ceased, and you may also have the beginnings of osteoporosis, a disease that makes your bones thin and weak.

You are at the highest risk for the female athlete triad if you

- are a competitive athlete;
- are involved in sports such as gymnastics or bodybuilding that require you to check your weight often;
- exercise more than you need to, without taking in enough calories;
- constantly diet for performance, appearance, or both;
- have perfectionist personality traits;
- have stopped eating with your family and friends; and
- have the attitude that amenorrhea (loss of your period), excessive exercise, and weight loss are positive attributes in athletics.

Some symptoms of the female athlete triad are weight loss, absent or irregular periods, fatigue and stress fractures, and increase in illness due to a weakened immune system. I have occasionally encountered the female athlete triad in my practice. For example, I once worked with a woman who was an ultraendurance athlete and did an extreme amount of exercise. She had begun to experience bone fractures all over her body, along with various illnesses. Her periods had become very irregular. Once we talked, it was apparent that she was consuming fewer calories than her body required to carry out all its activity. We corrected this situation through a higher-calorie diet with the correct percentages of protein, carbohydrate, and fat. Ultimately, she had to cut back on her exercise to regain her health. Once she was healthy again, she was able to return to her sport in much better shape than she left it.

Long before a woman or girl's condition advances to a full blown medical diagnosis of female athlete triad, she is measurably underfueling her body but might not be aware of it. As a sport nutritionist, my goal is to identify someone at risk before they have progressed so far down that path of ill health. Fifty years of research on female athletes has recently made it to the headlines of practice

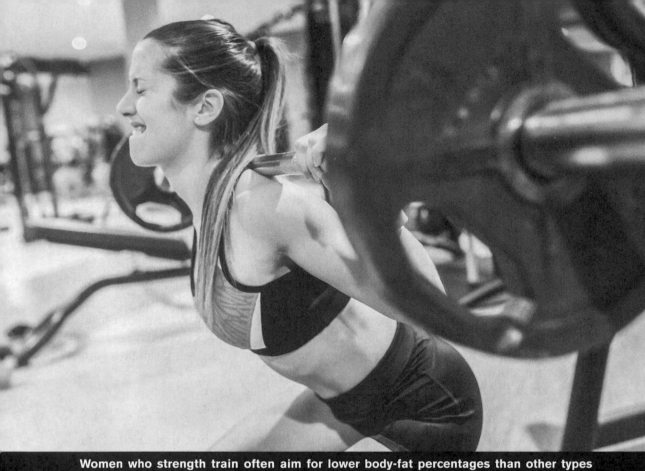

Women who strength train often aim for lower body-fat percentages than other types of female athletes.

Westend61/Getty Images

guidelines, and standards have now been set for identifying and guiding athletes with low energy availability (LEA), the more common condition that precedes the female athlete triad.

I will present a more in-depth discussion on LEA and the female athlete triad in chapter 7, but it is important here to note that the International Olympic Committee (IOC) has published recommendations to extend the conversation about LEA to males. Despite the fact that virtually all the data have been collected from females, the IOC has decided to include males because there are data that indicate problems with low-energy dieting in males and those risks should not be unaccounted for. This is a rare instance in which the data exist nearly exclusively on females yet is being extrapolated to males. In almost all cases in sport nutrition, the situation is the other way around.

The IOC expanded the concept of LEA and has branded their syndrome as relative energy deficit in sports, or RED-S, to recognize that males, as well as active individuals who may not necessarily self-identify as athletes, will be included in the at-risk population. According to the authors of the IOC Consensus Statement,

"The syndrome of RED-S refers to impaired physiological functioning caused by relative energy deficiency, and includes but is not limited to impairments of metabolic rate, menstrual function, bone health, immunity, protein synthesis, and cardiovascular health."

According to the IOC, the cause of RED-S is

"the scenario termed low energy availability, where an individual's dietary energy intake is insufficient to support the energy expenditure required for health, function, and daily living, once the costs of exercise and sporting activities are taken into account."

Here is the translation that I give to my clients: Active individuals who underfuel can often continue to participate in their sport at a high level for a period of time, and so it is difficult for them to understand that any of the symptoms that they are experiencing are from too few calories. However, our bodies will preferentially fuel the highest energy need first, leaving our foundational health needs only partially fueled. Exercise is fueled, but the rest of the body is not. When calorie intake is chronically low, health deteriorates. Common symptoms are loss of menstrual cycle, reproductive function, and libido; thyroid dysfunction; poor immune function; fatigue; headaches; structural loss in hair, skin, and nails; poor sleep; lack of mental alertness or focus (foggy brain); and a short temper. Athletes commonly report working out harder but declining in performance and eating less but getting softer. Injuries from poor balance and poor judgment are common, as are stress fractures and bone breaks.

I must emphasize that the data supporting the health consequences in men are limited, at best. We know, as stated above, what happens in women who chronically underfuel. However, I have had male clients who have suffered from a number of the consequences listed above, and so I want to make sure that men do not exclude themselves from this risk.

The goal of treatment for LEA or RED-S is to calculate the amount of energy or calories required to support an individual's athletic endeavors, called the energy of exercise expenditure (EEE). We then determine how much energy the individual is consuming, the energy intake (EI). Energy availability (EA) is all the energy that is left over to fuel the foundational health needs of the body, and it is normalized to fat-free mass (FFM) in kilograms because most of our energy expenditure is linked to our muscle, or fat-free mass.

Here is the equation:

$$EA = \frac{EI - EEE}{FFM}$$

EA is considered low when it is less than 30 calories per kilogram of fat-free mass per day. This low EA, or LEA, value (30 kcal/kg FFM) is linked to abnormal physiological markers of reproductive function and bone metabolism in women and girls.

Adequate or optimal EA is greater than or equal to 45 calories per kilogram of fat-free mass per day.

It is very important that you determine whether you are under-fueling your body to the point of LEA. When identified early, you can avoid the damaging effects of LEA on your health and ultimately on your performance. As I mentioned above, it is best to intervene early, before an athlete is far down the road of the female athlete triad. I have found that with good planning, all my clients are successful at sculpting their bodies while avoiding the LEA syndrome. Sometimes we need to fall between 30 and 45 calories per kilogram of fat-free mass per day for a short period of time, but we don't stay there as a rule.

While almost all the research on LEA has been done with women, I admittedly have also had male clients who have suffered with similar abnormal health consequences.

Muscle Dysmorphia in Men: Bigorexia

Women aren't the only ones who obsess about their weight and appearance; men can be just as preoccupied. Body dissatisfaction in men has nearly tripled over the last three decades. An obsessive dissatisfaction with one's body is termed *muscle dysmorphia*, but it is commonly known as bigorexia; it is seen largely in men and tends to manifest in athletes. Muscle dysmorphia (MD) is listed in the Diagnostic and Statistical Manual of Mental Disorders (DSM-5) as an obsessive–compulsive disorder.

Whereas women tend to believe that their bodies are bigger than they really are, men with this disorder tend to falsely believe that their bodies or their muscles are too small. They may have a poor body image and an obsessive desire to build muscle and avoid gaining fat.

Following are some of the signs of muscle dysmorphia:

- Excessive strength training (spending countless hours in the gym) and other compulsive exercising that interferes with work and life

- Body checking (looking in mirrors and other reflections more than 12 times per day) or avoiding mirrors altogether, and comparing oneself with others

- Concern about appearance not explained by body fat or body weight

- Obsessive weighing and dieting, and focusing on physical defects not observable or deemed unimportant by others

- Spending less time with family and friends or finding the time spent with them stressful, or feeling distressed in work situations

If you find that you're training excessively and you're worried about it interfering with your daily life, and if your joy in life has diminished at the same time, seek counseling, because this disorder is psychiatric. It does not respond to aesthetically oriented interventions such as exercise programs, diets, or plastic surgery to correct perceived bodily flaws. Some research indicates that antidepressants may help. See a qualified psychologist if you or someone you love may be suffering from this disorder.

A quick, easy-to-use, four-factor test from David Folgado De la Rosa Medical that could serve as a screening tool to determine if the user has a high risk of MD has been constructed, validated, and implemented in a mobile application. It is available as an app on Google Play, called the Bigorexia predictor, that you can download to determine if you have this syndrome.

Your Weight-Loss Goal Formula

Once you have determined your body composition through an appropriate method, you can figure out how much weight you need to lose to reach a lower body-fat percentage with the following formula:

1. Present body weight × present body-fat % = fat weight
2. Present body weight – fat weight = fat-free weight
3. Fat-free weight / desired % of fat-free mass = goal weight
4. Present body weight – goal weight = weight-loss goal

As an illustration, let's say you weigh 160 pounds (72.7 kg), with a present body-fat percentage of 15 percent. Your goal is to achieve 10 percent body fat. Your body-composition goal, then, is 10 percent fat and 90 percent fat-free mass. How many pounds do you need to lose?

Here's the calculation:

$$160 \text{ lb } (72.7 \text{ kg}) \times 0.15 = 24.0 \text{ lb } (10.9 \text{ kg}) \text{ current fat weight}$$

$$160 \text{ lb } (72.7 \text{ kg}) - 24.0 \text{ lb } (10.9 \text{ kg}) = 136 \text{ lb } (61.8 \text{ kg}) \text{ current fat-free weight}$$

$$136 \text{ lb } (61.8 \text{ kg}) / 0.90 = 151.1 \text{ lb } (68.7 \text{ kg}) \text{ goal weight}$$

$$160 \text{ lb } (72.7 \text{ kg}) - 151.1 \text{ lb } (68.7 \text{ kg}) = 8.9 \text{ lb } (4.0 \text{ kg}) \text{ or about 9 lb}$$
$$\text{of fat weight to lose}$$

To arrive at 10 percent body fat, you need to lose about 9 pounds (4.0 kg). Naturally, you want those 9 pounds to be fat pounds. Here's a look at how to maximize fat loss and minimize muscle loss.

Exercise and Fat Loss

Your objective is to lose body fat without losing muscle mass. You don't want to lose strength or endurance, either, and you don't want your performance to suffer. So how can you keep on the losing track? Forget about diet for a moment; the other key is exercise.

When it comes to burning fat, exercise is your best friend in three ways:

1. *The more exercise you do, the less you have to worry about calories.* By burning 300 to 500 calories a day through exercise, you don't have to cut those calories out of your meal plan, and you enhance the rate of calorie burning. As I noted previously, these caloric deficits have been tested in research and proven accurate.

2. *Exercise hikes your fat burning after exercise.* Scientists call this condition excess postexercise oxygen consumption, or EPOC. The more oxygen you use, the more fat you are likely to burn. We have known for years that all kinds of exercise can raise what I call your afterburn, the amount of oxygen you use for recovery, which can translate into the amount of fat calories you burn after exercise. The key has been to understand what kinds of exercise raise this value the highest for the longest period of time. The answers have been coming fast and furious, and the winner for how high EPOC can go is clearly high intensity interval training, known as HIIT.

With HIIT, your workouts will be shorter, but you'll actually be working out at a higher intensity than when you are doing steady exercise on the cardio machines at your gym. Basically, you work out in intervals—bouts of all-out effort at a rate of 80 to 90 percent of your maximal heart rate (MHR), alternated with short stretches of active recovery. You can do any kind of high-intensity exercise to meet the guidelines of HIIT all-out effort training (e.g., sprinting outside on a track, working out inside on a rowing machine, using a stationary bike or treadmill, or even performing plyometrics) for one to two minutes. On a 1 to 10 scale of perceived exertion, your high-intensity training should exceed a level of 7. Active recovery can be the same activity but at a lower intensity (e.g., from a sprint on a track to a jog, from a two-minute hill climb on an indoor bike to a three-minute flat at a level of 4 or 5, or from intense plyometrics to squats, sit-ups, and push-ups). This cycle is repeated for about 20 minutes. Plenty of research shows that HIIT is a super-effective way to burn fat.

Studies show that your afterburn rate rises exponentially with an increase in intensity during exercise. This is in contrast to a linear increase in afterburn as exercise duration increases. While steady state exercise at high intensity burns a higher EPOC compared to moderate intensity aerobic exercise or circuit training, high-intensity interval training leads to higher oxygen consumption per time during exercise, which results in the highest EPOC, afterburn. The length of afterburn has not been consistent among studies, ranging from 30 minutes to 4 hours, depending on the fitness level of the subject and the intensity and number of bouts of the training session. The more fit you are, the greater the physical challenge, but the very short duration of HIIT also limits the duration of EPOC, despite its high peak value.

And here's something else: HIIT is a great way to burn belly fat. In a study from the University of Virginia, researchers recruited 27 middle-aged, obese women with metabolic syndrome (a prediabetic condition) and had them complete one of three 16-week aerobic exercise interventions: (1) no exercise training (control); (2) low-intensity exercise training (LIET); and (3) HIIT. At the end of the experimental period, HIIT had significantly reduced total abdominal fat, and there were no such changes in the control or LIET groups.

This is not to dissuade you from doing moderate-intensity training, endurance training, or circuit training. Testing has shown that if you measure calories burned *during* exercise, a longer duration exercise session or even a steady state high-intensity exercise session will likely burn more calories. Cumulatively over time this may lead to more total calories burned. But if your time is limited and you need to be efficient with your training, the short duration of HIIT won't decrease your calorie-burning potential; you make some of it up in the afterburn. It's also a great way to change up your training and add variety, which keeps you interested and more likely to stick with exercise daily.

If you want to know what muscle groups create greater EPOC, just think about what it takes to recover from a leg/glute/lower body day compared to an arm/chest/upper body day. That's your clue to the fact that working big muscles like glutes create a higher afterburn than working smaller muscles likes biceps and chest. (Believe me, I'm not judging your chest or biceps!)

The big picture here is that exercise variety promotes all kinds of improvements in fitness and strength, speed, and power. Changing up your routine and adding in HIIT protocols on short days can make a big a difference to your cross-training and body-sculpting goals.

Now let's add in a little discussion about diet and HIIT, to demonstrate how recovery feeding can bump up your fat burn. Scientists in Japan wanted to know if HIIT would enhance the increase in oxygen consumption that comes from eating food, called the thermic effect of food (TEF). Ten subjects spent multiple 24-hour sessions in a metabolic chamber. HIIT exercise consisted of six or seven bouts of 20-second bicycle exercise (intensity: 170 percent $\dot{V}O_2$max) with a 10-second rest between bouts. HIIT was always preceded by 10 minutes of exercise at 50 percent $\dot{V}O_2$max. On two separate days, four subjects were fed lunch and dinner and EPOC was tested with and without exercise. Six different subjects fasted and were studied on two separate days with and without exercise. The researchers' main finding was that HIIT enhanced a small but significant increase in diet-induced (fed) TEF during the 10.5 hours after exercise, with no comparable increase with feeding but without exercise.

Eating is part of your daily routine. If you get in a HIIT workout before you eat, you capitalize on your fat-burning potential. That's an entirely new benefit from your recovery shake or meal, so don't skip it thinking that you'll lose more weight. That's like leaving money on the table!

3. *Exercise preserves muscle.* If you lose 10 pounds (4.5 kg) of body weight, you may be lighter, but if 5 pounds (2.3 kg) of that loss are muscle, you sure won't be stronger, and your performance can suffer. Appearance-wise, you can still look flabby when muscle tissue is lost. Exercise is one of the best ways to make sure you are shedding weight from fat stores rather than from muscle stores.

Researchers have put this principle to the test. In a study of 10 overweight women, half of the women were placed in a diet-plus exercise group and half of the women in an exercise-only group. The women in the first group followed a diet that reduced their calories by 50 percent of what it took to maintain their weight, and they worked out aerobically six times a week.

The women in the exercise-only group followed the same aerobic exercise program but followed a diet designed to stabilize their weight.

After 14 weeks, it was time to check the results. Here is what happened: Both groups lost weight. But the composition of that loss was vastly different between the groups. In the group that dieted and exercised, the weight lost was 67 percent fat and 33 percent lean mass. In the group that only exercised, the women lost much more fat—86 percent fat and only 14 percent lean mass! Not only that but RMR declined by 9 percent among the dieters, whereas it was maintained in those who only exercised.

What does all this tell us? Sure, you can lose weight by low-calorie dieting. But you risk losing muscle. Also, your metabolic rate can plummet, sabotaging your attempts at successful weight control. With exercise and a nonrestrictive diet, you preserve calorie-burning muscle and keep your metabolism in gear.

Other Intensity Strategies for Fat-Burning

If you don't do HIIT, there are other ways to burn fat through exercise. For example, try to work out at a level hard enough to raise your heart rate to 70 to 85 percent of MHR. MHR can be calculated by subtracting your age from the number 220. During low-intensity exercise (20 minutes or longer at around 50 percent of MHR), fat supplies as much as 90 percent of your fuel requirements. High-intensity aerobic exercise at roughly 75 percent of MHR burns a smaller percentage of fat (around 60 percent), but results in more total calories burned overall, including more fat calories.

To illustrate this concept, here's a comparison based on studies of aerobic intensity. At 50 percent of MHR, you burn 7 calories a minute, 90 percent of which come from fat. At 75 percent of MHR, you burn 14 calories a minute, 60 percent from fat. So at 50 percent intensity, at which 90 percent of the calories are from fat, you are burning only 6.3 fat calories per minute (0.9×7 calories per minute), but at 75 percent intensity, at which only 60 percent of the calories are from fat, you are burning as much as 8.4 fat calories per minute (0.6×14 calories per minute). In short, you burn more total fat calories at higher intensities.

Intensity in strength training refers to how much weight you lift. For your muscles to respond—that is, get stronger and better developed—you have to challenge them to handle heavier weights. That means continually putting more demands on them than they're used to, progressively increasing the weight you lift from workout to workout. The more muscle you can develop, the more efficient your body becomes at fat burning, because muscle is the most metabolically active tissue in the body.

If you have difficulty exercising at a high intensity, try increasing your duration—how long you exercise. You can burn just as much fat working out longer at a lower intensity as you can exercising at a higher intensity for a shorter duration.

POWER PROFILE: Fat-Burning and Muscle Building in a Competitive Master Bodybuilder

Blaine is a personal trainer in the province of Saskatchewan, Canada. His goal was to retain maximum lean tissue and reduce his body fat to 9 percent or lower, in order to compete in two bodybuilding contests. At the time I started working with him, he weighed 165 pounds (74.8 kg), and the last time he competed, he weighed in at 145 pounds (65.8 kg). Yet after looking at his competition photos, Blaine felt like he had lost too much muscle mass. The nutritional plan he had used to prepare was 2,600 calories—39 percent carbohydrate, 48 percent protein, 13 percent fat—which is different from what I usually recommend.

After analyzing Blaine's diet, I discovered that he was actually consuming a little over 1,900 calories, with 212 grams carbohydrate, 189 grams protein, and 35 grams fat. I felt that we definitely needed to increase all parts of Blaine's diet to get him building muscle, and then as the contests approached, burn off fat.

The first bump we made was to 2,670 calories (264 g carbohydrate, 165 g protein, 106 g fat) with a goal of rising to 3,300 calories, and maybe more. Calorie increases came from adding 70 grams of Vitargo before training, and 70 grams of Vitargo plus 25 grams of whey protein after exercise. He followed this nutritional advice to the letter.

After adding in all those calories and all that carbohydrate, just before his contest Blaine weighed 150 pounds (68 kg), and his body fat was 9.4 percent. Relative to his previous shows, his body fat was lower by 0.3 percent and his weight was 2 pounds (0.9 kg) heavier—exactly his goal.

He reported that he performed his workouts at 75 percent maximal effort, while feeling excellent with no signs of fatigue or lethargy. But the big news was that Blaine won both the Grandmasters and Lightweight categories during his competition. "I felt fantastic and am on top of the world," he told me.

There's more: Blaine competed in another contest one week later, a competition held by the INBF, one of the world's largest natural bodybuilding organizations. For that contest, his body fat was 9.1 percent and his body weight was 151 pounds (68.5 kg).

Blaine's results at the INBF show were equally as impressive: First place Masters (40+) and second place Lightweight (165 pounds max).

This all goes to show what increasing the amount of proper nutrients, including carbohydrate, can do to help you get cut and not lose precious muscle. You do not need to starve yourself down to competition size.

There is a connection between exercise and diet to burn body fat. You don't necessarily have to drastically cut calories; you can actually keep them somewhat high. You need to fuel your planned high-intensity training with enough carbohydrate to actually get to high-intensity levels. The coordination of a variety of exercise with enough of the right amounts of fuel at the right times will make all the difference when you are aiming to cut for an event, or even slowly burn off fat mass over time. Chapters 18 and 19 will demonstrate how you put these food strategies into action in your life around your training.

Antifat Diet Strategies

The old-fashioned way of figuring out how many calories you should eat to lose weight is to just chop off 500 to 1,000 calories from your current diet. One pound (0.5 kg) of fat is equivalent to 3,500 calories. According to the laws of thermodynamics, if you feed yourself 500 calories fewer than you need each day for seven days, theoretically you should lose 1 pound (0.5 kg) by the end of the week, week after week. Double that amount and you should lose 2 pounds (0.9 kg). But dietitians have known for years that it never works this way, and this strategy becomes more frustrating as the weeks of dieting wear on.

At Georgia State University, Dr. Dan Benardot wondered why these seemingly clear laws of physics don't hold true within the human body. His research has shown that once food enters the biological system of the body, there are more variables at work than the simple number of calories that are given off by a pound of fat when measured directly in a science lab. The human body is a living organism, and the drive for survival allows the rules of the system to change based on thousands of years of adaptation to the environment. Dr. Benardot tested two groups of female gymnasts and runners: One group ate a diet of 500 fewer calories than they needed to maintain their weight each day, and the other group ate 300 fewer calories. What he found was astounding: The group that ate 300 fewer calories had a lower percentage of body fat than the group that actually ate less food. His theory is that when too few calories are eaten, resting energy expenditure (REE) slows down to meet the energy available to the body.

The ability of the body to slow metabolic rate to meet available energy has long been understood by scientists. Called starvation adaptation, it is induced in extreme circumstances of famine to allow the body to survive far longer than would be predicted based on normal metabolic rates of energy use. Dr. Benardot proposed for the first time that even under mild states of energy deficit, energy use slows down. There is no benefit to eating far fewer calories than your body needs. In fact, he called a 300-calorie deficit the ideal metabolic window for women to lose the most amount of fat in the shortest amount of time.

This appears to be particularly relevant in people who really don't have that much weight to lose but may not apply when margins of intake and overweight are much larger. For example, if you are eating 1,000 calories more than you need and are 50 pounds overweight, you will certainly benefit from dropping the extra calories to boost your initial weight loss. That 500 to 1,000 calories dropped off your diet was completely surplus to begin with, and gets you to a calorie level that is still high enough to maintain your metabolic rate and allow for rapid weight loss.

On the other hand, for people with only 5 to 10 pounds to lose, who may only be eating 300 to 400 calories more than needed on a daily basis, and who are burning 500 to 1,000 calories during workouts, dropping 500 to 1,000 calories puts them into such a significant energy deficit that their body responds by slowing energy metabolism. That's why Dr. Benardot's work does not necessarily apply to a population of highly overweight or obese individuals but is highly applicable to many athletic individuals. In fact, it is a tenet of scientific research not to extrapolate research results from one demographic study group to a different study group. Unfortunately, when the mass media reports on research results, they will often do exactly this kind of extrapolation, mischaracterizing results and giving an ultimate impression that the strategy doesn't work.

So if you match the profile of a fit individual with a little bit of fat to lose, forget low-calorie dieting. When you reduce your caloric intake by 300 to 400 calories, you can keep your metabolic rate high enough to continue to burn fat at a good clip. Additionally, you want to have enough energy to perform at peak levels both physically and mentally. Finally, always check your total calorie intake against the healthy energy availability value of no less than 30 calories per kilogram of fat-free mass per day. Here's how to eat to give yourself the best chance at losing fat and saving muscle:

Don't Starve Yourself

Because you strength train and probably do aerobics as well, you actually need more food, not less. Researchers at Tufts University found that when older men and women began a strength-training program, they needed 15 percent more calories just to maintain their body weight. This finding is not so surprising, really. With strength training, the exercisers began to expend more calories. Plus, their RMR increased because they had built more muscle.

You can figure out exactly how many calories you need to lose fat. Based on my research with competitive bodybuilders, I have concluded that an intake of 35 to 38 calories per kilogram of body weight a day is reasonable for fat loss and muscle preservation in someone training five or more days per week. The minimum is 29 to 32 calories per kilogram for a rapid cut for the same level of training. If you are training only three or four days per week, then of course your calories will be lower. Typically, those who train fewer days per week are somewhat less muscular, so energy needs are lower as well. Anything less than that is too restrictive, and you won't be well nourished.

Again, at least in females, check that your energy availability is greater than 30 calories per kilogram of fat-free mass per day, and ideally 45 calories per kilogram of fat-free mass per day or more, even if you are calculating your diet using the Power Eating diet plan templates. The target ranges for energy intake that I recommend in the Power Eating meal plans are always based upon total body weight rather than fat-free mass, which is the basis of the energy availability calculation.

Let's say you are a man exercising five or more days per week and you weigh 180 pounds (82 kg). Here's how to figure your calorie requirements to lose fat: 82 kg × 38 kcal/kg = 3,116 kcal. For maintaining body weight, you should eat up to 42 calories per kilogram of body weight a day, or 3,444 calories a day. If you want to build muscle and you increase your exercise intensity, duration, or frequency, go even higher—to 52 calories per kilogram of body weight or more, or 4,264 calories a day.

If you still need a calorie deficit to continue losing fat or to break a plateau, get that deficit by increasing your activity level and modifying your calories slightly.

For example, restrict your calories by about 300 to 400 calories a day and increase your HIIT or aerobic exercise. This deficit, again, is the ideal metabolic window for weight loss.

Correct Your Dietary Fat

Be sure to include the right kinds of fat in your diet, including omega-3 fat from fish or algal supplements and monounsaturated fat from extra-virgin olive oil, avocados, nuts and seeds, and nut and seed oils. An Australian study showed that diets rich in monounsaturated fat helped premenopausal women preserve muscle while losing weight. Diets high in omega-3 fat may actually protect against obesity; many studies have observed the fat-burning effect of omega-3 fat. Include up to five fish meals in your diet each week (choose fish wisely). The more muscle you maintain while losing fat, the greater your chance of keeping the weight off for good.

Preserve Muscle With Protein

To lose mostly fat and keep your metabolism running in high gear with muscle mass preserved, you must have adequate protein in your diet. Protein also helps control your appetite. If you go on a diet that is too low in calories, there is a good chance that your dietary protein will not be used to build tissue but instead will be broken down and used for energy much like carbohydrate and fat are. As a reminder, for losing body fat, the nutrient profile of your diet should be at least 30 percent protein, 40 percent carbohydrate, and 30 percent fat.

There is some very interesting recent research that increasing protein intake during a calorie deficit while training may be even more helpful for muscle preservation and fat loss. This study exemplifies exactly the kind of scenario that many of you face. At McMaster University in Hamilton, Canada, 40 young, overweight, recreationally active men (23 years old, BMI >25) participated in a 4-week study in which they were given a 40 percent calorie-deficient diet equaling 33 calories per kilogram of fat-free mass. They were separated into two diet groups: the control group, which received 15 percent protein (1.2 g/kg BW), 50 percent carbohydrate, and 35 percent fat; and the protein group, which received 35 percent protein (2.4 g/kg BW), 50 percent carbohydrate, and 15 percent fat. Notice that the fat percentage changed based on the protein composition of the diet, but carbohydrate stayed the same.

The subjects followed identical high-volume exercise routines for 6 days per week including aerobic, circuit, and high-intensity or speed-intensity training. All outside activity was also tracked for comparison between groups. The results showed all subjects benefitted similarly from exercise training with advances in performance and loss of total body weight, but the protein group (2.4 g/kg/day) gained muscle mass (+1.2 kg; control maintained) and lost significantly more fat (-4.8 vs.-3.5 kg) compared to the control group.

This is really fantastic data, and gives us a template to follow. The other big news here is that we have a timeframe that demonstrates that 1- and 2-week studies don't give us the real picture. Had this study been shorter we may never have seen this measurable and significant difference.

On the other hand, one could say that four weeks is too short to see what the long-term effects might be. When it comes to any diet, the question is, can you stick to it? That is actually the most important factor. When diet studies are carried out to one year or longer, the key becomes whether the subjects stick to the plan. If they do, they lose weight and keep it off. If they can't stick to it, or to some version of the plan, they gain the weight back.

My goal with Power Eating is to guide you to a plan that can work for you. Although I wish I had the absolute answer, there is really not one single plan that works for everyone. If there were, we'd all know it and have this overweight problem solved already. I present you with all the important evidence; you decide what you think will work for you.

Lower Body Fat With Less Carbohydrate

In the past, I've hesitated to recommend lower-carbohydrate diets to highly active groups of people. I didn't think an active person or athlete could exercise hard under conditions of low carbohydrate intake. Don't miss that the very successful diet strategy above still had 50 percent of calories from carbohydrate and the subjects lost more weight based on more protein in the diet, not less carbohydrate. However, several new lines of research reveal that a low-carbohydrate diet with adequate vegetables, dairy, and small amounts of nuts and seeds can provide fuel for workouts, while still triggering weight loss. These days, if you are someone who does better with lower carbohydrate (notice I never say no carbohydrate), I now endorse the right kind of lower-carbohydrate dieting as an effective way to get lean.

The fat-loss diet I recommend is neither painful nor will it make you feel deprived. I've organized the plan to precisely time and combine foods to maximize your mood, mental focus, and physical energy. I also make sure that you have the right amount of calories and nutrients in a targeted way throughout the day to put all the necessary nutrients to work for you. Check out chapters 18 and 19 for menu plans that will support your training, physique, and fat-loss goals.

Reach for Veggies and Whole Foods

Whole foods are infinitely healthier than processed foods. Despite all of the science that has given us functional, engineered foods, we still have not outdone mother nature. Individual vitamins and minerals, phytonutrients and food factors, fatty acids, amino acids, and fiber never work as well as supplements as they do when combined in their natural form in whole food. Supplements are helpful, but only for convenience, for targeted action, and as extra nutritional insurance. I certainly use products and supplements in my diet and suggest them to my clients. But supplements, whether in food or pill form, will never replace whole foods.

Even though an athlete's life can be busy, hectic, and demanding, the choice to use whole foods makes a huge difference in physical and mental performance. It may take a little extra effort, but the effort is worth it. You'll need to plan ahead by creating shopping lists, meal plans, and recipes. If you travel, you'll need to think ahead and purchase the kinds of foods that stay fresh and are appropriate for an

- Think about this message: You are polluted, and we can clean you up! How appealing is that message?
- Now think about a completely different message: Your body is an amazing filtration machine, and here are some purification strategies to maximize your results!

The marketing angle of "your body is broken, and we know how to fix it" is, frankly, degrading. It is the tried and true strategy of advertisers in the diet world, tearing down your spirit as well as your body. Marketers position their product as the great savior for your ailing, dysfunctional body. This messaging is the antithesis of what appeals to the world of sports and fitness world, in which we emphasize that your body is awesome and that we can help build it up stronger and faster.

So it's not surprising that one of the biggest diet-marketing messages of the last decade has been that you are polluted, and we can clean you up. That message is virtually a myth with little supporting evidence. But the concept of using a more pure diet to destress your body and maximize performance is certainly supported by scientific evidence in the real world.

FACTS OVER HYPE

Detox diets eliminate most things that we know are unhealthy, increase inflammation, and make us feel bad: alcohol; foods high in sugar, refined carbohydrates, saturated fats, and trans fat; not to mention high intakes of caffeine, tobacco, and other recreational drugs. For some short period of time the dieter dramatically lowers calories, increases hydration, and takes tremendous control over their eating. The less health-promoting their diet and lifestyle was before the detox diet, the better they will feel from the cleanse.

There isn't, however, one bit of evidence to tell us that the ingredients of the cleansing ritual did anything, but there is plenty of data to help us understand that good hydration, lots of plant foods, and eliminating processed, packaged, and fast foods high in calories and low in nutrients will make you look and feel better.

Why not cleanse, even if it just tricks us into doing the right thing for a few weeks? Research on successful weight loss is quite clear: It takes learning how to eat well and exercise daily to healthfully lose weight and maintain the weight loss. Detox diets don't teach anything about how to eat well, and exercising during the cleansing ritual is discouraged. While there is data that people who have a good initial weight loss may have more motivation to stick with a program long term, quick weight loss without any information about changing food and exercise habits typically results in quickly regaining at least the weight lost, and possibly greater fat gains.

PURIFICATION OPTIMIZATION

Rather than an annual cleanse for one week, create a year-long purification ritual for lifetime health and fitness. A fluid-filled, plant-based diet is the natural sustenance for your body's amazing filtration systems and purification pathways.

The inside of your body meets the outside environment at the lining of your digestive tract. It is a high priority of the body to keep the intestinal membrane healthy to protect your body from environmental contaminants. The cells naturally turn over (die and are replaced) every 21 days. The scientific term is actually *exfoliation*. You can give your own intestines a facial of sorts by eating a high-fiber diet. The fiber is not digested and creates bulk as it works its way through the tract. As it pushes through it gently cleans up the lining, keeping it fresh and healthy. If you follow a purification diet that emphasizes lots of fruits and vegetables, grains and beans, nuts and seeds, you are by default increasing your fiber intake and cleaning up your intestines. At the same time the extra bulk helps things move through more quickly and efficiently, which usually helps to decrease intestinal discomfort and bloating and lowers the risk of toxin absorption.

Beneficial bacteria (probiotics) and yeasts in our gut are partnered with many of the fibers from plant foods to protect us from environmental assaults and toxins and support immune function. Probiotics exert their purifying effect by crowding out the unhealthy gut flora like yeasts, viruses, and bacteria that trigger illnesses and disease. They can transfer some of their genetic disease-fighting capacity to our own intestinal cells. And they can alter the pH balance of our gut to reduce virulent organisms, and even enhance our own essential mineral absorption.

Prebiotics are the fibers that feed the probiotic cultures so that they can prosper. Prebiotics may also inhibit the ability of unhealthy colonies to attach to the lining of the gut wall. The specific fiber lignin is a powerful prebiotic, found predominantly in flaxseed and other edible seeds (such as strawberries and kiwi), and in lesser amounts in root vegetables and fruits.

Psyllium seed and chia seed, commonly recommended additions to popular detox diets, contain lignins as well as mucilaginous fibers that work as natural laxatives. These same fiber properties are found in beans. When using a psyllium supplement, it is very important to drink plenty of fluids to avoid stool compaction. The large fluid intake explains the powerful effect of a liquid fast combined with psyllium seed supplements. You will certainly feel lighter after a few days of this regimen. But if you include a variety of high-fiber foods in your diet every day, you'll always be light on your feet.

YAY OR NAY TO JUICING

Fruit and vegetable juices are concentrated sources of nutrients and plant products. These natural biochemicals may prevent cancer development (carcinogenesis) by interfering with detrimental actions of mutagens, carcinogens, and tumor promoters, some of which can come from our contaminated environment. In fact, some of these products may actually detoxify cancer-causing compounds and tumor promoters. For example, glucaric acid, found in high amounts in apples, broccoli, Brussels sprouts, cabbage, and bean sprouts, may help to control and even prevent cancers by inhibiting beta-glucuronidase, an enzyme that can promote cancer.

Juicing with vegetables can be a great way to enjoy a lot of vegetable nutrition in a small amount of time, but the drawback is that juicing removes most of the fiber, so you consume less fiber. Whole foods give you greater purification power. Juicing with fruits is also a compact way of getting those nutrients, but it increases sugar intake dramatically. While you might take a whole day to eat five servings of fruit, you can easily consume five servings of fruit juice in one sitting. Despite the natural source of the sugar, it is still a stressful jolt to your system. It is ideal to eat whole foods. Juice occasionally if you enjoy it, with an emphasis on vegetables rather than fruits.

> continued

PURIFICATION RITUAL REALITY

Numerous enzymes produced naturally by the body work nonstop to purify our cells. A plant-based diet rich in deeply colored vegetables and fruits supports this activity. Staying well-hydrated keeps all your cells at functional capacity and helps flush toxins from cells and organs quickly. Diets that provide adequate protein and carbohydrate to build enzymes and fuel metabolism, and are at the same time low in added sugars, refined carbohydrate, and saturated fat to limit inflammation, are the best purification optimization rituals.

Some of the best purification optimizers are listed below:

- Broccoli
- Cauliflower
- Cabbage
- Kohlrabi
- Bok choy
- Brussels sprouts
- Kale
- Chard
- Mustard greens
- Spinach
- Onions
- Leek
- Garlic
- Chives
- Oranges
- Tangerines
- Cantaloupe
- Peaches
- Nectarines
- Grapefruits
- Lemons
- Berries
- Mangoes
- Papayas
- Kiwis
- Cherries
- Plums
- Watermelons
- Red grapes
- Apples
- Apricots
- Pineapple
- Tomatoes
- Peppers
- Chilis
- Carrots
- Corn
- Winter squash
- Sweet potatoes
- Yams
- Olives
- Fish
- Shellfish
- Nuts
- Flaxseed (ground)
- Psyllium seed
- Chia seed
- Extra-virgin olive oil
- Fish oils
- Lean protein
- Whey protein

If you eat a variety of these foods, day in and day out, your body will naturally purify itself—without any special detox diet—and you'll feel healthy and strong as a result.

on-the-go lifestyle. You'll also have to scope out restaurants and grocery stores that can meet your needs. And you'll have to understand food well enough to make adjustments to your food plan and still stay on track to meet your goals.

Remember, it is far more important to eat a diet abundant in vegetables and fruits than to avoid them because you can't find or can't afford organically raised produce. Whether conventional or organic, always wash your produce well.

Throughout the day you should eat plenty of nonstarchy vegetables. This results in a diet rich in anti-inflammatory nutrients, fluids, and fiber. These characteristics make vegetables filling, which helps when you're cutting back on calories and trying to control your appetite. The fibers from most nonstarchy vegetables are not gas forming, either; they create little to no discomfort and bloating in athletes.

Let me share my own personal story about ramping up the fiber in your diet. I have begun teaching in South Vietnam, at Can Tho University of Medicine and Pharmacy. My trips to Vietnam last about 2 weeks, and while there, I eat only local, cultural foods. Although I have eaten a lot of Vietnamese food from restaurants in my home city of Seattle, the amount of leaves and woody stems in the food from the Mekong Delta is on a whole different level. I also usually eat some sort of soup at two or three meals each day, and it is only one part of the meal. Because I am a guest of the university, the faculty love to take me out to their favorite food spots, and as an honored guest I never say no to any food that is offered. I am perpetually full while there, and by the time I board my flight home I am certain that I've gained at least 5 pounds. Don't get me wrong; Vietnamese cuisine is my favorite in the world, but I get my full up to my eyeballs each time I visit.

Here's the point: By my second day home, after losing all the extra water that I hold from the hot climate and extra sodium in the food, I am always 5 pounds *lighter* than I was when I left Seattle. It is the ultimate high-fiber and high fluid–volume diet. In fact, Dr. Barbara Rolls from Penn State University did research and wrote a diet book on exactly this concept, but it isn't part of our American standard cuisine. In Vietnam, if you love the food and want to lose weight, it's easy!

Monitor Added Sugar in Your Diet

This may not sound very politically correct, but sugar in your diet isn't really what makes you fat. If you control your calories and exercise regularly, a little sugar won't bother you. And if you eat a lot of sugar but stay in calorie balance, you may not be healthy but you won't automatically gain weight.

But there are issues with high sugar diets that can lead to overweight and obesity. The first problem goes back to idea of fiber in the diet helping to control the amount that you eat. Highly refined, high-sugar foods are very low in fiber and very low in other important nutrients and phytochemicals that help our bodies stay in metabolic balance. High-sugar foods are also typically also high in fat, making them very calorically dense but very nutritionally empty.

Highly refined foods, made up of simple sugars and refined carbohydrate and typically high in fat, are very low in the robust flavors found in whole foods. Instead, they are flavored with laboratory chemicals, regardless of whether their label says "natural." What seems to happen is that these highly refined, artificially flavored foods, by design, push every signal button in your body to encourage your appetite and decrease your inhibitions to control the volume of food that you eat. In other words, the makeup of foods that are high in added sugars means they are high in calories and most people tend to eat more of them. That definitely leads to weight gain. Once you are overweight, the hormonal systems in your body that help you burn energy and control appetite are overcome by the fat on your body sending out signals that further disrupt appetite control and metabolic processes. This is the point where your body becomes resistant to insulin and when you are no longer utilizing sugar for fuel but are instead automatically storing it as fat. While this process takes some time, it takes a long time to reverse, as well.

The lesson is this: Change the composition of your diet to keep the fat off. This means cutting down on high-fat, sugary foods. If you have a sweet tooth, choose dark chocolate or combine the sweet food with a whole protein and a healthy fat to increase satiety and decrease the amount of sweet that you eat. Stay away from sweetened beverages as they have been strongly linked to the high incidence of obesity. We don't seem to manage liquid calories and balance them out in our day like we do with solid foods.

If you are considering using artificially sweetened foods, proceed with caution. See the section on artificial sweeteners later in this chapter for more on the controversy over their use.

Don't Fast Prior to Exercise if Performance Is Your Goal

Fasting prior to exercise has been rumored to boost fat burning. This strategy is still controversial. While some studies confirm that there is no difference in fat loss between exercising on an empty stomach and exercising after having eaten, others disagree. In reality, fasting prior to exercise may slightly boost fat burning but will not improve exercise performance!

Additionally, if you exercise after fasting, your body doesn't have enough muscle glycogen for fuel—a precarious situation. The fact is, inadequate glycogen causes muscle protein breakdown, which is not the state you want to achieve for building muscle, strength, and power.

My advice is to always go into intense exercise well fueled. If you train early in the morning and feel that you can't eat a full breakfast prior to training, then have a small snack at least. Ideally, your snack would have 20 to 25 grams of protein and at least 35 grams or more of carbohydrate, depending on your own total carbohydrate needs and the intensity and duration of your workout, but even half of that is better than nothing. You might find that a liquid shake made from whey protein and a carbohydrate source such as fruit, juice, or a carbohydrate supplement is your best strategy. Yogurt is often well tolerated and is a natural carbohydrate–protein combo. Then have a full breakfast after your training. Timing for any preworkout meal or snack is highly individualized based on what you can tolerate. Some can eat and train; others need up to 60 or even 90 minutes before exercise. Experiment on your own, and remember that liquids empty most quickly from your stomach.

Also keep in mind that whatever you eat within an hour of training is probably still in your stomach when you begin training. If you have a long warm-up, that may work for you by allowing further digestion. Simply putting food (or carbohydrate supplement) into your mouth signals your brain that you've got fuel on board, so if you have a workout of only an hour, or that is moderate in intensity, your performance may not suffer. But if you expect to plunge right into a high-intensity workout with food in your stomach, that food won't be fueling your training. This is a time when a liquid carbohydrate supplement may be useful for you.

If you train later in the day, you'll have already been feeding yourself and fueling your muscles. So make sure that you have eaten within 90 minutes to 2 hours prior to exercise. Find the foods that work for you. Yogurt is a good choice; so are liquid shakes. If you're someone who enjoys a burger prior to training hard, that is fine too, but if you work out right away, it won't be fueling your training; it will still be digesting in your stomach. Do what works best for you.

Keep your fat intake to a minimum in your preworkout snacks and meals. It will slow digestion and make you feel fuller for longer. Avoid high-fiber foods around exercise for the same reasons.

Don't Skip Breakfast

Skipping breakfast is not a good way to lose body fat; in fact, it could even make you fatter! Most people who skip breakfast make up those calories, with interest, throughout the day. In Madrid, Spain, researchers found that overweight and obese people spent less time eating breakfast and ate smaller quantities and less varied types of food at breakfast compared with normal-weight people. Eating breakfast stokes your metabolic fires for the day. By contrast, going hungry in the morning is just another form of fasting, which slows down your metabolism. Plus, your physical and mental performance suffers when you are running on empty.

If you're like me, you're rushed in the morning, with barely enough time to shower and dress, let alone eat breakfast. If that is the case, eat what you can. Even on my busiest mornings, I plan ahead and never skip breakfast. Something is better than nothing. A study done in England found that because ready-to-eat cereals are high in vitamins and minerals and low in fat, they make a great choice for breakfast. When choosing cereals, those made from whole grains with low or no sugar and high fiber are the best bets. My favorite cereal breakfast is puffed kamut grains with freshly ground flaxseed meal, chia seeds, fresh blueberries and banana, and nonfat milk. And of course, a freshly brewed coffee! On my better days, I add a whole egg plus two egg whites.

The best breakfasts include a combination of carbohydrate, protein, and fat. If you are always on the go, you need some nutritious breakfasts that take minutes to fix. There are several breakfast recipes in chapter 20 to help you. Some of these can even go on the road with you—so there is no excuse to skip breakfast!

Limit Alcohol Intake

If your goal is to perform at peak levels, be aware that alcohol consumption will limit your progress. The data are quite clear that alcohol, a central nervous system depressant, diminishes athletic performance not only within hours but also within days of consumption. Alcohol also increases appetite and caloric intake, both of which are detrimental to losing body fat.

There is a broad misconception that calories from alcohol are not recognized by the body and so don't count. This is false. The calories are absolutely recognized by the body and metabolized. Just like protein, carbohydrate, and fat, alcohol calories are stored as fat when caloric consumption is above caloric needs. Current research shows that alcohol calories add to all of the other calories that you eat in the day, yet they are considered "empty" calories because they provide virtually no nutrients. Alcohol calories are also burned preferentially to the other macronutrients, so on an evening out drinking and eating you are most likely to burn your alcohol calories and store the rest of your calories as fat. And because alcohol lowers your inhibitions, when you drink and eat, all of your best intentions go out the window.

While few people drink alcohol before training, it is not an uncommon practice after training. But when you consume alcohol after training, carbohydrate metabolism is altered, so recovery is not as rapid. Endocrine function and sleep are disturbed, further disrupting recovery. If you expect to perform at high levels within a day or two of your last bout of exercise, ideally don't drink at all, or don't drink more than one or two alcoholic beverages between bouts.

Alcohol consumed before or with meals tends to increase food intake both by lowering inhibitions and enhancing the short-term rewarding effects of food. It is true that moderate alcohol intake may protect against obesity, particularly in women; however, increased alcohol consumption and dependence, as well as binge drinking, may increase risks of obesity. Most likely, you want to avoid obesity and stay as lean as possible. Except on special occasions, alcohol has no regular place in the diet of someone trying to achieve physique and performance goals.

Top 10 Fat-Loss and Performance Foods

Fitness, strength, power, endurance, and beauty come from beating the challenge. The higher the intensity of your workout, the longer you can sustain working out, and the more consistent your training day after day, the more sculpted your physique. The foods that support true fat-loss and performance are those that fuel your mind and body, and keep you feeling your best so that you can train hard, recover, and repeat!

1. Cultured foods

    These are not the foods that are part of your cultural heritage, but the foods that contain those all-important probiotic cultures. The significance of the symbiotic relationship between our human cells and our brethren of bacterial and yeast origin is becoming clearer every day. As each new research study is published, we find that these cells boost our health and prevent disease in more ways than we could have ever imagined. Recent data has shown that specific probiotic strains may even assist with fat loss and maintenance of a healthy body weight. If training on a daily basis is important to you, include cultured dairy foods like yogurt, kefir, and labne; fermented vegetables like sour pickles, sauerkraut, kimchi, tempeh, natto, and miso; Moroccan preserved lemons; and the beverages kombucha and amazake.

2. Flaxseed meal

You need food to stay strong and healthy, and so do the probiotic strains. Flaxseed meal is rich in inulin, a nondigestible fiber that feeds the beneficial flora in your gut. In all likelihood, diets rich in a variety of fibers, including inulin, create an environment in your gut to allow the healthiest biome to flourish, keeping you strong and healthy inside and out. Flaxseed must be ground, or else you don't get the benefit of the fiber.

3. Milk

Getting yourself to the gym or the field requires feeling like you want to go there. Mental focus, mood, and mental energy are all part of consistent training and the ability to sustain an intense workout. Milk is one of my all-time favorite "feel great foods." Milk is high in the amino acid tryptophan, a building block for the manufacture of serotonin in your brain. Serotonin is our primary "good mood" neurotransmitter, and without tryptophan, serotonin levels are low, meaning a bad mood, or even depression, isn't far behind. The natural combination of carbohydrate and protein in milk allows for the rapid transport of tryptophan into the brain; this transport is impeded without carbohydrate. Milk is fortified with vitamin D, also required for serotonin production. In addition, multiple studies have shown that whey protein and calcium from dairy foods is associated with fat loss, muscle gain, and better maintenance of a healthy body weight. If you can't drink cow's milk, then goat's milk is a close second. Soymilk fortified with vitamin D and calcium is good, but nut, seed, and grain milks are much lower in protein and have a completely different nutrient composition.

4. Eggs

Egg yolks are the primary source of choline, a B-vitamin, in our diets. Choline is half of the neurotransmitter acetylcholine, which is active every time we think or move: that's 24/7! Americans, fearful of cardiovascular disease risk, have been dumping egg yolks down the drain for the past 30 years, and our consumption of choline has been going down the drain with the yolks. As a nation, we are consuming barely one third of our dietary need for choline. The alarm bells have rung in the nutrition world, and we are now strongly recommending that everyone add at least one egg yolk a day back to their diets, especially since multiple studies have shown that an egg yolk a day does not raise cardiovascular disease risk, even in people with coronary artery disease. Choline is also critically important for the health of brain cells. So if thinking and moving are important to you, and you want to be able to train hard, then add at least one egg to your daily routine.

5. Fish

Fish oil has been widely touted as a way to fight inflammation, and the research is there to support the claims. Now we are finding that fish protein may have its own special effect: helping tamp down oxidative stress and allow for better overall fat loss. While taking fish oil supplements is certainly an important foundational health strategy, eating fish as a primary protein source is also important. I ask my clients to aim to eat five fish meals each week. All fish is better than a hot dog, so you can count whitefish like turbot along with fatty fish like salmon and mackerel. Fatty fish is also high in vitamin D, helping to keep you in the mood to exercise.

6. Iron-rich foods

A study of athletic women found that 50 percent had a compromised iron status but were not necessarily anemic. Recent research has shown that even without anemia, low iron status may increase fatigue and diminish exercise performance. Women with low iron status spend more time in a sedentary state, and the investigators in this study speculate this circumstance may lead to weight gain over time. Heme iron from animal sources has greater bioavailability compared to nonheme iron from plant foods. Even iron-enriched plant foods still contain only nonheme iron. Iron-rich animal foods include lean red meat and dark meat poultry, clams, mussels, mollusks, and oysters. To enhance nonheme iron absorption from plant foods, combine these foods with either a heme iron-rich animal food (all animal foods with iron) or a source of vitamin C. Plant sources of nonheme iron include iron-enriched breads and cereals. Good sources of nonheme iron are 1 cup of cooked beans; 1 ounce of pumpkin, sesame, or squash seeds; one baked potato; one medium stalk of broccoli; and 1 cup of dried apricots.

7. Beans and legumes

Beans are another one of nature's "feel great foods," with a built in combination of protein and carbohydrate. But that's just the beginning. Beans are rich in soluble fiber, which helps to fill you up and keeps you feeling satisfied for longer. While the starch refuels your muscles and the protein supports recovery, the magnesium, potassium, and calcium help to keep your electrolytes in balance. Beans are also rich in iron, zinc, folate, and vitamin B_6, nutrients that support your training, recovery, and overall health to keep your workouts consistent and your metabolism high, day in and day out. Include a wide variety of legumes in your recipes, such as garbanzo, black, navy, pinto, kidney, and lima beans; soybeans; black-eyed peas; yellow, red, and brown lentils; and yellow, green, and red split-peas.

8. Extra-virgin olive oil

   There is a notable difference between olive oil and extra-virgin olive oil (EVOO). The processing is different, the taste is usually different, and the use in cooking is different, yet they are both generally healthful additions to your diet. A significant health factor has also been identified that is exclusive to EVOO: oleocanthal. Oleocanthal is a natural phenolic compound that is a potent anti-inflammatory, similar to the nonsteroidal anti-inflammatory drug ibuprofen. Oleocanthal is responsible for the peppery finish often experienced when consuming EVOO alone or with just a bit of bread. When you train hard enough and long enough to get a training and sculpting effect, you may benefit from keeping your tissues bathed in this healthy anti-inflammatory that has no negative side effects and will only add a lovely flavor and texture to your meals.

9. Watercress

   Sometimes researchers have the most interesting ideas. Knowledge of the potential antioxidant capacity of the nutrients beta-carotene and alpha-tocopherol found in watercress led to a study where investigators fed subjects watercress two hours before an acute bout of tissue-damaging exercise. They continued for a period of eight weeks, feeding watercress two hours before chronic exercise that induced tissue oxidative damage. Both the short- and long-term protocols resulted in a protective effect in the watercress-supplemented subjects against the tissue-damaging effects of the exercise. Limiting tissue damage after exhaustive exercise may lead to more regular, daily bouts of hard training, allowing you to maximize your workouts for optimal sculpting.

10. Coffee

   The use of caffeine to enhance exercise performance is an age-old and evidence-based practice. Effective doses of caffeine work to lower the rating of perceived exertion (RPE) during aerobic exercise; in other words, you can work out harder for longer and not notice it. In the same amount of time your work output goes up, and so does your calorie burn. More recently a study was conducted to test whether an equivalent amount of caffeine from coffee has the same effect as caffeine alone. The researchers gave subjects a controlled dose of caffeine, a placebo, caffeinated coffee, or decaffeinated coffee equivalent to 2.27 milligrams of caffeine per pound of body weight. They found that the caffeine and caffeinated coffee gave equal benefit to the subjects' performance, and the placebo and decaf did nothing. So if you are a coffee drinker, put your coffee to work for you. Drink it before exercise to push for peak performance and maximum sculpting.

Sport Nutrition Fact Versus Fiction: Can You Cheat on Your Diet and Still Lose Weight?

One of the most typical diet questions that I'm asked while standing at the buffet table at a party is, "What do you think about having a cheat day?" Here's my answer (a little more detailed than you'd get at the party).

The idea of the cheat day came out of the world of bodybuilding. Although notorious for their ability to follow a very restricted diet before competitions, male bodybuilders observed that on the day after their competition they looked much better than when they were on stage for the event. Not surprisingly, although they were eating only tuna and chicken breast to get cut before competition, immediately after the competition the nearest ice cream parlor was packed with competitors. After the late afternoon indulgence, they'd awake the next morning to an incredibly buff body, showing more cuts and definition than the day before. It didn't take long for the cheat day to be incorporated into the standard dieting regimens of male bodybuilders.

But what about female bodybuilders? By self-report, the women I work with find that adding a cheat day every once in a while is fine. However, unlike their male counterparts, who seem to be able to return to their diet regimens with great control, women tend to have less restraint during the week following a cheat day.

Dr. Pamela Peeke confirms this idea in her book *Body-for-LIFE for Women* (Rodale, 2005). According to Dr. Peeke, women are more likely to binge during a cheat day. She recommends incorporating balance into your everyday diet to promote healthy relationships with food that can lead to successful weight loss.

Until recently, the concept of a cheat day was based on theory and anecdote. Now, however, there are data on what happens behaviorally and the outcome of that behavior. In 2005, a study published by researchers at the Center for Human Nutrition at the University of Colorado examined the common characteristics of successful long-term weight-loss maintainers on the National Weight Control Registry (NWCR). The NWCR lists over 10,000 people who have been successful in long-term weight-loss maintenance. Although the NWCR does not represent a random sample of all dieters, it does have value in identifying strategies that may help others become successful in keeping weight off.

One of the key results was that participants who maintained a consistent diet across the week were one and a half times more likely to maintain their weight within 5 pounds (2.3 kg) over the subsequent year than were participants who allowed themselves a cheat day during the week. The same was true for people who allowed themselves more flexibility during holidays and traveling. Both groups that had free time outside their diet plans had a greater risk of regaining their lost weight.

To my way of thinking, the whole concept of cheating exemplifies a negative approach toward food. Cheating, whether planned or not, implies guilt for a bad deed done. Because we experience ourselves as living through a week of deprivation during which our favorite foods are off limits, all we do is crave them while working hard at avoiding them. Then comes our cheat day, and rather than eating a normal serving size of chocolate cake, we binge and eat half the cake. Then the guilt sets in, and there goes the other half of the cake. What a waste of time and emotion!

Get rid of the idea of cheating. Build a positive approach to food and dieting by daily balancing your food with your exercise, and your favorite foods with all the foods that you eat to maintain your health.

The easiest way to maintain balance in your diet is to start with the big picture. What are your favorite foods that you think you should avoid, and which days are your most active days? By plugging in sweet treats after exercise, you put the sugar to work for you. Not only do you not feel guilty about eating it but also your body benefits from the sugar after exercise. You can feel good about rewarding yourself for a hard, sweaty workout. Whatever that sweet treat is, make sure to include a source of milk protein at the same time, to get the biggest bang for your buck. Is a sweet, blended milk-based drink at your neighborhood latté stand or smoothie bar a sweet? Or maybe a cookie and a glass of milk? What about a latté and a bagel? All of these contain the right ingredients to help your muscles recover, build, and refuel after exercise. Of course, keeping your serving sizes small will help contain your calories, but it will seem like plenty when you've never before allowed yourself to eat anything after exercise!

Is your weakest moment in the evening? Are you dying for chocolate? Plan to have a hot cocoa to help you relax and get you over the hump. The high tryptophan levels in milk combined with the few grams of carbohydrate will raise your serotonin levels and help your mind and body get ready for sleep. Non-Dutched, natural cocoa powder, or bittersweet chocolate containing at least 70 percent cacao, will do the same. This is a way to plan something good for you into your days.

What about the unplanned splurge? There will always be very special moments in life when we do something, or eat something, just because we feel like it at the moment. I say, celebrate those moments; don't disparage them. Don't ruin your wedding because the cake isn't in your plan for the day. Don't avoid the champagne toast on your birthday. And definitely don't forgo sharing food during a special moment with a loved one. Food plays a very intimate role in our lives, and restricting food during tender moments, happy occasions, and celebrations can make you feel left out. I'm talking about really special occasions that happen infrequently—not every holiday or day off from work.

When the day is done, look back on it with fondness. I hope the food and the moment were as good as you had hoped. Then tomorrow, go back to your plan. Cheating included; no guilt allowed!

Sport Nutrition Fact Versus Fiction: Do Sugar Substitutes Have a Place in a Fat-Loss Program?

Sugar substitutes are either natural or synthetic. For instance, the sugar substitute stevia is natural yet still highly processed, but the sugar substitute saccharine is artificial. Some sugar substitutes such as agave nectar and rice syrup are considered high-intensity sweeteners, because they are many times sweeter then sucrose or common table sugar. Because of the intensity of sweetness, only very small amounts are needed.

Most FDA-approved sugar substitutes are artificially synthesized, but there are some natural compounds, including stevia, sorbitol, and xylitol. Despite FDA oversight of these food additives, sugar substitutes remain controversial, and some question whether they pose health risks.

The most common reason people use sugar substitutes is to reduce calorie consumption to control body weight and body fat. Recent scientific studies indicate that this may not be quite so simple. Animal studies have shown that a sweet taste in the mouth induces an insulin response, causing increased fat storage from circulating carbohydrate. When a sugar substitute leads to this insulin response without an increase in blood sugar, there can be an increase in hypoglycemia or hyperinsulinemia as the result. These conditions lead to increased food intake, possibly cravings, no weight loss, and possible weight gain. Additionally, the body's usual response to sugar consumption in small amounts is to increase heat production and energy usage, and to blunt the appetite later in the day. With sugar substitutes, these responses never happen.

Sugar alcohols can cause terrible GI distress. These compounds are intensely sweet, calorie-free, and do not contain alcohol. They are calorie-free because we do not digest them, but the probiotics in our gut do digest them, and most people experience gas, bloating, discomfort, and even pain when these are consumed regularly and frequently.

Here is a list of sugar alcohols that you will find in sugar-free or no-added sugar sweetened products like beverages, candy, chewing gum, yogurt, cereals, cookies and others:

- Erythritol
- Glycerol (also known as glycerin or glycerine)
- Hydrogenated starch hydrolysates
- Isomalt
- Lactitol
- Maltitol
- Mannitol
- Sorbitol
- Xylitol

Population studies in humans have shown that increased consumption of artificially sweetened beverages leads to weight gain. Randomized controlled trials are very limited, however, and there is no strong clinical evidence to show a cause-and-effect relationship. My advice about all sugar substitutes is to keep these factors in mind and limit any use of added sweeteners in the diet, natural or otherwise.

6

Hydrating for Heavy-Duty Workouts

Quick: What's the most critical nutrient for growth, development, and health?

If you guessed water, congratulations! People frequently overlook the importance of water in their diet, and most don't even consider water an essential nutrient. Without enough water and other fluids, though, you'd die within a week.

Although water does not provide energy in the same way carbohydrate and fat do, it plays an essential role in energy formation. As the most abundant nutrient in your body, water is the medium in which all energy reactions take place. Thus, you need ample fluids for fuel and stamina. You get those fluids from a variety of sources—the foods you eat; the beverages you consume; and the plain, pure water you drink. Here's a closer look at the importance of water and other fluids in the diet.

Water: An Essential Nutrient

The fluids in your body form a heavily trafficked river through your arteries, veins, and capillaries that carries nutrients to your cells and waste products out of the body. Fluids fill virtually every space in your cells and between cells. Water molecules not only fill space but also help form the structures of macromolecules such as protein and glycogen. The chemical reactions that keep you alive occur in water, and water is an active participant in those reactions.

It's hard to say enough good things about water. It makes up about 60 percent of the body's weight in adults. As the primary fluid in your body, water serves as a solvent for minerals, vitamins, amino acids, glucose, and many other nutrients. Without water, you can't even digest these essential nutrients, let alone absorb, transport, and use them.

In addition to carrying nutrients throughout the body, water transports waste products out of the body. It is a part of the lubricant in your joints that keeps them moving. And when your body's temperature begins to rise, water acts as the coolant in your radiator. Enough said! You can see why water is so vital to health.

Temperature Regulation

Your body produces energy for exercise, but only 25 percent of that energy is actually used for mechanical work. The other 75 percent is released as heat. The extra warmth produced during exercise causes your body to heat up, raising your core temperature. To get rid of that extra heat, you sweat. As sweat evaporates, your blood and body cool. If you couldn't cool off, you would quickly succumb to heat stress caused by the increase in your body's core temperature.

Fat Burning

Drinking more water can actually help you stay lean. Your kidneys depend on water to do their job of filtering waste products from the body. In a water shortage, the kidneys need backup, so they turn to the liver for help. One of the liver's many functions is mobilizing stored fat for energy. By taking on extra assignments from the kidneys, the liver can't do its fat-burning job as well. Fat loss is compromised as a result.

Researchers from Basel, Switzerland, investigated the role that cellular hydration plays in fat-burning and protein synthesis by looking at well-hydrated versus poorly hydrated cells. They found that under conditions of hypo-osmolality—which is essentially hyperhydration (lots of hydration in cells)—the subjects burned more fat because their bodies tapped into fat, rather than carbohydrate, for fuel. They also found that dehydration prevents adequate protein synthesis.

If gaining muscle is your goal, you should care about the hydration state of your muscle cells (also called cell volumization). In a well-hydrated muscle cell, protein synthesis is stimulated and protein breakdown is decreased. On the other hand, dehydration of muscle cells promotes protein breakdown and inhibits protein synthesis. Cell volumization has also been shown to influence genetic expression (the process by which a gene carries out DNA instructions), enzyme and hormone activity, and metabolism. Bottom line: When you guzzle down that bottle of water, you're potentially boosting not only fat burning but also the maintenance of normal cell volume levels that are important for muscle protein levels.

In addition, water can help take the edge off hunger so that you eat less, and it has no calories. If you are on a high-protein diet, water is required to detoxify ammonia, a by-product of protein energy metabolism. And, as you burn off stored fatty acids as energy, you release any fat-soluble toxins that have been benignly stored in your fat cells. The more fluid you drink, the more you dilute the toxins in your bloodstream and the more rapidly they exit the body.

Muscle Strength and Control

Ever wonder why some days you're so pooped you can't pump iron? One reason may be dehydration. To move your muscles, you need water. Of all the places in the body, water is found in highest concentrations in metabolically active tissues such as muscle and is found in lowest concentrations in relatively inactive tissues such as fat, skin, and some parts of bone. Muscles are controlled by nerves. The electrical stimulation of nerves and contraction of muscles occur as a result of the exchange of electrolyte minerals dissolved in water (sodium, potassium, calcium, chloride, and magnesium) across the nerve and muscle cell membranes.

If you're low on water or electrolytes, muscle strength and control are weakened. A water deficit of just 2 to 4 percent of your body weight can cut your strength-training workout by as much as 21 percent—and your aerobic power by a whopping 48 percent. Your body's thirst mechanism kicks in when you've lost 2 percent of your body weight in water. But by that time, you're already dehydrated. To prevent dehydration, you must get yourself on a scheduled plan to drink often throughout the day.

Joint Lubrication

Water is the major component of synovial fluid, the lubricating fluid between your joints, and cerebrospinal fluid, the shock-absorbing fluid between vertebrae and around the brain. Both fluids are essential for healthy joint and spine maintenance. If your diet is water deficient, even for a brief period, less fluid is available to protect these areas. Strength training places tremendous demands on the joints and spine, and the presence of adequate protective fluid is essential for optimum performance and long-term health.

Mental Performance

Whether at the office or in competition, your hydration state affects your performance. Dehydration, in particular, decreases mental energy; causes fatigue, lethargy, light-headedness, and headaches; and can certainly make you feel down. In a study of subjects' abilities to perform mental exercises after dehydration induced by heat stress, a fluid loss of only 2 percent of body weight caused reductions of up to 20 percent in arithmetic ability, short-term memory, and the ability to visually track an object. Another study demonstrated that a minor loss of 1 percent of body mass as fluid led to impairments in both memory and attention. With that powerful proof, you should be motivated to stay well hydrated to keep your mental energy high and your focus sharp.

Disease and Illness Prevention

Probably the most surprising fact about water is the effect that chronic, mild dehydration has on health and disease. It was a practice of Hippocrates to recommend large intakes of water to increase urine production and decrease the recurrence of urinary tract stones. Today, approximately 12 to 15 percent of the general population will form a kidney stone at some time in life. Many factors can modify the risk factors for developing stones. Of these, diet—especially fluid intake—is the only one that can be easily changed and that has a marked effect on all aspects of urinary health.

A little-known fact is that low water intake is a risk factor for certain types of cancers. One study found that patients with urinary tract cancer (bladder, prostate, kidney, and testicle) drank significantly smaller quantities of fluid compared with healthy controls.

In another study, researchers discovered that women who drank more than five glasses of water a day had a 45 percent lower risk of colon cancer compared with those who consumed two or fewer glasses a day. For men, the risk was cut by 32 percent when they drank more than four glasses a day versus one or fewer glasses a day.

Why does adequate water intake appear to have an anticancer effect? One theory holds that the more fluid you drink, the faster you flush the toxins and carcinogenic substances out of your body, and the less chance there is for them to be resorbed into the body or to be concentrated long enough to cause tissue change.

Even more fascinating, a pilot study reported that the odds of developing breast cancer were reduced by 79 percent, on average, among water drinkers. In this case, maintaining a dilute solution within the cells possibly reduces the potency of estrogen and its ability to cause hormone-related cancers, according to the theory proposed by the authors of this research.

Mild dehydration can also be a factor in the occurrence of mitral valve prolapse, a defect of one of the heart valves that controls the flow of blood between the chambers of the heart. Mitral valve prolapse is a relatively harmless condition, but in a small percentage of cases, it causes rapid heartbeat, chest pain, and other cardiac symptoms. In a study of 14 healthy women with normal heart function, mitral valve prolapse was induced by mild dehydration and resolved with rehydration.

How Much Water Do You Need?

Nearly all the foods you eat contain water, which is absorbed during digestion. Most fruits and vegetables are 75 to 90 percent water. Meats contain roughly 50 to 70 percent water. And beverages such as juice, milk, and glucose–electrolyte solutions are more than 85 percent water. On average, you may consume about 4 cups (1 L) of water daily from food alone, but this is true only if you're eating an abundance of fruits and vegetables, which are the major food sources of water.

Most people are walking around in a moderately dehydrated state. You need 9 to 12 cups (2 to 3 L) of total fluids daily—even more to replace the fluid you lose during exercise. Of these 9 to 12 cups, make sure at least 5 of them (1 L) are pure water.

You lose about a quart (4 cups, or 1 L) of water per hour of exercise, depending on your size and perspiration rate. When you're working out moderately in a mild climate, you are probably losing 1 to 2 quarts (or liters), or 2 to 4 pounds (0.9-1.8 kg), of fluid per hour through perspiration. That means that a 150-pound (68 kg) person can easily lose 2 percent of body weight in fluid (3 lb, or 1 kg) within an hour. If exercise is more intense or the environment is more extreme, fluid losses will be greater. Thus, you see how easily you can become dehydrated.

If you don't replenish fluid losses during exercise, you will fatigue early and your performance will be diminished. If you don't replenish fluid after exercise, your performance on successive days will decay, and your long-term health may be at risk.

Moreover, according to the National Athletic Trainers' Association (NATA), dehydration impairs your physical performance in less than an hour of exercise—or sooner if you start working out in a dehydrated state—cuts your performance by as much as 48 percent, and increases your risk of developing symptoms of heat illness, such as heat cramps, heat exhaustion, and heatstroke.

In addition to exercise, many other factors increase water requirements, including high heat, low humidity, high altitude, high-fiber foods, illness, travel, and pregnancy.

What about you? Are you dehydrated? Table 6.1 lists the early and severe warning signs of dehydration and heat stress.

Following are easy actions you can take to monitor yourself for early signs of dehydration:

- Pay attention to how well hydrated you are going into exercise. If you were already dehydrated when you began your training session, then your fluid losses may be greater at the end of exercise. You will need to compensate for this every time it happens.

- Check your hydration status by observing how frequently you void, how much urine you pass, and the color of your urine. If you're urinating less frequently, the volume is markedly diminished, or the color is darker than usual, then you are dehydrated. The color should be no darker than straw; it should not be colorless, and it should not be as dark as brewed tea.

- Check your sweat rate. There's a really easy way to do this as a "back of the napkin" style of measurement, or a more complicated, scientific way. Although even the more scientific way isn't how we would do it in a research lab, it will get you closer to your real sweat rate number.
  - Really easy way: Weigh yourself without clothing before and after exercise. For every pound (0.5 kg) lost during exercise, you've lost 2 to 3 cups

TABLE 6.1   Signs of Dehydration and Heat Stress

Early signs	Severe signs
Fatigue	Difficulty swallowing
Loss of appetite	Stumbling
Flushed skin	Clumsiness
Heat intolerance	Shriveled skin
Light-headedness	Sunken eyes and dim vision
Dark urine with strong odor	Painful urination
Dry cough	Numb skin
Burning sensation in stomach	Muscle spasm
Headache	Delirium
Dry mouth	

Adapted from W.R. Johnson and E.R. Buskirk (eds.), *Structural and Physiological Aspects of Exercise and Sport* (Princeton NJ: Princeton Book Co., 1980).

(480-720 ml) of fluid. Any weight lost during exercise is fluid loss and should be replaced by drinking fluids as soon as possible after exercise.

- ○ The down side of the really easy way above is that it does not take into consideration any fluids that you consumed during exercise, any fluid losses from urination, or any weight that you added from food that you might have eaten during exercise. An actual sweat rate measurement will do that. This is the basic method that we use with serious athletes and athletic teams to get them closer to individual fluid needs. You can find more detailed instruction in table 6.2.

- Take note of a sore throat, dry cough, or hoarse voice, which are all signs of dehydration.

- Be aware that a burning sensation in your stomach can signal dehydration.

- Be aware of muscle cramps. No one knows for sure what causes muscle cramps, but a shortfall of water may be an important factor. Muscle cramps are more apt to occur when you're doing hard, physical work in the heat and don't drink enough fluids. You can usually alleviate the cramps by moving to a cool place, drinking fluids, and replacing electrolytes with a glucose–electrolyte solution, some salty foods, fruits, and vegetables.

- If you're a "salty sweater," you may need to drink saltier beverages during exercise and eat more salt throughout the day. You can check whether you are a salty sweater by wearing a dark or black T-shirt during exercise. If you see salt stains on the chest and under the armpits of the T-shirt where sweat has evaporated after exercise, then you are losing significant amounts of salt. This can lead to increases in muscle cramps. Replace salt lost during exercise by drinking beverages with slightly higher salt content during exercise and consuming salt with foods at meals and snacks.

Read through the table 6.2, and follow these guidelines:

1. Completely empty your bladder and intestines prior to beginning this test.
2. Begin the test fully hydrated.
3. Do not eat anything during the test. Only drinking is allowed.
4. Keep accurate records of the amount that you drink during the test. Premeasured water bottles work very well, but you'll need to know the weight of the empty bottle.
5. Weigh yourself pre- and postexercise, completely nude, ideally without any athletic tape or spandex that can absorb sweat.
6. Heart rate monitoring is optional.

TABLE 6.2 Estimating the Sweating Rate for an Athlete From Pre- and Postexercise Weight Changes

Date	Temp	Relative humidity	Weight pre	Weight post	Weight change	Fluid intake	Urine output	Total sweat loss[a]	Exercise duration	Hourly sweating rate	Weight change (%)	Thirst (1-10)	Heart rate	RPE[b] (1-10)
7/08	75 °F	50%	130 lb (59 kg)	128 lb (58.2 kg)	2 lb (0.8 kg)	12 oz (~0.350 kg)	0	0.8 + 0.350 = 1.15	1.5 h	1.15 / 1.5 = 0.75 kg (24 oz)	1.6	4	150	6

Comments for session: 7/08
Workout was running on flat terrain, it was windy, did not feel extremely thirsty, a bit dry at the end, felt I could pull it through well. Felt that my fluid intake was good. RPE was what coach wanted me to do. Felt comfortable.

Comments for session:

Comments for session:

[a]Total sweat loss: weight change + fluid intake.

[b]RPE: rating of perceived exertion.

Steps to estimate hourly sweating rate:
1. Make sure you are hydrated before the exercise session.
2. Warm up for 5 to 10 min or until you begin to sweat. Urinate if necessary.
3. Take nude body weight on a stable scale with an accuracy of 0.1 kg before exercise, and repeat the process after exercise.
4. Use a heart rate monitor, and measure your heart rate.
5. Subtract weight post from weight pre to calculate weight change; if you are converting from pounds to kilograms, divide pounds by 2.2.

> *continued*

TABLE 6.2 > *continued*

6. Measure and add fluid consumed (fluid intake) to weight change; if you are converting from ounces to grams and kilograms, multiply ounces by 28.4 to convert to grams (g) and then divide by 1,000 to convert to kilograms (kg).
7. If no urine was passed, leave this blank or it is equal to 0. If you collected urine, subtract it in kilograms from weight change (number 5 above: Use same conversion as in number 6 above, converting fluid ounces to grams and then to kilograms).
8. Divide total sweat loss (weight change + fluid intake − urine output) by exercise duration in hours to get an hourly sweating rate.
9. Convert your weight change from pounds or kilograms to % weight change. Did you exceed 2%?
10. Rate the thirst you perceived during exercise: 1 = not thirsty; 10 = highly thirsty with a dry mouth.
11. Record your heart rate.
12. Rate the effort you perceived during exercise (RPE); 1 = no effort; 10 = the highest effort)
13. Consider your fluid intake. Was it enough to maintain your effort?
14. Whereas thirst, heart rate, and RPE are not used to calculate your sweating rate, these factors are important for evaluating your fluid replacement strategy for this particular exercise session and environment. It may be that you exceeded a 2% body-weight loss by replacing fluid in an amount lower than the amount you lost through sweat but that you were able to complete your session with the RPE set by you or your coach. In addition, you did not feel thirsty and your heart rate responded normally to the intensity of the workout. As you can see, this spreadsheet could include more information such as total work accomplished, type of fluid, other energy sources from food or fluids, and possible sources of error to consider for this calculation. It's best to make your own spreadsheet that you can tweak in accordance with your needs. The goal of this spreadsheet is to monitor your fluid balance and to identify the range of fluid intake that best fits your sport in various environments. Ultimately, this should help you to optimize your race strategies!

Reprinted by permission from M.M. Manore, N.L. Meyer, and J. Thompson, *Sport Nutrition for Health and Performance*, 2nd ed. (Champaign, IL: Human Kinetics, 2009), 245.

Drinking Schedule for Strength Trainers, Heavy Exercise, and Competitive Events

If you are an elite athlete, you usually can't rely on thirst to tell you when to drink fluids. By the time your thirst mechanism kicks in during exercise, you've already lost 1 to 2 percent of your body weight as sweat. You need to drink water at regular intervals whether you're thirsty or not, and you need to do so every day. Remember, if you fail to drink enough fluids one day, your body can't automatically rehydrate itself the next. You'll be doubly dehydrated and possibly begin to show some signs of dehydration.

On the other hand, many average exercisers actually can rely on thirst because their sweat rates are lower and rehydration needs are more moderate. In fact, the latest recommendations from the National Athletic Trainers' Association emphasizes the individuality of fluid needs, and no longer posts a blanket rehydration recommendation for all exercisers. Even with elite athletes, individual variability is quite high. This is why we depend on sweat rate measurements for individual recommendations.

Before Exercise

Make sure that you have been drinking regularly up until exercise. Recreational exercisers should maintain healthy hydration levels going into a workout or competition. If you are an elite athlete, you might drink slightly more than you need prior to a heavy workout or competition in a hot environment. Do not increase your body weight by more than 2 percent.

During Exercise

For many recreational athletes, drink according to thirst. This should keep you fairly well hydrated. If you have calculated your sweat rate, then follow that data. Drink according to your sweat rate losses, and try not to go beyond the 2 percent loss of body mass goal.

As mentioned earlier, elite athletes may need to focus more on a drinking schedule, because "drink when you're thirsty" is not always a successful strategy during competition. Create a fluid plan based on your sweat rate losses, considering the conditions of your race compared to those when you conducted your sweat rate test. If possible, conduct a sweat rate test under close-to race conditions prior to the race so you have better data. Follow your fluid plan during the race. If you find that you cannot follow the plan, then at least drink according to thirst to avoid major problems with dehydration or hyperhydration.

After Exercise

This is the time to replace any fluid you've lost. Weigh yourself before and after exercise; then drink 2 to 3 cups (480 to 720 ml) of fluid within two hours after

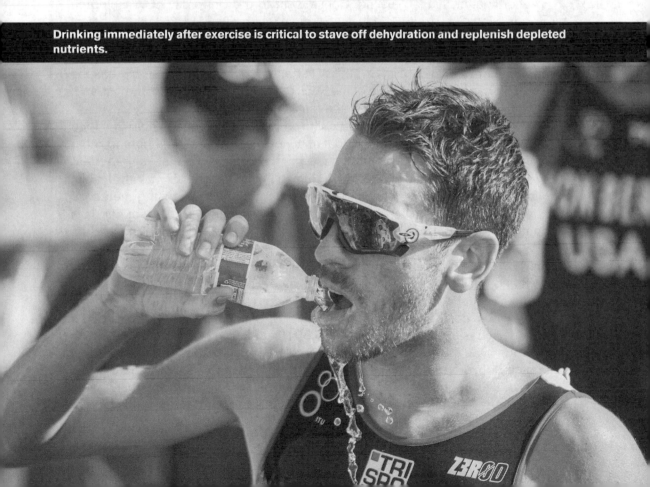

Drinking immediately after exercise is critical to stave off dehydration and replenish depleted nutrients.

exercise for every pound (0.5 kg) of body weight you've lost. Another way to calculate your postworkout fluids is to drink 150 percent of the weight that you lost during the event. Continue to drink an additional 25 to 50 percent more fluid for the next four hours.

POWER PROFILE: An Unusual Source of Hydration, Plus Mega-Nutrition, in a World Class Athlete

Sonya was planning to compete in Expedition Pacific, in which she would attempt to row from Japan to San Francisco and be the first woman to cross the Pacific nonstop. She felt like she had "winged her nutrition planning" for this grueling feat. I wasn't so sure. Sonya hadn't had any testing or done any nutritional planning prior to setting out on an enormous human-powered endeavor?

I scheduled Sonya for testing at the Seattle University Human Performance Lab where Sean Machak, lab supervisor, donated his time and facility to run Sonya through a series of tests to evaluate her metabolic needs both in and out of the boat, on dry land and in a water simulation. I'll describe the results of this testing below.

Shortly after that lab testing, Sonya went to the University of Washington Sports Medicine Center at Husky Stadium where Dr. Mark Harrast, Medical Director, gave Sonya a full exam to evaluate her health and make certain she was prepared for this ultra-athletic event. Last but not least, Sonya had an appointment with a dentist, Dr. Jeffrey P. Kanter, to make sure that a toothache wouldn't halt her in the middle of the Pacific Ocean. Dr. Jeff is also my husband, so this Expedition was now all in the family.

With a clean bill of health, we set out to prepare Sonya's shopping list for food and supplements to fuel her foundational health needs, her rowing and other athletic activities, as well as her recovery and comfort during the long journey.

The data that was collected at the Human Performance Lab was invaluable. We could see Sonya's foundational energy needs, or her resting metabolic rate (RMR), as well as her predicted energy usage during all parts of her days on the boat: sitting, lying down, rowing, trimming the boat, and pulling anchor.

Sonya's RMR was estimated to be 2,091 calories per day, equivalent to only 20 percent of her total estimated daily energy expenditure. Trimming the boat and pulling anchor made up an estimated 16 percent of her daily energy expenditure, and a whopping estimated 64 percent of her daily energy expenditure would come from rowing! Totaled, Sonya's estimated energy expenditure on a daily basis was approximately 10,501 calories!

Once I had those basic numbers, I needed to break down the caloric values into carbohydrate and fat needs for fueling Sonya's days. Carbohydrate is fast fuel, and it is required for performing high-intensity exercise. Unlike just rowing a boat over flat water, open ocean rowing is fairly intense exercise and greatly depends on available carbohydrate for fuel. The other physical activities on the boat also require high power outputs because the boat is constantly rocking, and depending on the weather, the energy expenditure can range quite a bit. Fat is used as fuel for low- to moderate-intensity activity levels, and fat has other essential structural and functional roles in the body.

Sonya's protein needs were predominantly tied to the structural and functional jobs that only protein can do. Because it would be very difficult for Sonya to actually eat enough calories every day to meet her energy needs, I increased the amount of protein in her diet to cover the possibility that she would be using some of her protein intake as energy.

I knew that it was very unlikely that Sonya would consume everything that I had planned for her to eat every day. She would have days when she ate well, and days when she didn't feel like eating very much. Nonetheless, her job every day was to eat as much as possible. The single biggest known biological risk to her successful completion of this ultra-event is loss of strength and power due to low calorie intake. It was well known that she would lose weight during the crossing, and this is why she had packed on some extra pounds prior to departure. But if her weight dropped too low from the high exertion and under-fueling, she wouldn't make it.

Designing a menu plan required knowing not only Sonya's estimated needs but also how much she could actually eat and how much weight and volume she could stow. Sonya methodically packed her food and supplements and separated them into waterproof bags of rations to create a daily routine. This is a breakdown of her typical daily nourishment:

Day Bag

Food for meals from backpacker's pantry

Pure starch carbohydrate supplement for rowing and recovery: Vitargo

Vitamins and mineral supplements: US AIVA Health Sciences, Inc.

Average calories: 3,908; fat: 99 grams; protein: 195 grams; carbohydrate: 580 grams

Snack Bag

An assortment of carbohydrate-rich and fat-rich foods that she could eat throughout the day (crackers, pretzels, trail mix, popcorn, nuts), sweets and canned foods (ginger snaps, jelly beans, fruit leathers, tuna, sardines, Spam, canned fruit)

Average calories: 2,358; fat: 131 grams; protein: 107 grams; carbohydrate: 188 grams

Other Bag

Comfort foods (peanut butter, Nutella, cookies) and extra-virgin olive oil and coconut oil to pack in the calories when it counts

Average calories: 876; fat: 68 grams; protein: 11 grams; carbohydrate: 63 grams

> continued

POWER PROFILE > continued

All Combined

Average calories: 7,142 to 7,258; fat: 298 grams; protein: 313 grams; carbohydrate: 831 grams

Hydration was absolutely essential to Sonya's health and the success of this expedition. Sonya had a desalination system on board, which would allow her to create drinking water along the way. It would have been impossible to carry enough drinking water with her for the voyage. There is sodium and other electrolytes in her food and her supplements to support her body's extra needs due to hard physical labor. Her hydration goal is to consume as much as she can, just like her food goal. Between rowing and maintaining the boat, and probable seasickness during the first few weeks of the voyage, eating and drinking enough would be one of Sonya's most difficult tasks.

Here's the end of the expedition story: Due to many weeks of obstacles—from shipping her boat to getting through customs to cultural issues in Japan—Sonya took off so late in the season out on the Pacific that the storms had begun. She was barely 300 miles off the Japanese coast when she had to call off her attempt due to the terrific storms that posed a life-threatening danger.

Best Sources of Water

The easiest way to get water is right from your faucet. But reports of contaminated tap water are of concern to many people—and with good reason. The water supply in some areas contains contaminants such as lead, pesticides, and chlorine by-products that exceed recommended limits. A good move is to buy a water purifier, which filters lead and other contaminants from tap water. Some filters attach right to the tap; others can be installed as part of the entire water system. One of the most convenient and economical filtering methods is the pour-through filter you can place in a special pitcher and put right in your refrigerator. If you use a filtration product that removes fluoride from your water, discuss this concern with your dentist, because fluoride can support good dental health.

Another option is to purchase bottled water. There are hundreds of brands, the most popular of which offer spring water and mineral water. Spring water is taken from underground freshwater springs that form pools on the surface of the earth. Mineral water comes from reservoirs located under rock formations. It contains a higher concentration of minerals than most sources. Well water is another type of bottled water, which is tapped from an aquifer. Spring, mineral, and well waters still may contain some contaminants. For this reason, federal regulations are tightening on the bottled water industry. Although bottled water is not the most environmentally friendly option, it is an option for regular hydration. Once you get in the habit of drinking water regularly, buy your own personal reusable water bottle that you can fill at home with pure water and take with you to support hydration.

Distilled water, also labeled as purified water, is another type of bottled water. It has been purified through vaporization and is then condensed. A drawback of distilled water is that it does not contain any minerals. In addition, fluoride is missing from many bottled waters. However, several brands now add back a mineral package, making it more nutritious and usually better tasting.

Some people like seltzer water. This is a sparkling water that is bubbly because of the addition of pressurized carbon dioxide. Many of these products are flavored and contain sucrose or fructose. Although carbonated waters are fine to drink throughout the day, they are not desirable during exercise. The gas from the bubbles takes up space in your stomach and makes you feel fuller, decreasing the amount of total fluid you will drink during and after exercise.

Regardless of what type of water you drink, be sure to drink the 9 to 12 cups (2-3 L) or more of fluids you need daily to stay well hydrated, and make at least 5 of these cups (1 L) pure water.

Designer Waters

Water now comes in more varieties than ever before. Today, there's fortified water, fitness water, herbal water, oxygen-enriched water, electrolyzed water—the list goes on. Welcome to the world of designer waters. Although they may taste great, watch out for unsubstantiated claims on the labels, and for what I call "clear soda pop" masquerading as water. Some sweetened waters have almost as much sugar as soda. I'm concerned not only about the amount of sugar added to many of these so-called waters but also about the amount of sugar substitutes. If you're drinking more than two of these beverages a day—namely, any that use sugar substitutes for sweetening—while also consuming sugar substitutes in other foods, then you're pumping your body with too many sugar substitutes.

One problem, too, is that you're training your palate to be satisfied with only very sweet flavors. And quite possibly, you're stimulating your appetite even though you're taking in low-calorie food and beverages. So, while drinking water, try to limit or eliminate altogether a need for sweetness in that water.

With any of the waters that include herbs, botanicals, or any ingredients that companies claim are functional, try to determine what the active ingredients are and how much the beverage contains. If the manufacturer won't list what is in the beverage, don't drink it. The reason for not listing ingredients is most likely either that manufacturers don't know the exact amount of ingredients because there is no serious quality control, or there's really nothing special about their ingredients, and they don't want you to know that their marketing claims are overblown. If you can't find that information, you can probably conclude that the dose is not effective. Otherwise, they'd be eager to tell you that they have an effective dose. Always read ingredient and nutrition labels to make informed choices.

Fortified Water

Featuring a splash of flavor and sweetness, these waters are fortified with predis-solved vitamins and minerals. Some are formulated for people who want to drink their supplements; others, for active people who drink water during workouts and want a little more flavor than plain water provides.

Fortified waters are not to be confused with sport drinks or glucose–electrolyte solutions, which are packed with more carbohydrate energy and higher amounts of electrolytes than specialty waters contain.

Fitness Water

These designer waters contain some vitamin but with only 10 calories per serving. They are meant to be used when you want some flavor in your water but don't need a glucose–electrolyte solution or extra calories.

Herbal Water

Fairly new on the water front are herb-enhanced waters. You can now swill water containing such popular herbs as echinacea, ginkgo biloba, Siberian ginseng, ginger, or St. John's wort. These beverages are a good option if you want the benefits of medicinal herbs without popping pills. Generally, herb-enhanced waters have a hint of flavor without sugar, calories, or carbonation.

Be aware of how many servings you consume of herbal or fortified waters, along with other sources of the same herbs, vitamins, and minerals. You might easily take in too much of these substances. And because the herbal part of the food industry is yet to be regulated, there's no guarantee that you're getting the ingredients listed on the label.

Oxygen-Enriched Water

These beverages are said to be enhanced with up to 40 times the normal oxygen concentration found naturally in water. Available flavored or unflavored, they claim to boost energy by increasing oxygen saturation in the red blood cells. To date, though, no published medical evidence has validated such claims. There appears to be no value in them other than as another good source of water.

Electrolyzed Water

This category describes water that has been separated into alkaline and acid frac-tions. The alkaline fraction is bottled for drinking with a pH of about 9.5, compared with other bottled waters in which the pH ranges from 6 to 8. The process removes contaminants and most of the total dissolved solids but leaves in electrolytes such as calcium, magnesium, potassium, sodium, and bicarbonates. Claims for electro-lyzed water include smoother taste, healthier water, improved hydration ability, electrolyte availability, and antioxidant properties. Aside from smoother-tasting water, the scientific research into most of these claims is in its infancy. Keep an eye on this research.

What About Coconut Water?

Coconut water—the liquid that sloshes around in coconuts—is positioned as a healthy alternative to sport drinks. One reason is that it is packed with 15 times the amount of potassium as the leading sport drink, plus it contains no fat, dyes, or added sugar. What's more, coconut water is a natural "isotonic" beverage, meaning that it contains the same levels of electrolytes as your blood.

Aside from the great taste, how does coconut water stack up against plain water and sport drinks for rehydration after exercise? A study published in 2002 looked into this. It evaluated the effects of three fluids: water, a carbohydrate–electrolyte drink, and coconut water. The researchers found that coconut water basically worked as well as a carbohydrate–electrolyte beverage and performed better than water for rehydration.

Another study regarding this issue, which appeared in 2007 in the *Southeast Asian Journal of Tropical Medicine and Public Health*, reached a similar conclusion after comparing the effects of plain water, sport drink, fresh coconut water, and sodium-enriched fresh coconut water on rehydration. The findings? The most effective rehydration occurred with the sport drink and the sodium-enriched coconut water.

To evaluate whether coconut water can enhance physical performance, a study was conducted in 2012 comparing the effects of two different forms of coconut water (concentrated and not from concentrate) and a carbohydrate–electrolyte sport drink on measures of hydration status and physical performance in exercise-trained men. The subjects underwent a dehydrating exercise protocol, followed by a moderate-intensity exercise performance protocol to exhaustion, and times were recorded. In this study, there were no differences in outcomes for rehydration or performance between all the beverages, including bottled water, both coconut waters, and the carbohydrate-electrolyte sport drink. However, the authors suggest two limitations to the study: (1) only marginal 2 percent dehydration and (2) an exercise protocol to volitional exhaustion rather than a time trial more similar to an actual competitive event.

Other health claims made by manufacturers about coconut water are absolutely unsubstantiated. These include claims that coconut water prevents cancer, slows aging, gives you smoother skin, normalizes blood pressure, lowers unhealthy cholesterol, and cures a number of kidney and digestive disorders. As for the cancer claim, some of the substances in coconut water, such as selenium, are antioxidants and fight cancer in the lab, but many fruits, vegetables, nuts, and whole grains contain the same cancer-fighting compounds. So far, only animal studies have hinted that coconut water may lower cholesterol and blood pressure. Honestly, no single food substance can do all these things, and we just don't have enough research to make such claims about coconut water.

Even so, coconut water can be a good choice for rehydration. Compared to other beverages, it is a healthy option, thanks to its content of potassium, vitamin C, antioxidants, and phytochemicals.

Are Sport Drinks Superior to Water?

In some cases, yes. For general types of exercise lasting less than one hour, water is still the best sport drink around. The nutrient you most need to replace during and after these types of workouts is water.

Carbohydrate drinks and carbohydrate–electrolyte solution drinks (also known as sport drinks) do have their place, mostly during high-intensity and heavy-weight exercise, high-intensity interval training, and exercise lasting more than 45 minutes; they are especially useful for endurance and ultraendurance athletes but are loved by lifters, too. These products can be carbohydrate alone, or a mixture of carbohydrate and electrolytes, either in powder form or a ready-to-drink beverage mixed in water. Electrolytes are dissolved minerals that form a salty soup in and around cells. They conduct electrical charges that let the minerals react with other minerals to relay nerve impulses, make muscles contract or relax, and regulate the fluid balance inside and outside cells. In hard workouts or athletic competitions lasting 45 minutes or longer, electrolytes can be lost through sweat.

Where carbohydrate–electrolyte solutions may have an edge over water is in their flavor. A lot of people don't drink much water because it doesn't taste good to them. Soldiers participating in a study at the U.S. Army Research Institute of Environmental Medicine were given the choice of drinking plain chlorinated water, flavored water, or lemon-lime carbohydrate–electrolyte solution drinks. Most soldiers chose the carbohydrate–electrolyte solutions or flavored water over plain water. If you don't need the extra carbohydrate and electrolytes, one way to sneak more water in and still get the flavor is to dilute your carbohydrate–electrolyte solution or use one of the new flavored fitness waters. But remember, you will not get the performance-enhancement effect for exercise over one hour if you do this.

If you're an avid water drinker and really like water, you'll benefit just as much from water as you will from using a carbohydrate–electrolyte solution, unless you're moderately exercising an hour or more, or exercising at a high intensity for longer than 30 to 45 minutes. But if you don't like water or tend to avoid it during exercise, try filtered or bottled water, which tastes different than regular water. Or try a carbohydrate–electrolyte solution that contains less than 8 percent carbohydrate and some sodium. Another idea is to put some (but less than a full dose) powdered sport drink mix into your water, although the powdered mixes sometimes don't taste as good as their premixed counterparts. Yet another low-calorie solution is to add a flavor packet to your water. There are many different brands, and you should experiment with them for taste.

Finally we shouldn't leave this section without a conversation about stacking your own sport drink. Many athletes like to titrate their own carbohydrate and electrolytes based on the needs of their body, rather than the manufacturer's formula. This allows you to choose a powdered carbohydrate and mix in the electrolyte pack of your choice. If you are doing long-distance, moderate-intensity exercise in a hot climate, you might use slightly less carbohydrate but more electrolyte, especially sodium, if you experience heavy salt losses. At the very least, if a carbohydrate–electrolyte solution, or any of these other suggestions, encourages you to drink more, it has done its job.

Is Juice a Good Sport Drink?

Juices are a source of fluids. Orange juice, for example, is nearly 90 percent water and is full of vitamins and minerals. Although juices count as part of your fluid requirement, you'll feel at your best if you base your daily fluid plan on at least 5 cups (1 L) of water and use small servings of juice to help you attain your minimum 9 to 12 cups (2-3 L) of total fluids.

There are some cautions to consider regarding juice as a fluid in your training diet. In recent years, there has been a lot of hype surrounding the health benefits of fruit and vegetable juices. The makers of commercial juicing machines claim that fresh juices are a panacea for all kinds of ills, from digestive upsets to cancer. But is it better to drink your five servings of fruits and veggies every day rather than eat them? No way!

In most juices, the pulp has been removed from the fruit or vegetables to make the juice. That means that the all-important fiber has also been subtracted, because the pulp is where you find the fiber. Granted, some juice machines boast that their process keeps the pulp in the juice to retain the important fiber and concentrate the nutrients. These products are excellent choices for a once-a-day juice. But they still do not replace whole fruit.

Freshly squeezed juice is often touted as a better source of nutrients than commercial juices. But commercially prepared juices that are frozen and refrigerated properly are only slightly lower in nutrients than fresh juice. If you don't buy fresh produce, don't store it properly at home, and don't drink your freshly squeezed juice immediately, your homemade juice may even be lower in nutrients than a well-made frozen or refrigerated brand.

Whether they are cooked, squeezed, dried, or raw, fruits and vegetables need to be a big part of your diet. If using a juice machine is one way of eating more fruits and vegetables and is enjoyable for you, go for it. But remember the drawbacks, and don't use juice as your only source of fruits and vegetables.

If you want to drink juice to rehydrate your body, dilute it with water by at least twofold. A cup (240 ml) of orange or apple juice plus 2 cups (480 ml) of water will provide a 6 to 8 percent carbohydrate solution, similar to a sport drink formulation. Don't use this combination during exercise, however, because of its fructose content. The body doesn't use fructose as well as the combination of sugars in a regular sport drink. In addition, some people are fructose sensitive and may experience intestinal cramping after drinking juice. As noted earlier, juice may interfere with fluid absorption if consumed during exercise. Instead, drink your juice–water mix as part of your fluids an hour or more after exercise. The addition of water will speed the emptying of the fluid from your stomach and thus rehydrate your body more rapidly, and the carbohydrate will help replenish glycogen.

Hydration Danger Zones

It's hard to imagine that water could be bad for you, but just like everything else, too much water at the wrong time can actually be harmful. Moderation is the key, even when we're talking about water.

Overhydration

When considering your water intake, you must also consider overhydration. Hydration is a delicate balance between fluids and minerals. The concentration of sodium and other minerals (collectively known as electrolytes) in the bloodstream must fall within a very narrow range, or it can affect muscle contractions. That includes those of the most important muscle: your heart.

When you take in too much water relative to the amount of electrolytes in your body, the result will eventually be a condition called hyperhydration or hyponatremia. The problem is that the blood has become too dilute, which is just as dangerous as dehydration. During dehydration there are high levels of electrolytes without enough fluids. Surprisingly, the symptoms of dehydration and hyperhydration are basically the same.

Hyperhydration occurs more frequently than you might think, particularly in endurance events such as marathons and triathlons. Not nearly as well documented is the possibility of bodybuilders hyperhydrating as a result of high intakes of purified water combined with very low food and sodium intakes during a cutting diet. Although no occurrences of hyponatremia have been documented in strength trainers not participating in another sport, you should be aware that very high intakes of purified water over an extended period of time may put you at risk. Whether you're training for an endurance event or preparing for a strength-training competition, you can avoid hyponatremia with a few simple precautions.

If you're training for your first marathon or triathlon, don't cut all salt out of your diet (though, as a general rule, most of us could get away with a lot less than we currently take in). If the day is cooler or less humid than you expected, compensate by drinking less than you'd planned during the event. You should never gain weight during an exercise bout or competition.

Go for sport drinks over pure water, especially if you're competing in endurance competitions. A 2006 study published in the *British Journal of Sports Medicine* looked into the fluid-intake behaviors of runners competing in ultraendurance events. The researchers concluded that runners could finish their competitions relatively dehydrated and hypernatremic—and that it was detrimental to performance to overdrink water. They also stated that the best way to prevent hyponatremia was to consume electrolyte-containing sport drinks.

If you're not an endurance athlete, don't think you have to match those more highly trained competitors drink for drink. Their sweat is different from yours; it contains more water and fewer electrolytes. Your body is leaking sodium, while theirs are holding on to it. If you see pretzels being handed out along the course of a distance race, help yourself, assuming you're not sodium sensitive and you don't have high blood pressure. The extra sodium will prevent you from becoming hyperhydrated.

When you are dieting to make weight prior to a competition, don't overdo the water. Drink water with minerals in place of purified water, or don't try to remove all the sodium from your diet. As long as you are eating, your risk of hyponatremia is remarkably diminished.

Water, Body Weight, and Competition

For years sport nutritionists, myself included, have recommended that athletes drink before they get thirsty and make sure that they don't lose more than 2 percent of their total body weight during an exercise session or race event. The assumption was that any body weight lost during exercise is completely fluid, and that these losses hamper performance.

A study published in the *Journal of Sports Medicine* refutes that assumption. The researchers found that, in two races, athletes drinking only in response to thirst lost more body mass than total body water. The researchers speculated that this loss in body mass confers a competitive advantage. If you can lose body mass during the race and weigh less, yet stay adequately hydrated, you have a better chance of winning.

In this study, the athletes stayed sufficiently hydrated. Thirst mechanisms appeared to be triggered to maintain electrolyte status, and sodium and potassium concentrations remained within healthy ranges. Therefore, the researchers recommended that athletes not drink based on body weight losses, but allow their natural thirst mechanisms to drive their hydration practices.

As for sodium, many athletes wonder whether they should supplement with this electrolyte to boost performance. The researchers of the preceding study examined this issue too with athletes competing in an Ironman Triathlon in South Africa. A third of the subjects received sodium tablets to use freely for the 12 hours of the race; another third received a placebo starch tablet to use freely throughout the race; and the final third did not supplement at all.

At the end of the race, there was absolutely no difference in performance or the concentration of sodium and other electrolytes in the athletes' bodies. The researchers concluded that the Institute of Medicine recommendation of 1.5 grams of sodium per day for the general population is adequate to maintain serum sodium concentrations during a 12-hour ultraendurance event. Although some people may have increased needs, in general, eating a standard Western diet should offer adequate amounts of sodium. On the other hand, do not reduce your sodium intake when preparing for an endurance event. Lastly, you know if you lose large amounts of salt by the way your clothes can stand up on their own after you finish a long training session. They are caked with salt. The key to hydration, electrolyte replenishment, and rehydration is to customize your intake to match your needs as closely as possible.

Caffeine, Creatine, and Glycerol

In addition to carbohydrate and electrolytes, you might find that other products can be added, or stacked, onto your sport beverage. Caffeine is the most popular and is no longer considered a diuretic (causing fluid loss) at levels that can enhance performance. Creatine, taken for strength and power enhancement, also enhances cellular hydration at the same dosages recommended for power building. Lastly, glycerol, which studies show can increase body water, shows equivocal responses in performance enhancement. Since glycerol can cause GI upset and headaches, most athletes bypass this supplement. To read more about supplements, see chapter 10.

Alcohol

It has been a long time since a client has asked me whether drinking beer is a good way to replenish fluids and carbohydrate. But clients frequently ask whether alcohol will hurt their exercise performance, and even more frequently, they want to know whether drinking a little bit of alcohol may actually be heart healthy. Thanks to an ever-growing body of scientific research and knowledge, here are some answers to those questions and more.

What is in Alcohol?

Alcohol is a priority fuel, which means that it is burned preferentially, or ahead of, any other energy source until it is cleared from the body. It is not converted into muscle or liver glycogen storage or muscle protein, and it is not stored as fat. However, since it receives priority fuel status in the body, it might divert the use of carbohydrate and fat as fuel sources and send them down the path to fat storage. So if you drink and train, alcohol puts fat burning on hold and may ramp up fat storage. It's not your friend if you're trying to stay lean.

Pure alcohol supplies 7 calories per gram and nothing else. In practical terms, a shot (1.5 ounces, or 45 ml) of 90-proof gin contains 110 calories, and 100-proof gin contains 124 calories. Beer has a little more to offer but not much. On average, a 12-ounce (360 ml) can of beer contains 146 calories, 13 grams of carbohydrate, traces of several B-complex vitamins, and, depending on the brand, varying amounts of minerals. Light beer and nonalcoholic beer are lower in calories and sometimes carbohydrate. All table wines have similar caloric content. A 3.5-ounce (105 ml) serving of table wine contains about 72 calories, 1 gram of carbohydrate, and very small amounts of several vitamins and minerals. Sweet or dessert wines are higher in calories, containing 90 calories per 2-ounce (60 ml) serving.

What Are Alcohol's Side Effects?

Today, alcohol is the most abused drug in the United States. Ten percent of users are addicted, and 10 to 20 percent are abusers or problem drinkers. Alcohol is a central nervous system depressant. Compared with other commonly used substances, alcohol has one of the lowest effective dose–lethal dose ratios. In other words, there's a small difference in the amount of alcohol that will get you drunk and the amount that will kill you. The reason more people don't die from alcohol intoxication is that the stomach is alcohol sensitive and rejects it by vomiting.

Acute alcohol intoxication results in tremors, anxiety and irritability, nausea and vomiting, decreased mental function, vertigo, coma, and death. In chronically large amounts, alcohol causes the loss of many nutrients from the body, including thiamin, vitamin B_6, and calcium. Furthermore, chronic alcohol abuse has negative effects on every organ in the body, particularly the liver, heart, brain, and muscle, and can lead to cancer and diseases of the liver, pancreas, and nervous system.

Don't drink alcohol in any form if you're pregnant. It can cause birth defects. Drinking alcohol in large amounts can also lead to accidents, as well as social, psychological, and emotional problems.

How Does Alcohol Affect Exercise Performance?

Because alcohol depresses the central nervous system, it impairs balance and coordination and decreases exercise performance. Strength and power, muscle endurance, and aerobic endurance are all zapped with alcohol use. Alcohol also dehydrates the body considerably.

To be a little more specific, if you knock down a few alcoholic beverages after a strength-training workout, you're likely to increase damage to your muscles, experience greater muscle soreness, and diminish strength and power. Your muscle-glycogen and tissue-rebuilding recovery from exercise will absolutely be diminished, and you certainly won't fully rehydrate. These effects have been observed in research.

As for endurance athletes, a study of trained cyclists given a small amount of alcohol after 60 minutes of cycling showed a significant decrease in average cycling power output, oxygen consumption, carbon dioxide production, and glucose oxidation. Their heart rates increased, and they felt more fatigued and less energetic when they consumed alcohol. So basically, drinking alcohol has a negative effect on endurance performance. Also, alcohol use increases the risks of sport injuries.

The bottom line: Alcohol will clearly put your training on the skids. It has no place during tournament play, when training occurs the day after a game, or when several games or events are played weekly. Although celebrating with alcohol may appear to be fun, it puts you and your teammates at risk.

Is Alcohol Really Heart Healthy?

Research has found that daily consumption of one drink per day can do your heart good by positively affecting the levels of good cholesterol (HDL) in your blood. The higher your HDL levels, the lower your risk of heart disease.

However, excessive alcohol intake increases your chance of developing heart disease. More than two drinks a day can raise your blood pressure and contribute to high triglycerides, a risk factor for heart disease. Drinking large amounts of alcohol on a habitual basis can also cause heart failure and lead to stroke.

Alcohol consumption contributes to obesity, another major risk factor in the development of heart disease. Extra pounds are hard on your heart, and the higher your weight climbs, the greater your risk. Being overweight also raises blood pressure and cholesterol, which are risk factors themselves.

Women and Alcohol

Women's drinking patterns are different from men's—especially when it comes to how much and how often they drink. Women's bodies also react differently to alcohol than men's bodies do. That means women who drink beyond moderate levels face a variety of health risks from alcohol. Some specific reasons for this increased risk follow:

- Women typically start to have alcohol-related problems at lower drinking levels than men.
- Women typically weigh less than men.
- Pound for pound, women have less water in their bodies than men do, and alcohol resides predominantly in body water.

These health risks can include the following:

- **Liver damage**. Women who drink are more likely to develop liver inflammation than men.
- **Heart disease**. Women are more susceptible to alcohol-related heart disease than men.
- **Breast cancer**. Women who have about one drink per day also have an increased chance of developing breast cancer compared to women who do not drink at all.
- **Pregnancy**. Any drinking during pregnancy is risky. Heavy drinking can put a fetus at increased risk for learning, behavioral, and other problems.

Reprinted from "Alcohol and Your Health," National Institute on Alcohol and Alcohol Abuse, National Institutes of Health, U.S. Department of Health and Human Services, accessed April 5, 2018, https://www.niaaa.nih.gov/alcohol-health/special-populations-co-occurring-disorders/women.

Is a Drink a Day Good Prevention?

The risks of alcohol outweigh its positives. If you drink alcoholic beverages, do so in moderation, with meals, and when consumption does not put you or others in harm's way. Moderation is defined as no more than one drink per day for women and no more than two drinks per day for men. One drink is 12 ounces (360 ml) of regular beer, 5 ounces (150 ml) of wine, and 1.5 ounces (45 ml) of 80-proof distilled liquor. However, exercising, getting adequate sleep, stress reduction, quitting smoking, and lowering your blood cholesterol with a healthy diet are better ways to prevent heart disease without any added risks.

Sport Nutrition Fact Versus Fiction: Do Soft Drinks Rehydrate the Body?

If given the option, many people would choose a soft drink over water to rehydrate themselves following workouts. And who can blame them? Soft drinks taste good, seem to quench thirst, and are generally refreshing.

But soft drinks are among the worst choices for rehydration. Soft drinks are laced with huge amounts of sugar—roughly the equivalent of 10 teaspoons or more per can. Because of their sugar content, soft drinks are absorbed less rapidly than pure water. The sugar in them keeps the fluid in your stomach longer, so less water is available to your body. Rather than rehydrating your system, soft drinks can make you feel even thirstier. Also, the sugar can trigger a sharp spike in insulin, followed by a fast drop in blood sugar. This reaction can leave you feeling tired and weak. In addition, the sugar in soft drinks is high-fructose corn syrup, and fructose does not replenish glycogen as rapidly as other forms of carbohydrate. Fructose also can cause cramps in people who are sensitive to it.

What about sugar-free soft drinks? These beverages contain artificial sweeteners, which don't do anything for refueling your muscle cells and remain controversial regarding whole body and mind health. Furthermore, all soft drinks are, of course, carbonated, and carbonation produces gas. Who wants a gassy stomach, which will limit the amount that you drink and fully rehydrate?

Diluting a soft drink isn't a good option, either. Even diluted, soft drinks have nothing beneficial to offer. As far as rehydration is concerned, no fluids—including artificially sweetened soft drinks—have yet been proven to do a better job than plain old water or a good carbohydrate—electrolyte solution.

7

Fueling the Female Athlete

If you're like most highly active women, you're probably hungry for sport nutrition advice, especially since most dietary recommendations are geared toward male athletes. And I'm sure you want to know what differentiates the way women fuel from the way men do. This chapter will help answer those questions, focusing on helping women like you fuel correctly, get the most out of your workouts, and perform athletically at your very best.

There's no question that women have made great strides in sports since the passage and implementation of Title IX. Research shows that girls who play team sports are more likely to graduate from college, find a job, have a higher salary, and be employed in male-dominated industries.

But when it comes to research on sport injury and performance, the real "meat" of creating a winning strategy, females are vastly underrepresented, making up only about 2 to 3 percent of the research subjects. We don't even have data on how many female subjects are part of sport nutrition research studies. The numbers are undoubtedly growing, but up until very recently, virtually all sport nutrition recommendations for women were based on data collected on men. Even now most recommendations still depend on male-focused data.

Why does this matter? Because women are not small men or men with hormone issues! The anatomy and physiology of women and girls differs greatly from that of men and boys, and some parts are unique. Transferring sport nutrition and training recommendations based on males to females is as inappropriate and ineffective, and perhaps dangerous, as is the application of male-centric pharmaceutical research results to females.

In my opinion, the void in the data on the needs of female athletes has allowed weight-loss marketers to swoop down with information that masquerades as sport nutrition for women. Most of this misinformation has to do with "cut calories," "slash carbs," and "get thin." Such recommendations often lead to poor sport performance, and, for athletically active women, can cause dire health consequences; namely, increased risk for injury and illness, deficiencies in key nutrients such as iron, vitamin D, and calcium, and fatigue. Many female athletes shoot for 0 percent body fat, eat zero dietary fat, and avoid carbohydrate. These "fat phobia" and "carb phobia" phenomena are due in large part to what I mentioned above: The emphasis on thinness that is so prevalent today and a reliance on information that comes out of the "diet world."

Fortunately, within the halls of science and academia, a call for change is now being heard. Institutional review boards are beginning to highlight a requirement for female, as well as male, subjects in study designs. Journal editors and reviewers are starting to call foul when studies neglect to include females. Although there are currently a handful of scientists focusing their research on the needs of the female athlete, most of these scientists are men. Their contributions are wonderful, and I applaud nearly all of them for fostering lab environments in which female students are being mentored to take their place among the community of full-fledged faculty members and primary investigators.

We also need more female scientists to be role models to enlarge the ranks of female investigators in the fields of sport science and nutrition. By nature, scientists

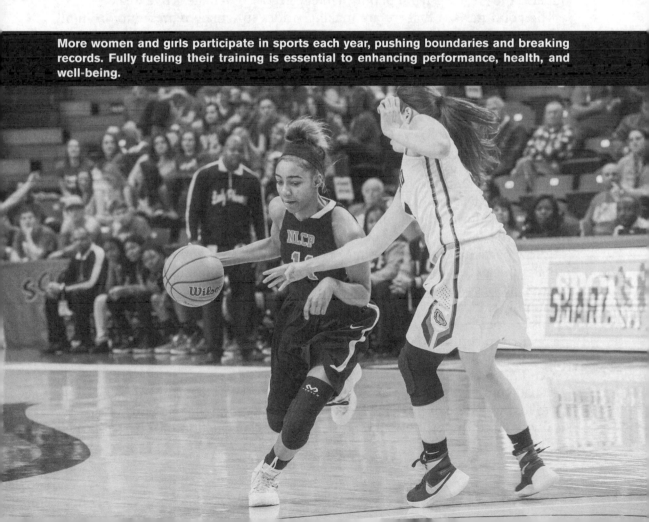

More women and girls participate in sports each year, pushing boundaries and breaking records. Fully fueling their training is essential to enhancing performance, health, and well-being.

typically study what they find to be personally interesting, and therefore female scientists will more likely have the desire and drive to study female athletes.

With more female-centric data, we will have more female-centric recommendations, and more female-centric products and guidelines. Athletes want what works. Women and girls know that what is out there for them today hardly works, and in more than a few cases can actually hurt their health and performance.

Female athletes also want to be the most that they can be, not the least. Skinny and sexy are not athletic goals, and that messaging repels athletic female consumers. They want to be stronger, faster, and more powerful—all to support their goals of winning. If accomplishing those goals leads to outcomes that also include being leaner and sexier, that's okay. But those are generally not the athletic goals they are seeking.

As in science, we need women in decision-making roles in product ownership, research and development, manufacturing, marketing, and sales, who have a personal interest in athletics and sport to create the change that women desire and the authentic products and stories that appeal to the athletic female consumer. The companies that pioneered the female athletic wear brands of Title Nine and Athleta have demonstrated this to the big brands of Nike, Under Armour, and Adidas, creating an enormously successful new market trend of not only female athletic wear but also the greater general public market category of female active wear.

The good news is that we are making strides in female representation in all areas of research and business. However, the most important issue facing women athletes today is nutrition—what to eat, when to eat, and how to supplement for a winning performance. Let's dig a little deeper.

Optimal Body Fat Percentage in Female Athletes

Normally, a healthy range of body fat for women is 20 to 25 percent. Many elite female athletes have less than 10 percent body fat, however. Female strength trainers and bodybuilders can range from 10 to 18 percent for most of the year, and then drop further during their competitive season. Competitive female runners may have as little as 5 to 6 percent body fat, according to some studies.

A low percentage of body fat may be perfectly normal and desirable for some female athletes because it enhances sport performance. As long as you don't severely restrict calories while training for a sport, there is nothing unhealthy about having a naturally lean figure. There are active people with bodies that can naturally land at this low percent body fat due to their genetics, not severe dieting. However, calorie restriction combined with overexercising depletes body fat stores to unhealthy levels, which elevates the risk of a syndrome known as the female athlete triad, which I discussed in chapter 5.

What typically contributes to the female athlete triad is that women deliberately try to lose weight to improve their performance or appearance, so body fat is drastically reduced. In response, the ovaries cut back production of estrogen. When estrogen is reduced, menstrual periods become irregular or cease altogether. With poor diet and low calcium intake along with low estrogen levels, osteoporosis, which increases fracture risk, becomes a serious concern.

The following recommendations will help to prevent, and treat, the female athlete triad (for more information and resources on the female athlete triad, visit www.femaleathletetriad.org):

- Follow a healthy, energy-rich diet adequate for the demands of your sport.
- Increase your caloric intake and make sure you get adequate calcium and vitamin D to help guard against osteoporosis.
- Cut back on your training intensity.
- See a sports medicine physician, who may prescribe hormone replacement therapy temporarily to replace lost estrogen and to stop your body from losing any more bone strength. However, your goal is to be able to have a regular menstrual cycle without exogenous hormone replacement.

You, Your Performance, and Your Menstrual Cycle

Increasingly, the often secretive nature of female physiology has fallen away, and there is more public discussion of the health and well-being of girls and women—including issues of their menstrual cycle. When things are kept under wraps and cannot be openly discussed, there is no recognition of the issues and no scientific effort to develop an understanding or discover solutions.

Take the menstrual cycle, for example. No topic within female biology has been more taboo than this. Yet without it, none of us would be here. The historical way female athletes have dealt with their monthly cycles has been to either sit out from play during their periods, or try to stop their periods altogether, because of both the discomfort as well as the assumption that it hindered performance.

Let's get right to the heart of the matter: Women and girls who compete during their periods do not show performance deficiencies. In fact, an elegant study conducted by Dr. Jaci VanHeest and her colleagues at the University of Connecticut looked at junior national elite female swimmers during their grueling 12-week competitive season. The researchers observed that those swimmers with similar training loads but higher energy availability maintained their full menstrual cycles with measured functional ovarian steroids and metabolic hormones throughout the season, and significantly outperformed the matched athletes who suppressed ovarian function and menstrual cycles through lower energy availability in the final meets at the end of the season. This study proves that the common and widespread practice of underfueling and overtraining female athletes to halt the menstrual cycle with the goal of enhanced performance is a failed strategy. The low metabolic state and altered hormonal environment negatively affect physical performance.

However, female athlete physiology does change throughout the month based on the biology of the menstrual cycle. If you try to fight that biology, you might underperform. But if you understand it and work with it, you can really maximize your potential. This is the information that all female athletes, and coaches and trainers of female athletes, should know.

The monthly menstrual cycle lasts an average of 28 days but can range from 20 to 45 days and still be considered normal. A healthy cycle has two phases: the first half between the first day of the period and ovulation, called the follicular phase, and the second half between ovulation and the first day of the period (or pregnancy), called the luteal phase. Each phase is typically labeled as days 1 through 14 and days 15 through 28, but since this is nature it's rarely exact, but it's close.

Your reproductive hormones estrogen and progesterone are mainly in charge of your changing phases, but luteinizing hormone and follicle stimulating hormone play important roles delineating the two phases. This is where your athletic performance begins to be more related to the discussion. These hormones affect more than just your periods. If you are paying attention throughout the month, you may have noticed that you can't explain why you have better or worse training days, or why your nutritional needs seem to change from week to week. Your reproductive hormones are at work on your athletic body. Knowing how and when they are working can give you an advantage to the weekly focus of your diet and training regimens.

Estrogen and progesterone levels are lower during the follicular phase (days 1-14), allowing an increase in carbohydrate utilization. Carbohydrate should be more prominent in the diet, and during this time high-intensity, power, and speed training will be advantageous. During the luteal phase (days 15-28), estrogen and progesterone levels rise, which helps maintain muscle glycogen storage, preserve liver glycogen, and increase fatty acid oxidation. Dietary carbohydrate can decrease slightly during this phase, and to take advantage of better fat burning, the training focus should turn to moderate-intensity endurance.

Female athletes are better than males at burning fat most of the time, but this is particularly true during the luteal phase. During endurance exercise, females have more efficient access to stored triglyceride droplets within the muscle fibers, which can be transported quickly into the cell to the mitochondria where energy metabolism and fat oxidation take place. Females are also better at recovery of these fat droplets from the diet back to the muscle cells after exercise. This explains the success that many female athletes have in ultraendurance events. However, when females perform high-intensity training, their need for carbohydrate is equally as high as that of a male athlete, and they have just as much capacity to utilize and store carbohydrate as a male athlete.

So carbohydrate and fat recommendations for female athletes should be periodized to reflect not only their training but also their monthly menstrual cycle. Therefore, female athletes should plan their diet and training with their monthly menstrual cycle in mind.

A final word here about the menstrual cycle is the issue of heavy bleeding. It is absolutely clear that women with heavy periods are at higher risk for iron deficiency, with or without anemia. While iron supplementation is helpful, it is not always comfortable due to GI discomfort, and sometimes it is not terribly effective. A focus on dietary solutions is important. Diets that include animal sources of heme iron help athletes recover more quickly and successfully compared to plant-only diets containing only nonheme iron. Refer to the section on iron in chapter 9 for a full discussion of good sources and best strategies for iron-rich diets.

How to Determine Your Energy Needs

The classic method to calculate energy needs has been to determine energy balance, the point at which calorie outgo balances with calorie input—in other words, calories in, calories out. However, even though a female athlete is in energy balance, this may not reflect her optimal energy needs. When an athlete's calorie intake is low, a low output reflects the low intake. The low output is not necessarily her optimal, achievable output. Therefore, energy balance may not be a useful concept for managing a female athlete's diet.

As I discussed in chapter 5, energy availability (EA) is a new method of calculating individual calorie recommendations. It refers to the energy obtained through what you eat minus the energy expended during exercise:

- EA equals dietary energy intake (EI) minus energy expended in exercise with a high metabolic demand (energy of exercise expenditure or EEE) per kilogram of fat-free mass (FFM).
- To determine EI, you can use any number of online apps. To determine EEE, you can use a very general calculation:
  - 0.1 calorie per kilogram of body weight per minute as an average for all sports worldwide. You can also look up energy expenditure for specific sports at targeted intensities for more specific data.
- Energy availability is the energy left over that is available to support fundamental physiological processes. You must fuel your foundational health first in order to enable the systems that support enhanced training effects and performance improvements.

EA should be no lower than 30 calories per kilogram of fat-free mass per day and is best at more than 45 calories per kilogram of fat-free mass per day.

I can almost always tell whether a female athlete has low energy availability just by the list of complaints that she has when she comes into my office: I'm training harder but my performance is worse; I'm eating less but getting softer; I have brain fog; I don't sleep well; I can't focus; I have frequent headaches; I keep getting injured; I don't have any energy; I've got nothing left for my partner and family; my hair is thinning and my skin looks terrible.

If you have low energy availability (LEA; defined as less than 30 calories per kilogram of fat-free mass per day), this means you do not have enough calories (energy) for your body's basic needs. Ultimately, your exercise performance, and your health, will go downhill!

Low energy availability may

- impair your body's ability to use glucose effectively for energy;
- increase fat stores in the body;
- increases cholesterol;
- slow down your metabolic rate;
- decrease your body's production of growth hormone (an important hormone for growth and repair);
- impair immune function; and
- impair reproductive function.

In women, LEA may cause periods to cease, which is a main characteristic of the female athlete triad (see above) and impairs bone health and development.

Your Carbohydrate Requirements

You need adequate fuel from carbohydrate in order to prevent LEA and fuel your performance. Carbohydrate can even help you stay lean. Yet despite these benefits, a substantial number of female athletes have some degree of carbohydrate phobia, or a fear that carbohydrate will make them fat. Despite my best attempts to educate them about their physiological demand for carbohydrate to perform their sport at high levels, adding starch-rich foods to their diets is often psychologically difficult.

They also have concerns about stomach upset and bloating from typical carbohydrate supplements. This is why I recommend they supplement with a high-molecular-weight carbohydrate starch called Vitargo, which does not produce these side effects. It's easy to titrate the amount you use based on your actual training needs for carbohydrate around exercise.

There are also a lot of myths floating around about carbohydrate requirements for female athletes. You may have heard, for example, that women burn more fat and less carbohydrate than men during exercise. While that is true that females are better fat-burners than males during lower- to moderate-intensity exercise, scientific evidence is not so clear during all-out maximal exercise. You most likely burn the same proportion of carbohydrate as guys do when you lift heavy, climb hills, or train at high-intensity levels.

Another myth exists that female athletes can't store and use carbohydrate as well as men can. This myth arose as a result of flawed studies using underfueled female athlete subjects. But when you are fully fueled, your muscle physiology and metabolism are similar to that of male athletes during high-intensity training and competition. You can indeed load glycogen and burn glycogen like men when you are fully fueled and you consume optimal carbohydrate per kilogram of body weight. The key here is to understand that your carbohydrate need is high during intense athletic challenge (high-intensity training), and you must have a plan to fuel it.

Dancers Are Performing Athletes

The life of a professional dancer makes enormous performance demands throughout practice, rehearsal, and performances. For this reason, dancers must consume sufficient quantities of energy from the major food groups to boost metabolic function, support hormonal and growth regulation, and meet the huge demands required by their activity.

Unfortunately, disordered eating and eating disorders are prevalent in dancers because of the pressure to stay thin. I define disordered eating, as attempts to lose or gain weight through starvation-type dieting, bingeing/purging, or excessive or compulsive exercising to control weight—all of which hurt health, well-being, and performance. There are psychological problems as well, including feeling shameful, guilty, and anxious about food and eating—and being in these mental states hurts performance, too. Anyone dealing with disordered eating should definitely seek professional help.

In general, the fuel in a dancer's diet should be composed of about 50 to 55 percent carbohydrate; 15 to 20 percent protein; and 25 to 30 percent fat. However, these values are based on about a 2,000-calorie diet. Personalized plans should be based on the macronutrient gram amounts described in the menus in chapters 15 through 19. Before a performance, fuel up with carbohydrate or a carbohydrate supplement. Carbohydrate sources such as fruits, vegetables, or grains are actually converted into energy faster than fats or protein.

Dancers also need to stay well hydrated. Without proper fluid intake, fatigue and injury can result. Also, dehydration can cause cramps, nausea, light headedness, or fainting and may severely impair performance. Ideally, you should drink water a few hours before extensive activity so that the fluid will get into your system. To tell if you are hydrating well, monitor your fluid level by checking your urine. You should be urinating a significant volume every two to four hours, and it should be light-colored.

Research has shown that like many other female athletes, dancers are often deficient in iron, vitamin D, and calcium, so it is a good idea to eat foods high in these nutrients, including meat, fish, and dairy products. Supplementation with extra iron, calcium, and vitamin D can also provide benefit.

Other supplements to consider are turmeric, an anti-inflammatory substance used as a spice in cooking or taken as a supplement; vitamin C (crucial for muscle repair) if you're not eating enough citrus fruits; and omega-3 fatty acids, for easing inflammation and supporting mental health.

Long rehearsals and demanding performances subject dancers to many physical and mental stresses. As with any female athlete, proper nutrition and supplementation can be your best ally when it comes to high performance and enjoying a long dance career.

Are you taking oral contraceptives? Then your body may burn fat even more preferentially over carbohydrate, particularly during low-intensity exercise. That mix changes, however, to favor carbohydrate metabolism when you increase cardio- or strength-training intensity.

If your training goal is to enhance physical performance, your total daily carbohydrate need falls within a large range:

Moderate duration training at low to moderate intensity: 5 to 6 grams carbohydrate per kilogram body weight per day

High duration training at high intensity: 7 to 12 grams carbohydrate per kilogram body weight per day

Your needs may change from day to day as your training regimen changes. Don't hesitate to periodize your carbohydrate and calorie intakes based on each training session. That's what I do for my clients. High, heavy days get more carbohydrate placed right around exercise—before, during, and after. Low- to moderate-training or endurance days may get fewer carbohydrate because it is fat that fuels that training. It's easy to modify from day to day by just adding or deleting your carbohydrate around exercise. The rest of your daily diet may stay pretty much the same.

Your Protein Requirements

Protein is also linked to energy availability and is necessary for complete muscle recovery, repair, and growth. When energy is fully available, protein is used primarily for the specific functions that require nitrogen, which are unique to nitrogen-containing amino acids. But when energy availability is low, protein is also used to meet energy needs by removing and excreting the nitrogen, and the requirement for protein increases to stay in nitrogen balance. While in an energy deficit, protein is called in by proxy to provide energy, as a kind of nutrient pinch-hitter.

As for protein, you'll utilize it most efficiently in amounts of approximately 20 to 25 grams per serving. This is the equivalent of about 4 ounces of animal protein or 1.5 cups of beans (which contain a plant protein). If you include this much protein at every meal and snack, four to five times a day, you will consume very close to the amount of protein a woman's body requires to build lean muscle. If you are in an energy-deficient state, however, increase your protein intake by 10%. These are just round numbers. You can personalize your needs by using the calculations below.

More specifically, your total daily protein requirements fall in the following ranges, depending upon your sport:

Endurance Athlete

1.4-1.6 g/kg/d

Strength Athlete in a Maintenance Phase

1.5-1.6 g/kg/d

Strength Athlete in a Building Phase

1.8-2.0 g/kg/d

Strength Athlete in a Sculpting Phase

2.2-2.5 g/kg/d (this may be decreased for a small athlete)

Some women are afraid that a high-protein diet might cause their body to lose minerals (such as calcium) from their bones. However, there is no direct evidence to show that this actually happens. In a six-month study, 24 exercise-trained women were recruited to determine whether a high-protein diet would negatively affect minerals in the lower spine and full body. Half of the group served as a control and followed their habitual diet. The experimental group ate 2.2 grams of protein per kilogram of body weight daily—considered a higher-protein diet. In fact, the higher-protein diet bumped up the women's protein intake by 87 percent. All the women maintained their regular exercise programs.

At the end of the study, six months of high-protein eating had no effect on mineral density anywhere on the women's bodies, as measured by DEXA scans. The take-home message is to not worry about protein depleting your bones of minerals.

Your Dietary Fat Requirements

Fat plays a critical role as a source of fuel during low- to moderate-intensity levels of training. The functions of fat in the body go beyond fuel for training, however. Fat supports conditioning; recovery and tissue growth; the immune, reproductive, endocrine, and nervous systems, and joint mobility functions.

Choosing the right fats—which I call high-performance fats—will help you train at peak levels. These include fats from fish, avocados, nuts, seeds, olives, olive oil, and plant butters and oils. All of these offer important structural materials for your brain and central nervous system. They also are the building blocks of key hormones and enzymes.

Your actual requirement for fat is based on the need for essential fatty acids, which is quite low relative to the rest of your diet. Recommendations for fat intake are best made as a proportion of total energy intake. The overall fat recommendation for female athletes is 25 to 35 percent of total daily energy intake.

Your Hydration Needs

Female athletes do not sweat as much as men do, because you generally have a smaller body mass and lower metabolic rate. In low temperatures or hot, dry environments, this difference disappears when measured relative to body surface area. However, in hot, humid environments, females sweat less than males, losing less fluid and reducing their risk of hypohydration, or dehydration.

If you're having your period, your menstrual cycle also alters the handling of fluid and electrolytes by the kidneys. But despite the hormonal regulations, there does not appear to be a need for altered hydration recommendations based on the phase of the menstrual cycle.

In women, there is a higher risk of hyponatremia (the lack of sodium in the blood caused by excessive sweating, excessive water drinking, persistent diarrhea, or overuse of diuretic drugs), although the risk of dehydration is the same in men and women. The increased risk of hyponatremia in females occurs for several reasons: smaller body size, altered sweat rates, and behavioral factors leading to increased water consumption. Some women are more likely than men to be obsessive about drinking enough water during athletic training and competition, leading them to drink more than they need. This dilutes the blood and leaves too much water in proportion to sodium. Standard recommendations are to consume 0.4 to 0.8 liter per hour.

If you compete in endurance events, choose fluids containing carbohydrate and an appropriate mix and level of electrolytes to decrease the risk of hyponatremia. If the electrolytes, including sodium, are in the fluid that you are drinking, your

Is Milk the Ideal Recovery Food for Women?

Milk is often touted as the best recovery aid for athletes due to the generous amounts of calcium, vitamin D, and other bone-building nutrients, particularly for women. While it is absolutely a healthy food and a good choice for supporting bone health, a very recent study showed that it might not be the best choice for exercise recovery.

Ten trained female team sport athletes participated in a study in Carlow, Ireland, to test 500 ml of milk versus 500 ml of a carbohydrate-only, energy-matched product in a randomized crossover study to determine the impact of milk on numerous factors of exercise recovery 24, 48, and 72 hours following exercise.

According to the authors, "consumption of 500 ml of milk after repeat sprint cycling had little to no benefit in minimizing losses in peak torque or minimizing increases in soreness and tiredness and had no effect on serum markers of muscle damage and inflammation."

What would be better? First, let's examine the amounts of carbohydrate, protein, and leucine in 500 ml, or 2.1 cups, of milk:

- 24 grams carbohydrate
- 16 grams protein
- 1.6 grams leucine (an important amino acid for synthesizing muscle)

Based on all recommendations for nutritional needs to support exercise recovery, this formula is too light. Ideally, after an intense team sport training session, an athlete would need to consume at least 1.0 gram per kilogram body weight of carbohydrate and 0.5 gram per kilogram body weight of protein (minimum 20 g), along with 2.4 g leucine. I sometimes lower the amount of carbohydrate when I know that the athlete will get right to a meal of food, enabling the athlete to eat more whole-food carbohydrate sources rather than drink liquid sources. But the protein, and especially leucine, should be higher. These are the amounts that have been shown in studies time and again to show enhancement of exercise recovery.

But don't eliminate milk, add to it! Use 1 to 2 cups of milk as the liquid base for adding some whey protein and whole fruit, or even a few scoops of a protein-carbohydrate recovery shake. Milk has so much more to offer than water!

blood is far less likely to become diluted. Recommendations for fluid consumption are broad and should be individualized to your own sweat rates. A good goal to shoot for is to minimize fluid losses during training or competition to no greater than 2 percent of your body weight.

Fueling for Training and Sculpting

Both male and female athletes strive to sculpt their bodies, along with improving performance. It is possible to support both goals, using specific diet strategies that encourage you to eat well and fully fuel your training.

However, athletes are notoriously accustomed to being underfueled, so it is very difficult for them to eat enough food to fully fuel the needs of training yet still be empty enough to feel comfortable while training. The most common complaint of athletes who try to fully fuel their training with whole food is stomach or gastrointestinal discomfort.

Be sure to emphasize whole-food consumption throughout the day, and focus carbohydrate supplementation around training. This allows for healthy food choices and helps you view your training fuel as an essential part of your workout, rather than extra calories that will limit the aesthetic benefits of your training. More frankly, it takes away the stigma of carbohydrate in your diet as "making the athlete fat" and changes carbohydrate to a positive that fuels your training to enhance your performance and your body sculpting. The message, then, is to *never underfuel training,* or you will not reach high-intensity levels of work output. This is my Power Eating paradigm:

- Eat more
- Gain energy
- Train hard
  - Build muscle
  - Burn fat

In that order! If you restrict fueling, you will never optimize your muscle training, and the only way you will maintain your fat loss is to continue to restrict calories. If you fully fuel your training and maximize your training efforts to optimize muscle, your calorie needs will increase and you will burn off fat and keep it off.

Interestingly, when carbohydrate is not available, the rate of perceived exertion increases. In other words, you'll think you're working out harder than you really are, when in fact, your performance is decreasing. Also important, the excess postexercise oxygen consumption (EPOC) is lower with lower-intensity training. Fat oxidation is high during EPOC, so the higher the intensity and duration of training, the higher the level of fat oxidation and the longer the duration of the afterburn. Therefore, carbohydrate-fueled exercise should lead to an increased training effect and enhanced body sculpting.

Focus your carbohydrate consumption around exercise—before, during, and after—because carbohydrate provides extra fuel to your muscles and to your central nervous system to support high-intensity training. Fueling around exercise also enhances daily energy availability for the immune system, the reproductive system, bone metabolism, and other functions throughout the rest of the day. Carbohydrate-rich foods and supplements can both be used. Your choice should be driven by what feels best and supports the best performance. Then, if you want to lose weight, you can remove 300 to 400 calories from your menu during the rest of the day. This strategy never underfuels your training but allows for a small caloric deficit at another time of day to lead to fat loss.

Another important issue is to never train on an empty stomach or while fasting. Unfortunately, this is a common practice among female athletes, who mistakenly think that they can enhance their performance *and* decrease body fat. But the data are clear: Fasting impedes performance goals. Over time, the well-fueled athlete will develop a more sculpted physique.

Here are effective carbohydrate fueling strategies for high-intensity exercise:

Duration of Exercise	Recommended Intake
1-2 hours	1 gram per kilogram body weight per hour
>2 hours	1+ gram per kilogram body weight per hour (upper range depending on elite status and intensity zone of athlete)

You have to be careful about oversupplementing with most carbohydrate supplements, because they can cause gastrointestinal (GI) distress. In fact, more female than male triathlon and ironman competitors complain about GI distress, and more females use whole foods rather than supplements out on the race course compared to males. Eating whole foods out on the course may satisfy your need to chew, but that food is sitting in your stomach for most of your race and not fueling your performance.

Here is where supplementing with evidence-based products becomes key. It is easy for marketers of sport nutrition products to claim that their products work great because they use science published on an ingredient from another manufacturer or lab, but do not do research on their own product. When it comes to stomach-emptying time, gut comfort, speed of entry into the bloodstream, insulin response, muscle-glycogen replenishment, and impact on performance, you want to know whether research has been done on a specific product so you don't waste your time and money on unfounded marketing claims. Look for products that contain multitransport carbohydrates or high-molecular-weight carbohydrates with product research to back up their claims. These will be the easiest on your gut and give you the best results. However, you may still find that you have to get used to fully fueling yourself as part of your regular training program. Never try something new on competition day.

A Food Plan for Performance and Sculpting

To meet the dual goals of performance and sculpting, you can slightly reduce your food intake to allow for loss of body fat while maintaining lean muscle and performance. If you cut your calorie intake by only 300 to 400 calories per day (less than 500 calories per day), you can reduce fat without lowering your resting metabolic rate. You should not create this deficit during exercise fueling. Instead, you can make it part of the food plan.

I tell my clients that we put their carbohydrate to work for them during exercise, and then extract 300 to 400 calories of foods from their food plan, depending on which macronutrient amounts can be lowered. This is easy and makes sense to the athlete. Athletes should eat all the other foods, listed below, that are important to fuel their body and mind.

Following are the major nutrition concepts and diet strategies that will make an enormous difference in your health and performance:

- Eat breakfast. This ensures proper fueling after the seven to eight hours of fasting while sleeping and keeps metabolism elevated throughout the day.

- Use a carbohydrate supplement to support training early in the day. If there is a window of several hours between eating and training, eating food is an important choice for preparing the body for total daily health and performance. If training is very early in the morning and you cannot eat and be empty enough to train, fuel with a carbohydrate supplement according to the product label. Most products (my choice is Vitargo) can be consumed comfortably within 30 to 45 minutes preexercise. Use less carbohydrate if training will last less than one hour, but do not go into training in a fasted state.

- Fuel frequently throughout the day. Eat every three to four hours throughout the day. Combine sources of protein, carbohydrate, and high-performance fat to ensure a broad range of nutrients each time you eat.

- Recover with nutrition. Combine carbohydrate with high-quality protein after you exercise to enhance recovery.

- Avoid fat and fiber around exercise to speed stomach emptying.

- Throughout the day, choose nutrient-dense carbohydrate sources:
  - Watery vegetables (typically foods such as greens and salad-type veggies)
  - Starchy vegetables (primarily sweet potatoes, white potatoes, and winter squash)
  - Fruit
  - Whole grains
  - Beans
  - Dairy

- Throughout the day, choose nutrient-dense protein sources:
  - Meat
  - Fish and seafood
  - Eggs
  - Dairy

POWER PROFILE: A Young Athlete Who Knows Her Nutrition

In fifth grade, Athena, who had been training as a figure skater, was looking for a different kind of summer sport camp and tried Seattle Derby Brats, a camp known for taking a strong stand for girls, empowering them to be strong, healthy, and confident. They accomplished through a supportive, inclusive community teaching junior roller derby.

At camp, Athena found an environment that supported individual performance as well as team mentality. Right away, though, Athena knew that she had to step up her training and diet to keep up with the power of her teammates. Fortunately, she had learned from her mom, Alice, a former hockey player and current roller derby coach, how to train hard and fuel her body.

Athena says that she's been successful in her sport because she has a positive attitude, an open mindset, and she stays in shape and eats well. Here is Athena's daily food plan, which fits well into her school day, along with the adjustments she makes for tournament days. She's definitely done a great job figuring out her needs and fueling her body.

DAILY

Breakfast (at home):

3 eggs, sunny side up

Or

Yogurt and granola

When she has time, she eats both options together *and* always a lot of water.

Lunch (carried in her backpack):

Salad with lettuce, cucumbers, carrots, chicken, goat cheese and vinaigrette dressing.

Dried apricots and almonds.

Dinner (around 5:00 p.m. before practice):

Cauliflower, Brussels sprouts, or broccoli

Chicken

Pasta

Practice (around 5:45 to 7:45 p.m.):

Water

Snacks (carried in her backpack for use throughout the day):

Almonds, apples, bananas, almond butter, water

No juice or soda: "It offs my game…I lose focus."

Athena doesn't like milk, but she eats yogurt to keep dairy in her diet.

TOURNAMENT DAY DIET

Pregame Breakfast ("lots of carbs"):

Oatmeal

Eggs

Fruit

Then she goes back to sleep, wakes up and has lunch.

Lunch:

Pasta

Some kind of meat

Water

Around game time, Athena prefers not to eat anything because she senses that she will have an upset stomach. But she has learned that if she doesn't fuel herself, she tires easily, loses focus, and gets a headache. So knowing that she plays better when she's fueled, she has trained herself to have snacks and use Gatorade drinks and gummies.

Tournament Pregame Snacks:

Bananas

Apples

Almond butter

Granola

Water

Gatorade

Tournament Half-Time Snacks:

Oranges

Nuts

Postgame Recovery Meal (at restaurant but still during tournament day):

Salad

Pasta or potato (some kind of carbohydrate)

Chicken or other protein

END OF TOURNAMENT CELEBRATION MEAL: PIZZA!

- ◦ Vegetable proteins
- ◦ Grains, beans, nuts, seeds
- • Throughout the day, choose nutrient-dense, high-performance fat sources:
  - ◦ Fatty fish (such as salmon and tuna)
  - ◦ Nuts
  - ◦ Seeds
  - ◦ Avocado
  - ◦ Olives
  - ◦ Extra-virgin olive oil
  - ◦ Vegetable oils

As you probably know, women have much lower levels of testosterone in their bodies than men do. However, they partially make up for these low levels by having much higher growth hormone (GH) levels. GH helps with fat-burning and muscle-building. But while men's GH levels rise when they exercise, women's GH levels don't. For this and other reasons, women should combine their training with a diet like that outlined above, since it will support elevated GH levels.

Female Athletes and Supplements

You have probably wondered about supplementation: Which supplements should I take to help with sports performance? Are they different from what male athletes take? These are important questions, because you definitely have supplementation needs unique to your gender.

Two minerals that women should consider supplementing are calcium and iron. Decades of research have shown that female athletes are commonly marginally deficient in these nutrients. Supplementation for antioxidants, muscle-building, and energy is also discussed below.

Calcium Deficiencies in Women

Female athletes, particularly those in weight-control sports, are often at risk of losing bone calcium. In a study I conducted at the 1990 National Physique Committee (NPC) USA Championships in Raleigh, North Carolina, female bodybuilders recorded their diets; were weighed and had their fat measured; and answered questions about their training, nutrition, and health. None of the women ate or drank any dairy products for at least three months before the competition, and most of them never used dairy products at all. None of them took calcium supplements, either.

Of these women, 81 percent reported that they did not menstruate for at least two months before a contest. The physical stress of training, the psychological stress of competition, the low-calorie diet, and the loss of body fat can all lead to a decrease in the body's production of estrogen. As in menopause, without enough estrogen, a woman stops menstruating. What's worse, no calcium can be stored in the bone when estrogen levels are low. Of course, these women were very lean, too. On average, they had 9 percent body fat. Extremely low body fat is another risk factor for loss of calcium from bones. Also, in women who develop the female athlete triad (disordered eating, menstrual irregularities, and weakened bones), low calcium intakes are common.

Female athletes are often low not only in calcium but also in vitamin D, which works with calcium to build bones and perform other functions. Being low in both nutrients can increase your risk of osteoporosis as well as stress fractures.

It is important to know that if you have irregular menstruation, no menstrual cycle, or stop menstruating before a contest, you should see a good sports medicine physician or a gynecologist who is familiar with your sport. Loss of estrogen production at an early age can have a critical impact on your bone health. It's possible for osteoporosis to develop at a very early age.

Take care of your inside while you are taking care of your outside. Add some dairy to your diet, and you'll be standing straight and tall for many years to come.

Iron Deficiencies in Women

Menstrual blood loss is one of the major causes of iron deficiency in women, and there is an inverse relationship between menstrual blood flow and serum ferritin, the major iron storage protein in the body. Daily iron requirements are higher for women than for men, yet women consume considerably less food, and less iron-rich food, compared to men. With a high risk of iron deficiency you can experience poor athletic performance as well as impaired cognitive functioning.

Iron deficiency causes anemia, a condition in which your blood has a lower-than-normal amount of red blood cells or hemoglobin. Hemoglobin is an iron-rich protein that helps red blood cells carry oxygen from the lungs to the rest of the body.

Some people can have an iron deficiency without anemia, and this is particularly prominent among athletic and physically active women. This is characterized by normal hemoglobin but reduced levels of ferritin (<12 ng/ml), a storage form of iron in the body. When iron is in short supply, your tissues become starved for oxygen. This can make you tire easily and recover more slowly. Several studies from Cornell University indicate that when untrained, iron-depleted women received an iron supplement during exercise training, they experienced greater increases in oxygen use and endurance performance. This goes to show how important iron is to performance. Taking iron supplements, however, will not enhance your performance if you have normal hemoglobin and iron status.

A study of Israeli Army female military combatant recruits found that 29.8 percent had iron deficiency without anemia, and 12. 8 percent were frankly anemic. The incidence was similar among noncombatant female recruits, as compared to 5.2

percent and 0 percent among male combatant recruits. There was no significant difference in total energy or iron consumption between any of the groups. However, plant sources constituted 85 percent of the iron sources for females and only 73 percent for males. Red meat made up 2 percent of the daily iron source for females but 20 percent for males. There is not a strong correlation between total iron intake and iron status in females. Rather, there is a more direct correlation between the dietary source of iron and menstrual iron losses.

Because women are more prone to low iron than men are, the United States Olympic Committee (USOC) recommends that female athletes undergo blood testing periodically to check hemoglobin and serum ferritin status. If you think you might be deficient in iron, talk to your physician or a registered dietitian who specializes in sport nutrition. Self-medicating with large doses of iron can cause big trouble and is potentially dangerous.

Prevent Deficiencies

To guard against the deficiencies discussed above, focus on foods rich in calcium, iron, and vitamin D. If you can't eat enough food, supplement your diet so that your intake is roughly equal to

- 1,000 milligrams of calcium daily,
- 18 milligrams of iron daily, and
- 2,000 to 4,000 IU of vitamin D per day (this can be lowered with sun exposure during summer months, since the sun helps produce vitamin D in your skin).

Antioxidant Supplements

It may also be a good idea to supplement with antioxidant vitamins, minerals, and other factors. These protect you against free radicals, which cause DNA damage and increase in number during and after exercise—a condition called oxidative stress. Oxidative stress can also interfere with important muscle adaptations that come with exercise, hurting your efforts in the gym. Taking antioxidants can counter the effects of this exercise-induced increase in oxidative damage and therefore help your progress in the gym. However, be careful not to megadose, or go beyond the upper limit of the dietary reference intake (DRI). I suggest taking a multivitamin that contains antioxidants with food each day. Avoid taking antioxidants just before or after training.

Creatine for Female Athletes

My female clients often ask me whether supplementing with creatine is good only for guys. Researchers from Kent State University in Ohio report differently in the journal *Nutrition*. They recruited 10 male and 10 female Division I athletes and randomly assigned half to supplementation with 0.2 gram of creatine per pound of fat-free mass and the other half to a similar amount of the placebo maltodextrin for three days. MRIs of both thighs and six 10-second, all-out stationary cycle sprints were conducted before and after supplementation.

Those MRIs revealed that the creatine group had statistically significant increases in body mass, and these athletes performed better in the 10-second cycle sprints, compared to the placebo group. Total work and peak power values for the creatine-supplementing males were greater than those for the women during the initial sprint. Yet the reverse was true during the last three sprints, where the women performed better than the men. Bottom line, if you frequently do interval training, taking a creatine supplement may help you go harder and longer, and this can lead to greater overall fat loss in the long run.

Caffeine

Many of my female clients include caffeine in their everyday diet but not around their training. They may be regular coffee or tea drinkers, but they have never put their caffeine to work for them. They either never thought to, or they worried that it wasn't good for training. However, the opposite may in fact be true: Caffeine appears to be a good ergogenic aid for female athletes—particularly those taking birth control pills. Why is this significant? Well, oral contraceptives have been rumored to limit muscle strength, but do they really? Not according to a study of 10 healthy female athletes on low dose birth control pills. Caffeine supplementation significantly increased the strength of their knee flexors and extensors—a very important outcome, since women athletes are so often plagued with a high incidence of ACL injuries.

You have to be careful with how much caffeine you take, however. Women who consume caffeine regularly (4 or more cups [1 or more L] of coffee a day or 330 milligrams of caffeine) and have a low intake of calcium in their diet (fewer than 700 mg a day) may run a greater risk of developing osteoporosis, or brittle bone disease.

POWER PROFILE: Going for the Gold

In February of 2016, I worked with a 25-year-old female Olympic gold medal swimmer preparing for the Summer Olympic Games in Rio. She was concerned about her body weight. When she competed at the previous Olympics, she had weighed less than her current weight, and she worried that she was too heavy to compete. During the past three years, she had added resistance training to her regimen and was currently 24 percent body fat. In order to lose weight, she had put herself on a very restricted diet of 1,535 calories, 195 grams of carbohydrate, 77 grams of protein, and 50 grams of fat. She had read that she needed to decrease carbohydrate to lose weight. She especially avoided fueling around training to increase weight loss. However, she reported feeling exhausted, irritable, and so hungry that when she returned home after practice she couldn't stop eating. Her performance had diminished significantly.

This athlete's resting metabolic rate was 1,700 calories a day. Her general calorie usage during training was 600 to 800 calories an hour, or sometimes more, depending on the training sessions. She trained an average of four and a half hours a day, six days a week. However, because she was so dramatically underfueling, she was not optimizing her training, nor did she have the fuel to support her foundational health needs.

Her regimen needed some serious overhauling. So that she could continue to train intensely, I added food in to her diet slowly, along with supplementation that would rapidly empty from her stomach and not cause gastrointestinal distress. Specifically, I increased her daily food intake to 2,050 calories, 200 grams of carbohydrate, 157 grams of protein, and 64 grams of fat. This allotment allowed for wiggle room so that she could add her favorite foods—which amounted to an average of 500 extra calories a day, bringing her food total to 2,500 calories per day.

I had her supplement with up to 300 grams a day of carbohydrate (another 1,200 calories) supplementation (Vitargo), depending on the intensity and duration of each workout. She would take a preexercise dose, a dose during exercise, and a dose afterward. Her postexercise dose was combined with 20 grams of whey protein isolate. This was often a morning and an afternoon supplement regimen around training.

By April, this athlete lost 3 pounds of body weight, maintained her muscle mass, and had regained her Olympic caliber swimming performance. She went on to make the Olympic team and win again in Rio.

I see this same scenario day in and day out in my office, in female and male athletes, but most dramatically in females. Female athletes typically underfuel by 1,000 calories per day. In this case, with this Olympian, she was below her final competition level calorie intake by nearly 2,000 calories a day.

8
Tapping Into Brain Power

When I worked for the great coach Pat Riley, he said that 50 percent of athletic performance is the result of mental focus—the ability to concentrate throughout an athletic event all the way to the final moments. This ability is what differentiates any athlete from a champion.

I became even more interested in what Coach Riley said after I moved to Seattle many years ago. The Seattle area sporadically gets some of the world's greatest weather in the spring, summer, and fall. But the payback is having to endure wet, gray, and short days—dark until 8:30 a.m. and dark again by 4 p.m.—during November, December, January, and part of February. Lack of sunlight can darken not only the skies but also people's moods.

After years of creating meal plans for hundreds of clients, including many professional athletes in the Seattle area, I found that my diets not only helped them lose weight but also improved their moods dramatically—no more feeling blue or sluggish. The athletes performed better physically and mentally, and happily for fans, they decided to keep playing for Seattle teams rather than run off to sunnier climates.

I have seen these results in pro football linebackers, pro basketball point guards, and Olympians in sports ranging from rowing to softball. Without that food-inspired feeling of exuberance, winning is just a pipe dream. A depressed athlete may as well sit on the sidelines. Placed on any of the popular weight-loss diets on the market today, most champions wouldn't get out of the locker room.

Most diets are inherently depressing. The way they are put together and the foods they dictate be eaten trigger chemical changes in your brain that actually make you feel depressed. Add that to a plan too low in calories to fuel a day's worth of energy to satisfy even a small pigeon, and you've got a prescription for feeling just exactly how you must have felt: lousy, no energy, and craving the foods that give you instant fuel and naturally elevate your mood.

My experience proved to me that one key way to enhance the mental alertness, focus, and mood of athletes and other active people is through food. Nutrition can affect cognitive processes and emotions, and studies confirm that brain health relies on many factors, including nutrients from our everyday diets. So, while you spend countless hours training and meticulously monitoring your eating and workout programs to maximize muscle, don't forget that cerebral fitness is within your control, too.

The Neurobiology of Food

What and when you eat, even at a single meal, can influence whether you feel happy, moody, irritable, alert, or calm. I refer to these responses as the neurobiology of food, which relates to how the cells of your nervous system are affected by nutrition. Choose the wrong foods (or skip meals altogether), and you might worsen an already stressful or emotional day, plus impede your performance.

A pervasive problem with many popular diets is that they slash carbohydrate. Your brain is almost entirely fueled by glucose, the end product of the digestion of carbohydrate from foods such as grains, fruits, vegetables, milk, and legumes. Glucose is a fast-acting fuel, easily conveyed in and out of cells; just the sort of action your brain needs to do its work rapidly and with laser-like focus.

How much carbohydrate do you need to boost your mental focus? Most studies on the subject agree that at least 40 percent of your total daily calories should come from carbohydrate sources to promote mental alertness and mood.

In addition to carbohydrate, your diet must include the right balance of protein and fat. Choose the right mix of these nutrients, and you set yourself up for cognitive success. This is partially due to an array of natural chemicals called neurotransmitters, which circulate throughout the brain and body, transmitting messages to and from the many nerves that help govern mood.

One of the best-known of these neurotransmitters is serotonin, low levels of which are a contributing factor in many types of depression. In fact, many prescription antidepressants help elevate serotonin activity in the brain. Your diet has a profound influence on serotonin secretion. Without certain nutrients (protein to produce its precursor, tryptophan, and carbohydrate to trigger its uptake into the brain), serotonin levels can become erratic (more on this process below). The result is irritability, plus cravings for carbohydrate. So carbohydrate and protein, working together, play a very important role in helping you maintain your mental focus and equilibrium.

Serotonin is just one of many brain chemicals that manipulate your mood. Another is neuropeptide Y (NPY), thought to be involved in how the brain regulates behavior and mood. It tends to be high when serotonin levels are low and when blood sugar plummets. You crave carbohydrates as a result. The best way to keep it in balance is to eat consistently all day long from a variety of healthy foods. Having enough good fat in your diet activates galanin, another feel-good brain chemical. In addition, B vitamins, including folate, help build the amino acids that create mood-influencing brain chemicals, such as dopamine. Vitamin D regulates the conversion of the essential amino acid tryptophan into serotonin, and omega-3 fatty acids, which boost levels of serotonin, play a role in supporting mood, focus, decision-making behaviors, and alertness.

The Gut-Brain Axis

Your gut (stomach and intestinal tract) and brain are tightly connected and in constant communication with each other in what scientists call the gut-brain axis. The brain talks to the gut, and the gut talks to the brain—bidirectional communication that plays a key role in physical and mental health, according to an accumulating amount of research compiled by scientists.

You have collections of microbes in your body (about a trillion), referred to as microbiota. In total, the microbiota weigh about twice as much as your brain. The brain influences gastrointestinal and immune functions that control the populations of good and bad bacteria in the gut, and these same good and bad bacteria influence the creation and regulation of brain neurotransmitters that affect brain function, mood, and behavior. For example, a study published in 2015 in *Biological Psychiatry* involved the transfer of gut bacteria from the intestines of obese mice to normal-weight mice. The recipients, whose weight remained unchanged, developed neuropsychological symptoms characteristic of obese mice, such as anxiety and changes in cognition and behavior.

Studies in humans have suggested that introducing certain foods and restricting others can help change the microbiota and reduce levels of anxiety or depression. Many of the dietary changes they suggest—which mirror the new Power Eating recommendations you will find in this book—are generally healthy overall and offer a way to protect and enhance brain health. Overall, these studies suggest that you can positively affect the health and diversity of good gut bacteria by taking the following actions:

- *Avoid a high-fat, processed, and sugary Western-type diet.* This appears to boost levels of unhealthy gut bacteria and significantly increases the risk for inflammation and depression.

- *Focus on whole foods.* These include plenty of fiber-rich whole grains, fresh fruits and vegetables, fish, and healthy fats such as olive oil, all of which have been linked to the promotion of beneficial gut bacteria.

- *Eat fermented foods.* These foods contain probiotics, which are living microorganisms that improve health by adding to the beneficial bacteria in your gut. Research suggests that regularly consuming the probiotics found in fermented foods such as yogurt, sauerkraut, kimchi and pickles, or taking probiotic supplements, may alter the nature of the microbiota in the gut, resulting in the production of compounds that are associated with positive brain changes. An important study published in 2013 in the journal *Gastroenterology* found that women who ate a cup of yogurt containing probiotics twice a day for

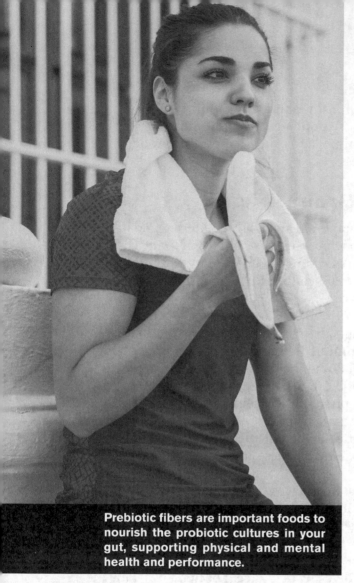

Prebiotic fibers are important foods to nourish the probiotic cultures in your gut, supporting physical and mental health and performance.

Antonio_Diaz/Getty Images/iStockphoto

one month reacted with less stress and anxiety to images of angry or frightened faces than did similar women who did not eat probiotics.

- *Eat soluble fiber.* This naturally contains "prebiotics," dietary fiber that stimulates the growth and activity of healthy bacteria in your gut. Good sources of prebiotics include whole grains, flaxseed, onions, bananas, and garlic. Among other beneficial effects, preliminary research suggests prebiotics may help you better manage stress. In a study published in 2015 in *Psychopharmacology*, three weeks of prebiotics consumption significantly suppressed levels of the stress hormone cortisol and shifted volunteers' thought processes from a negative focus to a more positive focus.

- *Always combine your training with a healthy diet.* This is another way to keep your intestinal bacteria in balance. A 2014 study comparing healthy nonathletes with 40 Irish soccer players revealed that the soccer players had about twice as much diversity in their gut microbiota; in other words, a higher ratio of good bacteria to bad bacteria, a sign of good health.

Supplements and Your Brain

There is a growing body of evidence regarding the use of many different supplements, including botanicals, to support brain health and function. Rather than giving them short shrift here, we have added a lengthy discussion in chapter 11.

Feel-Great Foods

An overall healthy diet, followed consistently, will definitely boost your mood and mental focus. In addition, there are certain foods, which I call feel-great foods, which specifically fuel upbeat moods and chase away depressive symptoms. Take a look.

Turkey

Turkey contains a lot of tryptophan, the amino acid that is the chemical precursor to serotonin. The production of serotonin in your brain is limited by how much tryptophan is available in your bloodstream. Because tryptophan is an amino acid, it is found in protein-containing foods.

I thus recommend eating the dark meat of turkey a couple times a week. Not only does this give you a steady supply of tryptophan, it also boosts your iron content better than white meat will. Adequate iron in your diet prevents physical and mental fatigue. Some of my clients have made turkey jerky one of their regular on-the-go snack foods, and this is a very smart move.

Milk

If you have been off milk for whatever reason—and I find clients who have plenty of reasons for the abstinence—then be open to including it in your diet again. Like turkey, milk is also very high in tryptophan. The reason is that milk contains whey protein, the actual source of the tryptophan. Studies indicate that whey can decrease physiological responses to stress, enhance mood, and even improve memory performance. People who are mildly depressed seem to get the most benefit.

Cow's milk is also one of the very few foods in our diet that is a good source of vitamin D because it is typically fortified with vitamin D. Vitamin D is a hormone that controls about 1,000 genes in the body, some of which regulate the release of serotonin. Scientists have found vitamin D receptors in the same regions of the brain that are associated with depression. One cup (8 ounces, or 244 g) of fortified milk contains approximately 115 to 124 IU of vitamin D. Cow's milk substitutes and other dairy foods may or may not be vitamin D fortified; make sure to read labels to know for sure.

Other dairy foods are high in whey protein, too. The best sources are reduced-fat and fat-free milk, yogurt, cottage cheese, and dairy beverages like kefir. Yogurt and kefir are excellent sources of probiotics. Another great source is a flavored whey powder, which can be blended into smoothies and taken as a midmorning, midafternoon, or postworkout snack.

Whole Grains, Fruits, Vegetables, and Legumes

Just when everyone is taking aim at carbohydrate and eliminating it from weight-loss diets, these carbohydrate sources are some of my most critical feel-great foods. For all its positives in your diet, the tryptophan in turkey, dairy, or a good whey protein powder can become a building block of serotonin only once it crosses the blood-brain barrier. But oddly enough—and significantly—it isn't the protein but the dietary carbohydrate in your diet that effects the crossing.

In the bloodstream, tryptophan competes with other structurally similar amino acids, called the large neutral amino acids (LNAA), for a spot on the carrier molecule that transports them across the blood-brain barrier. When protein intake is high,

Supplementing With BCAAs May not Be a Good Mood Performance Strategy

BCAAs compete with tryptophan, as well as tyrosine uptake in the brain. This lowers not only serotonin production but also dopamine synthesis. Increasing dopamine production is a hallmark of performance enhancement, suggesting that increasing BCAAs may be a poor strategy for improving performance. Carbohydrate may be particularly important if you choose to supplement with BCAAs.

---

there is an abundance of LNAAs, notably tyrosine and the BCAAs, and similar amino acids. Competition for spots is high, limiting tryptophan's access into the brain.

When protein intake is lower and carbohydrate intake higher, however, there is less competition for space on the carrier molecule. In addition, carbohydrate gives tryptophan another advantage by stimulating a series of biochemical events that remove most of the LNAA, except for tryptophan, from the bloodstream and move them into muscle cells. So carbohydrate-rich diets give tryptophan a competitive edge to cross the blood-brain barrier, elevating brain concentrations of serotonin and enhancing mood. Bottom line: Carbohydrate is good for your brain, not only because it provides the brain's favored fuel but also because it does the advance work for the utilization of protein.

Several studies have confirmed what I mentioned above: Diets containing at least 40 percent of calories from carbohydrates can have mood-improving effects on clinically depressed subjects. These diet-induced alterations in mood are less pronounced in healthy subjects since it is more difficult to show the impact of a mood change in someone who isn't markedly depressed. But in my practice, the first thing I hear after clients have followed my program for only one week is, "I have so much more energy, and I feel better than ever!"

The best feel-great carbohydrate sources are those found in whole grains, fruits, vegetables, and legumes. I recommend a meal plan where you get almost all of your bread servings from the whole-grain group; include starchy vegetables like winter squash, potatoes, and peas; and have at least one fruit daily from each of the citrus and berry families (use frozen berries when they are not in season). Also, eat at least one serving each day from the carotene (carrots, dark leafy greens, tomatoes), brassica (broccoli, cauliflower, cabbage, Chinese cabbage, Brussels sprouts) and allium (garlic, onions, shallots, chives) families.

You will always want to combine carbohydrate, protein, and fat in any meal or snack. For instance, a midafternoon snack of almonds, dried fruit, and V-8 juice is an ideal pick-me-up and quite satisfying. To boost your protein a little more, you can add string cheese to the snack.

My friends and family all know they can count on me for healthy snacks. I carry bags around in my car, purse, and even briefcase. Planning your snacks and taking them along with you can change your mood and drop pounds.

Fish, Flax, and High-Performance Fat

Sixty percent of your brain consists of fat. Polyunsaturated fatty acids (PUFAs) in the membranes surrounding brain cells play a role in every step of serotonin function, including boosting mood and keeping it elevated. Serotonin carries messages between brain cells. The term that scientists use to describe a healthy brain cell membrane is *fluid*. We're not talking about water here but about the ability of brain cell membranes to send messages efficiently and effectively from one to the next. The better the ability to send messages, the higher the fluidity.

The concentration of PUFAs in brain cells determines the fluidity of the membrane. High concentrations of omega-3 fats (specifically the type of PUFA found predominantly in fatty fish) are critical to fluidity. So eating wild salmon and low-mercury tuna is good for your brain as well as your heart. Forget the high fat content. This is healthy fat for your brain.

The same goes for adding a tablespoon of ground flaxseed to your diet. You can use flax oil if you prefer (it costs considerably more) or packaged flax meal (much more reasonable), but don't settle for eating the whole seed (about a dollar per pound in bulk). We can't digest the seed hull; the seed's inner goodness and fat-busting qualities will pass right through you. I prefer the seeds to the oil because the fiber in the seeds is a great prebiotic. Whole flaxseeds are easy to grind in a coffee-bean grinder. I have a small grinder solely dedicated to flax. Some people don't like the taste of flaxseed or flax meal, while others love the nutty flavor mixed right into a bowl of cereal or yogurt with fruit. If you don't like the taste, it is easy to mask in a smoothie, or even a scrambled egg or hamburger patty.

Here's where home recipes meet science. A recent study examining the association between depression and selected nutritional factors found lower levels of PUFAs in the red blood cells of depressed women when compared to healthy women. It also found significantly lower levels of alpha-linolenic acid (ALA) and linoleic acid, two essential fatty acids found in flax. These study results support the results of several earlier studies. Flax, fish, and eggs put you back in balance.

A study conducted in 1998 investigated the influence of total dietary fat on mood. During the first month of the study all subjects ate a diet consisting of 41 percent of the calories from fat. During the second month half of the subjects switched to a 25 percent fat diet. Following the second month, levels of anger and hostility increased dramatically in the low-fat group. Tension and anxiety was decreased in the higher-fat group.

There was another benefit beyond the mood upswing of those who consumed more fat: HDL cholesterol (the good cholesterol) levels improved on the higher-fat diet and declined on the low-fat diet. Remember, salmon, tuna, and other cold-water fish (sardines, anchovies, mackerel, herring, shellfish) are good for the brain *and* the heart.

Eggs

I have been on the bandwagon for returning egg yolks to the diet for more than 15 years. It all started when I worked with athletes who were having trouble with mood and mental focus. At that time, I went into the neurobiology literature and discovered that the essential B-vitamin choline played two very important functions in the body (among others that I'll get to below). First, choline is half of the most abundant neurotransmitter in the body, acetylcholine. Acetylcholine is utilized by our nerves every time we think or move—that is, constantly—so it is profoundly important. Second, as part of the phospholipid complex phosphatidylcholine, in partnership with phosphatidylserine, choline is required to create the channels in brain cell membranes that allow for nutrients to pass in and toxins to pass out. So choline is essential for healthy brain function, memory, how you feel, and how you think.

The major source of choline in the American diet is egg yolk, and we have been dumping yolks down the drain for decades due to the misconception that dietary cholesterol raises blood cholesterol levels. Americans in general, and women in particular, especially if they are on weight-loss diets, are consuming less than half of our dietary need for choline. In fact, there has never been a study to show that an egg yolk a day raises cholesterol levels, and several studies have shown that, in fact, an egg yolk does not raise cholesterol levels. Just one egg yolk each day (eat the whole egg; don't start dumping the whites down the drain) will raise choline intake by nearly 50 percent. But that's still not quite enough.

Recent research is showing the further importance of choline. A research group in Norway published a study investigating the role of choline in bone health in women. Those women with the lowest intakes of choline had the lowest bone mineral density measures and the greatest risks for hip fractures. Women smokers were at an even greater risk. The researchers encouraged more research on the connections between choline, bone mineral metabolism, and nicotine.

A research article in the *Journal of Clinical Lipidology* (2013) confirmed the health benefits of whole eggs and increased choline consumption. Women and men in the study group with metabolic syndrome were fed controlled carbohydrate diets along with three whole eggs per day. Similar subjects with metabolic syndrome in the control group were fed the same diet but with yolk-free egg substitute. Both groups lost weight. The study group did not have any rise in blood cholesterol levels, but they did have a significant lowering of markers of systemic inflammation; the control group had no inflammatory change.

So I'm ringing the alarm bells! We all need more choline in our diets. Most people, women in particular, will still need to supplement to get the healthy daily dose to support mind and body health. You will feel the difference.

Water

Brain cells need to be well-hydrated in order to work properly. Not surprisingly, then, brain function and mood state are affected by how much fluid you drink. When it comes to peak mental capacity, your hydration state will affect your performance. In a study of subjects' abilities to perform mental exercises after becoming dehydrated, a fluid loss of only 2 percent of their body weight caused reductions in arithmetic ability, short-term memory, and the ability to visually track an object by 20 percent compared to their well-hydrated state.

That's one major vote for filling up your water bottle, carrying it with you, and emptying it often. If you weigh 150 pounds, 2 percent of that is only 3 pounds or 6 cups of fluid. When you consider all the fluid turnover that your body goes through in a day, it's easy enough to be down 6 cups without being aware of it. (For detailed information about proper hydration, see chapter 6.)

My Other Top Picks for Brain-Boosting Foods

The fruits, vegetables, and spices in this list contain phytochemicals and antioxidants that protect brain cells, plus help maintain mental alertness and reaction time during athletic performance. Carbohydrate sources such as popcorn and whole grains are crucial for manufacturing key neurotransmitters. Others such as garlic are prebiotics. High-performance fat found in cocoa powder, flaxseed, nuts and other seeds, fish and seafood, and oils supply fatty acids that boost brain function. Protein, from turkey to pork to soy, helps manufacture tryptophan, a building block of serotonin. Yogurt, of course, supplies the body with gut- and brain-healing probiotics. And caffeine, found in tea and coffee, has long been known to naturally increase mental alertness.

- Air-popped popcorn
- Bananas
- Beans
- Blueberries
- Broccoli
- Caffeine-containing beverages (1-2 servings)
- Cocoa powder (or chocolate in small amounts)
- Dark, leafy greens
- Edamame (soy)
- Egg yolk
- Fish and seafood
- Flaxseed (must be ground or meal)
- Garlic
- Ginger
- Grapefruit
- Grape juice
- Green tea
- Lean pork
- Low-fat or fat-free dairy
- Mango
- Nuts
- Olives, olive oil
- Oranges
- Pomegranate
- Soy
- Spinach
- Strawberries
- Sunflower seeds
- Turkey
- Unrefined vegetable oils
- Water
- Whole grains
- Yogurt and other probiotic foods

Timing: The "When"

Earlier I mentioned that when you eat certain foods is critical to mental focus and performance. A successful strategy for fueling your brain incorporates the critical elements of timing and combining of nutrients so that you get the biggest bang for your buck both for performance and mood control. Eating five to six meals daily, including three main meals and snacks, supports brain fueling.

Let's be clear and practical about food timing and combining. Every meal and snack needs a balance of carbohydrate, fat, and protein. Never snack on only carbohydrate, even the fabulous choices of fruits and veggies. Add some nuts or a piece of delicious cheese. Put protein powder in your smoothies, and add flaxseed meal to your cereal or even on top of toast with some jam.

As for timing, a daily routine that includes eating every two to three hours takes planning and forming the habit. You will notice a dramatic rise in energy within the first week of more consistent eating—"no meal skipping" is your credo. It will take maybe two to three weeks to make it a habit, but it is well worth the adjustment. Some of my clients have lost significant pounds based almost entirely on no longer skipping meals or not loading up on the day's calories only at dinner time and into the evening. It's all about how you feel!

Here's another major lesson I've learned from working with pro and elite athletes across more than a dozen sports. Without enough calories in your diet, you will crash and burn early in the day, long before you maximize the amount of food you are eating for peak performance. Athletes who play late-afternoon or evening games need to eat throughout the pregame part of the day.

So what, and when, should you be eating to incorporate all the information I've given you about keeping your brain healthy? Using a one-day menu as an example, table 8.1 shows you what a day of eating to adequately fuel your brain and mental processes looks like.

Organic Food and Brain Health

Toxins can sneak into food through many different sources, including crops grown with herbicides and pesticides. Some toxins disturb neurological function, and there is emerging evidence that they can harm the brain, lead to cognitive decline, and perhaps contribute to the development of neurodegenerative diseases such as Alzheimer's and Parkinson's.

The body is naturally designed to protect vital organs (like the brain) against toxins by walling them off inside fat cells. Unfortunately, the brain is constructed mostly of fat, so many of these harmful substances cross the blood-brain barrier and lodge in the fat cells of the brain. This situation is potentially injurious to health if toxins are allowed to build up in fat cells over time.

One way to protect yourself is to purchase organic produce, which is free of pesticides and may be higher in brain-healthy omega-3 fatty acids. Although the research is ongoing as to whether organically raised foods are nutritionally healthier than those grown with pesticides and herbicides, or even do the least damage to you or to the environment, I think it is a good idea to consider organic foods in light of the pesticide connection to brain health.

An economical way to purchase organic produce is to visit local farmers' markets. What we do know is that when you shop at a farmers' market, or you meet the farmer who raised your food, you have a direct connection to the person who put time and effort into creating the food you eat. By buying local produce, you contribute to the livelihood of your community and to the physical care of your environment. Research shows that these positive connections enhance immune function, overall health, and quality of life.

TABLE 8.1   Sample Brain-Fueling Menu

Food group servings	Menu
Breakfast	
1 bread/starch	1/2 cup shredded wheat or 1 cup Kashi cereal
1 fruit	2 tbsp raisins (or 3/4 cup blueberries in season)
1 milk	1 cup fat-free milk
1 medium fat protein	1 egg (prepared any way without fat)
1 fat	1 tbsp ground flaxseed (sprinkle over cereal)
	Water*
Snack: Homemade smoothie	
1 milk	1 cup fat-free milk
2 lean protein	14 g flavored whey powder
	3 ice cubes blended with milk and whey powder
Lunch	
1 bread/starch	1 cup chicken/vegetable noodle soup
2 vegetable	2 cups mixed green salad
3 very lean protein	3 oz turkey
1 fat	2 tbsp olive oil and balsamic vinegar dressing drizzled over salad
	Water
Snack	
1 fruit	1 apple
1 vegetable	1/2 cup vegetable or tomato juice
1 fat	10 peanuts (ballpark style in shell)
	Water
Dinner	
2 bread/starch	1/2 cup brown rice 1/2 cup sweet potato
1 fruit	1 orange, sectioned
2 vegetable	1 cup steamed broccoli sprinkled with balsamic or raspberry vinegar
4 lean protein	4 oz grilled or broiled wild salmon
2 fat	8 large black olives 1 tsp extra-virgin olive oil rubbed on salmon
	Water

*I didn't list coffee, but trust me, it is OK to include one to two cups, or one to two shots of espresso, any time during the morning.

Enjoy Your Food

Your pet may selfishly wolf down its food, but as anthropologists tell us, humans are the only ones who intentionally share food, prepare it with the intention of nurturing one another, and socially interact while we eat it. (This of course is not referring to the instinctual feeding of young by adult animal parents.)

While the value of eating nutritionally balanced meals has been drummed into us, there is a really important factor that has been overlooked: Food strengthens the bonds of intimacy with those we love. Mealtimes can, and should, be wonderful opportunities to interact with the people in your life and to enjoy together the food you are eating.

Why is this important? Yes, we eat to train, and some people train to eat, but I feel we should embrace the enjoyment of food, and how it forms bonds of intimacy and creates closeness with our loved ones. When you have a food attitude like this, your health will be enhanced, as will your ability to manage your weight and energy. You'll enjoy your food even more and appreciate how it fuels and supports your body.

If we always focus on what we shouldn't eat, on the "science-ness" of food, or on why we can't enjoy our meals, a dysfunctional relationship is created not only between ourselves and our food but also between ourselves and others who may be the closest and most important people in our lives; namely, our family and friends. Nature has designed us to enjoy food so that we look forward to eating and we receive satisfaction in mind and body from eating.

I have a motto: "Think about what you need to eat, not what you can't eat next." Focus on nourishing your body, feeding your brain, and sharing your sustenance with others. Think about these things as you prepare meals and break bread with others. Even when eating alone, think about what your body needs to thrive. Doing so will help you thrive, in your personal, professional, and athletic lives for a lifetime.

PART II

Supplements

Beyond the natural foundation of a well-balanced, healthy diet, everyone wants to know what nutritional elements can enhance specific performance areas. Contemporary scientific thought on this looks at nutrients such as vitamins and minerals, food factors such as fiber and botanical phytochemicals, and supplements such as L-carnitine and beta-alanine, as possible ways to enhance training and performance. But can a vitamin, supplement, or food factor really help?

Many athletes believe supplements are capable of improving performance, so they megadose. Megadosing, however, is not always the correct strategy. In fact, it may be exactly the wrong strategy. If your goal is to coax along an energy-producing process in your cells, you may need just a very small amount of a certain nutrient or food factor to do so. More than what is required might trigger the opposite effect.

Fortunately, we know more than ever before about supplements and how to choose them, and that information is featured in this edition. Thus, part II reviews the most popular supplements used by strength-training athletes and gives you a guide to choosing the safest and highest-quality products. Using the most current scientific research, I evaluate the usefulness of these supplements. You can use my rating system to decide for yourself which products meet their marketing claims and which have promise. Because the category of products that *don't* work has grown so enormously, I no longer include it in this book.

Finally, it is more important than ever to expect purity in the products that you buy. You look for the best foods in the grocery store, and you should have the same expectations of your supplements. What are they made of? Where do the ingredients come from? Can you trust the source? Is there anything in the product that is not on the label, and is everything that is on the label really in the product? The only way to have confidence in these manufactured products is to know that they are certified free of banned substances and other contaminants by an independent, third-party laboratory. Every batch should be tested and certified for purity. If a product label doesn't proclaim that it has been tested, it probably hasn't been. To confirm that the product has been tested and certified, you can call the manufacturer and then follow up with a call to the testing lab and ask the lab to verify that they certified the product.

The three top independent labs that currently test for banned substances in dietary supplements are Banned Substances Control Group (bscg.org), Informed Choice-Informed Sport (informed-sport.com), and NSF Certified for Sport (nsf-sport.com). The testing strategies are not equivalent among these 3 or any others that you might find. For a comparison list see www.bscg.org/third-party-dietary -supplement-certification-comparison.

9

Vitamins and Minerals for Strength Trainers

Want to get sleeker, faster, stronger? Want to get ripped, shredded, striated, and vascular? Every supplement company says it's got the product for you. If only it were true! Only a small fraction of supplement products have had research done on them to confirm their manufacturers' claims. The other producers are either using someone else's ingredient-research data, or they're just making it up altogether. That's a fact, but hardly anyone in the industry talks about it.

But don't worry. I'm going to walk you through what we know and how certain supplements can help to support your physical performance goals. Scientists know much more about the nutritional requirements of muscle building and the development of power and speed than they did even 10 years ago. This chapter will limit the discussion to the products that work and to those that show considerable promise based on the science at hand.

Essential Vitamins and Minerals

Among the many pills and potions on store shelves are the well-known essential vitamins and minerals. Quite possibly, you may need extra amounts of both. Research shows that most Americans fall short of the requirements for many key nutrients, including vitamins C, D, E, and B_{12} as well as folic acid, calcium, iron, zinc, and magnesium, which is why a growing number of Americans are turning to supplements. A survey conducted by Ipsos Public Affairs on behalf of the Council for Responsible Nutrition (CRN) in 2016 shows that more than 71 percent of U.S. adults take supplements daily, and 75 percent of these users take a multivitamin. We know that people who are deficient benefit from supplementation. But what about people who eat fairly well? Can they benefit too? That is more difficult to ascertain.

Studies have looked at populations of people who report taking supplements and have run correlations between their intakes and incidence of disease over time. The problem is there is no standard protocol. Everyone is taking a different brand and a different amount. We don't know how rigorous they are about daily supplementation. We usually don't know much about their overall diet, although sometimes we do have dietary data on subjects. Therefore, there are only a handful of good studies to help us understand the impact of multivitamin-multimineral supplementation in people who are not already deficient in nutrients.

A 2013 meta-analysis (a study that reviews multiple other research studies), found that daily multivitamin-multimineral supplementation did not improve the risks for cardiovascular disease, cancer, or death from all causes in men or women who were well nourished. When the authors selected the two most substantial studies among those reviewed and evaluated those results separately, they found that both multivitamin-multimineral trials revealed a decreased incidence of cancer in men who took the supplements, but no similar effect in women.

Some data even suggest that taking supplements may help you live longer. A study published in 2009 in the *American Journal of Clinical Nutrition* analyzed data from 586 older women. The researchers drew the women's blood and assessed the length of telomeres, which are pieces of DNA on chromosomes. As we age, our telomeres shorten. So the longer they are, the better our bodies are at maintaining our youth. In women who took multivitamin-multimineral supplements, telomeres were longer, indicating that these basic supplements may promote longevity.

The American Medical Association (AMA) recommends that everyone take a multivitamin-multimineral supplement daily in order to help prevent chronic illnesses such as cancer, heart disease, and osteoporosis. Even people who eat five daily servings of fruits and vegetables may not get enough of certain vitamins for optimum health. Most people, for instance, cannot get the healthiest levels of folate and vitamin D and E from their diets.

Hard workouts increase your nutritional needs, as does dieting. That's why you may want to add certain vitamins and minerals to your nutritional arsenal. From a sport science perspective, if you are deficient in vitamins and minerals, your performance can suffer. Research shows that if you've taken in less than one third of the daily required amounts of certain B vitamins (B_1, B_2, and B_6) and vitamin C, you can lose aerobic power and strength in a matter of weeks. Taking a multivitamin-multimineral supplement isn't going to help you lift more, run faster, or build more muscle, but it will help prevent deficiencies that could impair your performance. This is particularly relevant when you are on a low-calorie weight-loss diet. To lose weight, you are taking in fewer calories than you are burning off, but you are also taking in less nutrient-dense food and therefore less of the vitamins and minerals that you need to eat every day.

Keep in mind that vitamin and mineral supplements should not replace food. With the right planning, your body can get almost all the nutrients it needs from a balanced diet. Notice that I said *almost*. What's more, your body absorbs nutrients

Choosing the Right Supplement

Following are the three most important issues to consider when selecting a vitamin or mineral supplement (or both):

1. ***Is the supplement pure and safe to take?*** Purchase products that are tested and certified for purity by third-party, independent agencies. This is the best way to be certain that what is listed on the label is actually in the product, *and* that there is nothing contaminating the product that is not on the label. This is very important for banned substance and drug testing! Don't just look for the certification badge on the website. Check to make sure that the product you are taking has been certified. Is the batch number of the product that you are using tested, especially for any drug-tested clients? In order to be certain, call the manufacturer and call the testing lab to ask if every batch is tested, or if testing is done once or a few times each year. There are currently 3 well-recognized third party independent labs that test for ingredients and banned substances: Banned Substances Control Group (BSCG.com), Informed Sport (informed-sport.com) and NSF Certified for Sport (nsfsport.com).

2. ***Does the supplement get absorbed?*** Supplements can pass through the digestive tract partially or completely unabsorbed. Make sure that the supplement meets USP standards for potency, uniformity, disintegration, and dissolution to ensure that you are getting all that you expect from it.

3. ***Is the formulation science based, and is the company credible?*** Expect to see studies proving the quality and research of the product. Look for studies that are done by a credible and independent third-party source. The company should also have a team of scientists that work on product research and development, and someone that you can talk with to answer your questions about the science, not marketing mumbo jumbo. Ideally the company should manufacture the products itself, rather than outsourcing the production. The manufacturer should voluntarily meet the highest manufacturing standards, known as Pharmaceutical Good Manufacturing Practices (Pharma GMP).

Finally, don't believe everything you hear or read in the media about supplements. The media try to interpret scientific studies, and they are not trained to do so. When looking for specific information on how to take care of your own personal health and needs, turn to the nutritional experts for advice.

---

best from food. However, if you would like the insurance of closer to 100 percent nutritional coverage, a good move is to take a daily multivitamin-multimineral supplement containing at least 100 percent of the daily values for vitamins and minerals. These formulations help you cover your nutritional bases and contain nutrients that have special value to strength trainers.

Dietary Reference Intake

An updated way of rating the amounts of the nutrients we need for good health is the dietary reference intake (DRI). It expands on and includes the familiar RDA (recommended dietary allowance), but whereas the RDAs target nutrient deficiencies, the DRIs aim to prevent chronic diseases (see chapter 1).

Applied to vitamins, minerals, and protein taken by men and women in specific age groups, the DRIs contain three rating sets appropriate for discussion here: the RDA, the amount that helps us maintain our health; the tolerable upper intake level (UL), the established ceiling amount to help us avoid taking too much of a nutrient; and the adequate intake (AI), which is an estimate of the average intake that seems healthy and won't harm health. For the purposes of this book, I place all nutrient recommendations under the heading of DRIs.

Antioxidants

There has been a lot of research done in strength sports about antioxidants—beta-carotene, vitamin C, vitamin E, and the minerals selenium, copper, zinc, and manganese. Antioxidants help fight free radicals, which form reactive oxygen species (ROS). These chemicals are produced naturally by the body and have historically been thought to cause irreversible damage (oxidation) to cells. Free radical oxidative damage can leave your body vulnerable to premature aging, cancer, cardiovascular disease, and degenerative diseases such as arthritis. The exercise-related functions of the key antioxidants are summarized in table 9.1.

Certain environmental factors such as cigarette smoke, exhaust fumes, radiation, excessive sunlight, certain drugs, and stress can increase free radicals and, ironically, so can the healthy habit of exercise. During respiration, cells pick off electrons from sugars and add them to oxygen to generate energy. As these reactions take place, electrons sometimes get off course and collide with other molecules, creating free radicals that roam throughout the body and create ROS. Exercise increases respiration, which produces more free radicals. Scientists have been intensely studying why this happens and may have discovered that the point of free radical production is not destruction, but a signal to the body to repair and grow—bigger, faster, and stronger. Interestingly, exercise not only increases production of ROS, it also induces the production of enzymes that fight ROS. Real damage occurs when the signaling system breaks down.

Body temperature, which tends to rise during exercise, may be another factor in generating free radicals. A third possibility is the increase in catecholamine production during exercise. Catecholamines are hormones released in response to muscular effort. They increase heart rate, let more blood get to muscles, and provide the muscles with fuel, among other functions.

Another source of free radical production is the damage done to the muscle cell membrane after intense exercise, especially eccentric exercise such as putting down a heavy weight or running downhill. In a domino-like series of chemical reactions, free radicals hook up with fatty acids in cell membranes to form ROS substances called peroxides. Peroxides attack cell membranes, setting off a chain reaction that creates many more free radicals. This process is called lipid peroxidation and can lead to muscle soreness. The point is, several complex reactions occur with exercise, and each one may accelerate free radical production.

Antioxidants and Inflammation

Chronic inflammation occurs when the damage from ROS is not halted by natural defenses built into our bodies. When the signals get crossed, or we don't have the ability to respond, inflammation begins to build and will chug along unchecked, creating greater tissue damage and soreness, and perhaps even at the genetic level, leading to premature aging and increased disease risk.

Antioxidants help guard against that unchecked inflammation in the body. But here's the rub: Scientists have lately questioned whether it is beneficial to tamp down training-induced inflammation completely. Initial inflammation, it turns out, is necessary for muscle building, so loading our bodies with an overabundance of antioxidant and inflammation-fighting compounds may disrupt the signaling and limit the body's ability to repair and grow. Without this inflammatory response, the muscle won't rebuild to the same level. Thus, you won't get as great a training effect from a hard workout.

Australian researchers looked into this issue by analyzing an assortment of studies that examined both acute and chronic antioxidant supplementation, primarily focused on vitamin E. They also looked at a number of other popular compounds, which we will discuss further in chapter 10. Their overall conclusion was that for athletes, chronic consumption of antioxidant supplements may be harmful to performance. However, they also concluded that chronic intake of 400 mg daily of vitamin E for athletes at high altitude is most likely a very helpful strategy. Acute intake of vitamin E may be helpful in fighting inflammation and enhancing performance during tournament play, but this was only seen in human subjects with intravenous supplementation, not with oral supplementation. Any other studies that show positive impact of oral supplementation were in animals. We cannot make conclusive recommendations when studies are not on human subjects.

My take away is that to get the best results from training, you should limit antioxidant supplementation to not much more than the DRI. Be aware that researchers do caution that if you're involved in very intense competition such as endurance sports, supplementing moderately with antioxidants is a good idea, because these sports can severely deplete the body's natural supply of antioxidants, compromising health. Therefore, never rely on antioxidant supplements alone. Get your antioxidants through a whole-foods diet that is rich in these nutrients. Food has never been shown to cause interference with tissue growth and repair.

Also, timing may be important because supplementation may be a good idea when your body has high demands. Plan your daily antioxidant and anti-inflammatory supplementation regimes at times during the day other than for several hours around exercise. We will discuss nonvitamin-mineral products in this category in chapter 10.

TABLE 9.1 Key Antioxidants

Vitamins	
Beta-carotene	
Exercise-related function	May reduce free radical production as a result of exercise and protect against exercise-induced tissue damage; complements antioxidant function of vitamin E.
Best food sources	Carrots, sweet potatoes, spinach, cantaloupe, broccoli, any dark green leafy vegetables, and orange vegetables and fruits.
Side effects and toxicity	None known because the body carefully controls its conversion to vitamin A. Daily intakes of 20,000 IU from either food or supplements over several months may cause skin yellowing. This disappears when the dosage is reduced.
DRIs for adults	No established limits. 2,500 IU daily from supplements is safe. You can get the same amount from a large carrot.
Vitamin C	
Exercise-related function	Maintains normal connective tissue; enhances iron absorption; may reduce free radical damage as a result of exercise and protect against exercise-induced tissue damage.
Best food sources	Citrus fruits and juices, green peppers, raw cabbage, kiwi fruit, cantaloupe, and green leafy vegetables.
Side effects and toxicity	The body adapts to high dosages. Dosages between 5,000 and 15,000 mg daily may cause burning urination or diarrhea.
DRIs for adults	Women, 75 mg; pregnant women, 85 mg; lactating women, 120 mg; men, 90 mg. Also, 110 mg for female smokers and 130 mg for male smokers.
UL* for adults	2,000 mg.
Vitamin E	
Exercise-related function	Involved in cellular respiration; assists in the formation of red blood cells; scavenges free radicals; protects against exercise-induced tissue damage.
Best food sources	Nuts, seeds, raw wheat germ, polyunsaturated vegetable oils, and fish liver oils.
Side effects and toxicity	None known.
DRIs for adults	15 mg; lactating women, 19 mg.
UL* for adults	1,000 mg.
Minerals	
Selenium	
Exercise-related function	Interacts with vitamin E in normal growth and metabolism; preserves the elasticity of the skin; produces glutathione peroxidase, an important protective enzyme.
Best food sources	Cereal bran, Brazil nuts, whole-grain cereals, egg yolks, milk, chicken, seafood, broccoli, garlic, and onions.
Side effects and toxicity	5 mg a day from food has resulted in hair loss and fingernail changes. Higher dosages are linked to intestinal problems, fatigue, and irritability.
DRIs for adults	Women, 55 mcg; pregnant women, 60 mcg; lactating women, 70 mcg; men, 55 mcg.
UL* for adults	400 mcg.

Copper

Exercise-related function	Assists in the formation of hemoglobin and red blood cells by aiding in iron absorption; required for energy metabolism; involved with superoxide dismutase, a key protective antioxidant enzyme.
Best food sources	Whole grains, shellfish, eggs, almonds, green leafy vegetables, and beans.
Side effects and toxicity	Toxicity is rare.
DRIs for adults	Women and men, 900 mcg; pregnant women, 1,000 mcg; lactating women, 1,300 mcg.
UL* for adults	10,000 mcg.

Zinc

Exercise-related function	Involved in energy metabolism and immunity.
Best food sources	Animal protein, oysters, mushrooms, whole grains, and brewer's yeast.
Side effects and toxicity	Dosages higher than 20 mg a day may interfere with copper absorption, reduce HDL cholesterol, and impair the immune system.
DRIs for adults	Women, 8 mg; pregnant women, 11 mg; lactating women, 12 mg; men, 11 mg.
UL* for adults	40 mg.

Manganese

Exercise-related function	Involved in metabolism; involved with superoxide dismutase, a key protective antioxidant enzyme.
Best food sources	Whole grains, egg yolks, dried peas and beans, and green leafy vegetables.
Side effects and toxicity	Large dosages can cause vomiting and intestinal problems.
DRIs for adults	Women, 1.8 mg; pregnant women, 2.0 mg; lactating women, 2.6 mg; men, 2.3 mg.
UL* for adults	11 mg.

Lipids

Coenzyme Q10

Exercise-related function	A coenzyme for mitochondrial enzymes of the oxidative phosphorylation pathway essential for ATP production; a potent antioxidant that decreases oxidative damage to tissues.
Best food sources	Organ meats, beef, soy oil, sardines, mackerel, and peanuts.
Side effects and toxicity	None known.
DRIs for adults	No established limits. Doses of 30-300 mg per day have been used in clinical studies of heart failure patients.
UL* for adults	No established limits.

*UL refers to tolerable upper intake levels, which have been established for vitamins and minerals. These levels represent the maximum intake of a nutrient that is likely to pose no health risks.

Beta-Carotene

Beta-carotene is a member of a group of substances known as carotenoids. There are hundreds of carotenoids in nature, found mostly in orange and yellow fruits and vegetables and dark green vegetables.

Once ingested, beta-carotene is converted to vitamin A in the body on an as-needed basis. As an antioxidant, beta-carotene can destroy free radicals after they're formed, and it has been shown to reduce muscle soreness by minimizing exercise-induced lipid peroxidation. With less soreness, you may be able to work out more times a week.

However, most clinicians now advise against supplementing with beta-carotene. Here is why: People who took supplemental beta-carotene while enrolled in a large cancer-prevention trial called the Carotene and Retinol Efficacy Trial, or CARET, continued to have increased rates of lung cancer six years after the trial was stopped early and the supplements discontinued, according to a long-term follow-up of trial participants. The results add to earlier evidence from this study and a second large prevention trial that, contrary to earlier expectations, not only do beta-carotene supplements not prevent lung cancer in people at high risk for the disease but also appear to increase rates of the disease, particularly among smokers. These findings hint that some adverse reaction is going on in the body. Therefore, it is wise to get your beta-carotene from vegetables instead.

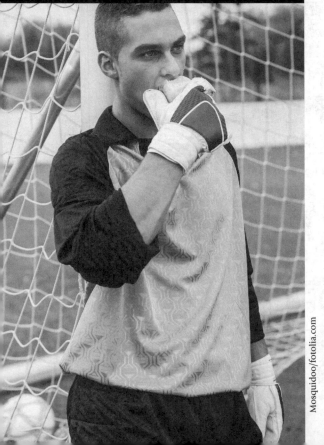

Aim to satisfy vitamin and mineral needs with plant foods such as fruits, vegetables, and whole grains.

Mosquidoo/fotolia.com

Vitamin C

Vitamin C, or ascorbic acid, is a nutrient that can be synthesized by many animals but not by humans. It's an essential component of our diets and functions primarily in the formation of connective tissue such as collagen. Vitamin C is also involved in immunity, wound healing, and allergic responses. As an antioxidant, vitamin C keeps free radicals from destroying the outermost layers of cells. When paired with a plant-based iron source, vitamin C enhances the absorption of this hard-to-absorb form of nonheme iron. Adding lemon juice to your spinach can give a better boost to your iron stores.

If you work out regularly or train for athletic competition, you know that a cold or respiratory infection can sideline you pretty fast. Fortunately, researchers have found that supplementing with 500 milligrams daily of vitamin C appears to cut the risk of upper respiratory tract infections. This benefit may be due to the antioxidant effect of vitamin C or to its overall immune-boosting capability.

Supplementing with vitamin C will improve your performance but only if you are deficient in this nutrient. Supplementation does not enhance performance if you already eat a healthy, nourishing diet that is high in citrus fruits (which are high in vitamin C) and other fruits and vegetables. In fact, a review of 12 studies showed that in 4 of those studies, daily doses of 1 gram (1000 mg) of vitamin C may lead to decrements in performance. The conclusion of the authors was that consuming vitamin C at levels that are naturally found in foods every day (250 mg) is best for supporting training effects and athletic performance.

My recommendation is that you should first and foremost make plant foods, which are often naturally high in vitamin C, the mainstay of your diet, ensuring a vitamin C–rich diet. During cold and flu season you might experiment with supplementation if you don't consume at least 500 milligrams of vitamin C in food alone. If you choose to supplement, stay below 1 gram (1000 mg) daily in food and supplements.

Vitamin E

Many studies on antioxidants and exercise have focused on vitamin E, which resides in muscle cell membranes. Part of its job is to scavenge free radicals, as I discussed above. There is so much research in this area in addition to the particular area of muscle tissue damage that I'd like to summarize some of the findings for you. (First, a quick note: Avoid taking supplemental vitamin E if you are taking anticlotting drugs such as low-dose aspirin or Coumadin, because vitamin E can further thin your blood.)

A few studies on vitamin E have found the following benefits of supplementation:

- Supplementation (at a daily dose of 800 mg) protects against muscle damage and free radical production in subjects aged 55 and older who exercised by walking or running downhill.

- Supplementation appears to prevent the destruction of oxygen-carrying red blood cells. Therefore, your muscles benefit from improved or sustained oxygen delivery during exercise.

- Supplementation may improve exercise performance at high altitudes; however, this benefit has not been observed at sea level.

However, based on other studies, vitamin E supplementation may have some drawbacks:

- Vitamin E may actually increase oxidative stress and levels of homocysteine (a protein in the blood that can have heart-damaging effects). This was shown in triathletes who took 800 IU a day for two months.

- Vitamin E is not effective at preventing muscle damage or oxidative stress in untrained men who performed strength training for the first time. Several studies have found the same results.

- Vitamin E does not appear to decrease exercise-induced lipid peroxidation (damage to the fatty membranes of cells).
- Vitamin D failed to reduce the risk of heart disease and cancer and actually may have increased the risk of heart disease in people with diabetes or pre-existing heart problems who were taking 400 IU daily. In another study, the same dose of vitamin E nearly tripled the risk of new cancers among 540 patients undergoing cancer treatment.

So what should you do? Sport nutritionists now assert that taking 200 IU of vitamin E appears safe. This is the dosage now being recommended, although consuming vitamin E from foods rich in high-performance fat is still the best strategy. Some people can get the recommended daily intake of 30 IU by eating foods rich in vitamin E, including nuts, sunflower seeds, and vegetable oils.

If you supplement your diet with vitamin E, choose a natural form of the nutrient over a synthetic version. Labeled as d-alpha tocopherol, natural vitamin E is isolated from soybean, sunflower, corn, peanut, grapeseed, and cottonseed oils. Synthetic vitamin E, labeled as dl-alpha tocopherol, is processed from substances found in petrochemicals. A review of 30 published studies on vitamin E concluded that the natural version is absorbed better by the body than the synthetic version.

Coenzyme Q10

Coenzyme Q10 (CoQ10) is actually a lipid that acts like a vitamin and is an essential component in the body's production of energy. But it is also an antioxidant that has been widely studied. CoQ10 is present in every cell in the body and is found in the greatest concentration in tissues with high energy turnover like the heart, brain, liver, and kidney, where it acts as an antioxidant in the mitochondria and lipid membranes by itself or in conjunction with vitamin E. CoQ10 supplementation has been effective in the treatment of heart failure.

Because of its role as an antioxidant in high energy turnover tissues like muscle and heart, CoQ10 has been theorized to decrease exercise-induced inflammation and possibly increase immune function. A Japanese study published in 2015 of 18 male Kendo athletes found that those who supplemented with 300 milligrams of CoQ10 daily for 20 days, while training strenuously, had lower inflammation and stronger immune function compared to those who received a placebo. Whether coenzyme Q10 is an effective supplement for sports performance is still unknown. The research is continuing and very interesting to watch. The amount of supplemental CoQ10 for the treatment of disease is often 150 to 200 milligrams daily but can vary within a range of 90 to 390 milligrams.

Antioxidant Supplements and Performance

If you take antioxidants, will you be able to work out longer and harder? Whether any antioxidant supplementation really improves performance hasn't been adequately nailed down by research. If you are undernourished—that is, you have a vitamin deficiency—you will definitely feel better and perform better by correcting that deficiency. But if your diet is already high in antioxidants, supplementing with extra antioxidants may not make much of a difference in your performance, and may possibly diminish the benefits of your hard training.

Many fitness-minded people I have worked with follow diets that are marginally deficient in vitamin E and other antioxidants. One of the reasons is that active, health-conscious people typically go on diets that are low in fat, but dietary fat from vegetable oils, nuts, and seeds is one of the best sources of vitamin E. What's more, some active people, particularly physique athletes, limit their intake of fruit. They incorrectly believe that the fructose in fruit will end up as body fat. But by cutting out fruits, they cut out foods that are loaded with beta-carotene and vitamin C.

The amounts of vitamin C and beta-carotene that seem to be protective are easily obtained from food. To get enough of these two vitamins, follow my Power Eating recommendations in chapters 14 through 19 and throughout the book. Strive to eat five or more servings of vegetables and three or more servings of fruits every day.

B-Complex Vitamins

There are nine major B-complex vitamins—thiamin, riboflavin, niacin, vitamin B_{12}, folic acid, pyridoxine, pantothenic acid, biotin, and choline—that work in accord to ensure proper digestion, muscle contraction, and energy production. Although these nutrients do not enhance performance, training and diet do alter the body's requirement for some of them. If you are active and you restrict your calories, or if you make poor nutritional choices, then you put yourself at risk for deficiencies, particularly of thiamin, riboflavin, choline, pyridoxine, and vitamin B_{12}. Table 9.2 summarizes the exercise-related functions of the B-complex vitamins.

Thiamin

Thiamin helps release energy from carbohydrate. Thiamin, along with pyridoxine and vitamin B_{12}, is believed to be involved in the formation of serotonin, a feel-good chemical made in the brain. Serotonin helps elevate mood and induce relaxation. Large doses of these vitamins (60 to 200 times the daily requirement) have been shown to help fine motor control and performance in pistol shooting. It remains to be seen whether supplementation with these vitamins would affect performance in precision sports that depend on fine motor control.

A study published in 2011 looked into supplementation with dietary thiamin and riboflavin in college swimmers (men and women) undergoing intensive training. The study found that during intensive training, swimmers had an increased need for thiamin but not for riboflavin.

The amount of carbohydrate and calories in your diet determines your dietary requirement for thiamin. By eating a well-balanced, carbohydrate-dense diet, you generally get all the thiamin you need. The best food sources of thiamin are unrefined cereals, brewer's yeast, legumes, seeds, and nuts.

There is one possible exception, however. Are you taking a carbohydrate supplement to increase calories? If so, you may need extra thiamin, particularly if your

TABLE 9.2   B-Complex Vitamins

Thiamin (B₁)

Exercise-related function	Carbohydrate metabolism; maintenance of nervous system; growth and muscle tone.
Best food sources	Brewer's yeast, wheat germ, bran, whole grains, and organ meats.
Side effects and toxicity	None known.
DRIs for adults	Women, 1.1 mg; pregnant women, 1.4 mg; lactating women, 1.4 mg; men, 1.2 mg.

Riboflavin (B₂)

Exercise-related function	Metabolism of carbohydrate, protein, and fat; cellular respiration.
Best food sources	Milk, eggs, lean meats, and broccoli.
Side effects and toxicity	None known.
DRIs for adults	Women, 1.1 mg; pregnant women, 1.4 mg; lactating women, 1.6 mg; men, 1.3 mg.

Niacin

Exercise-related function	Cellular energy production; metabolism of carbohydrate, protein, and fat.
Best food sources	Lean meats, liver, poultry, fish, peanuts, and wheat germ.
Side effects and toxicity	Liver damage, jaundice, skin flushing and itching, nausea.
DRIs for adults	Women, 14 mg; pregnant women, 18 mg; lactating women, 17 mg; men, 16 mg.
UL for adults	35 mg.

Vitamin B₁₂

Exercise-related function	Metabolism of carbohydrate, protein, and fat; formation of red blood cells.
Best food sources	Meats, dairy products, eggs, liver, and fish. Because 10 to 30 percent of older people may malabsorb food-bound B₁₂, it is advisable for those older than age 50 to meet their DRI mainly by consuming foods fortified with B₁₂ or a supplement containing B₁₂.
Side effects and toxicity	Liver damage, allergic reactions.
DRIs for adults	Women, 2.4 mg; pregnant women, 2.6 mg; lactating women, 2.8 mg; men, 2.4 mg.

Folic acid

Exercise-related function	Regulation of growth; breakdown of protein; formation of red blood cells.
Best food sources	Green leafy vegetables and liver.

Side effects and toxicity	Gastric problems; can mask certain anemias.
DRIs for adults	Women, 400 mcg; pregnant women, 600 mcg; lactating women, 500 mcg; men, 400 mcg.
UL for adults	1,000 mcg.

Pyridoxine (B_6)

Exercise-related function	Protein metabolism; formation of oxygen-carrying red blood cells.
Best food sources	Whole grains and meats.
Side effects and toxicity	Liver and nerve damage.
DRIs for adults	Women aged 19-30, 1.3 mg; women aged 31-70, 1.5 mg; pregnant women, 1.9 mg; lactating women, 2.0 mg; men aged 19-30, 1.3 mg; men aged 31-70, 1.7 mg.
UL for adults	100 mg.

Pantothenic acid

Exercise-related function	Cellular energy production; fatty acid oxidation.
Best food sources	Found widely in foods.
Side effects and toxicity	None known.
DRIs for adults (AI)*	Women, 5 mg; pregnant women, 6 mg; lactating women, 7 mg; men, 5 mg.

Biotin

Exercise-related function	Breakdown of fat.
Best food sources	Egg yolks and liver.
Side effects and toxicity	None known.
DRIs for adults (AI)*	Women, 30 mcg; pregnant women, 30 mcg; lactating women, 35 mcg; men, 30 mcg.

Choline

Exercise-related function	May lessen fatigue and improve performance in aerobic sports.
Best food sources	Egg yolks, nuts, soybeans, wheat germ, cauliflower, and spinach.
Side effects and toxicity	None known.
DRIs for adults (AI)*	Women, 425 mg; pregnant women, 450 mg; lactating women, 550 mg; men, 550 mg.
UL for adults	3,500 mg.

If sufficient scientific evidence is not available to establish a DRI, an adequate intake (AI) is usually developed.

carbohydrate formula contains no thiamin. For every 1,000 calories of carbohydrate you consume from a formula, you need to add 0.5 milligram of thiamin to your diet.

Dieting, very low carbohydrate diets, and erratic eating patterns can leave some nutritional gaps, too. To be on the safe side, be sure to take a daily multivitamin that contains 100 percent of the DRI for thiamin or up to 1.2 milligrams of the nutrient. It is not a good idea to exceed the UL recommendation for any B vitamins.

Riboflavin

Like thiamin, riboflavin helps release energy from foods. Also as with thiamin, your dietary requirement of riboflavin is linked to your caloric and carbohydrate intake. As a strength trainer, you need to consume at least 0.6 milligram of riboflavin for every 1,000 calories of carbohydrate in your diet, and some athletes may need even more. Riboflavin is easily lost from the body, particularly in sweat. In a study of older women (aged 50 to 67), researchers at Cornell University discovered that exercise increases the body's requirement for riboflavin. An earlier study at Cornell found that very active women required about 1.2 milligrams of riboflavin a day. However, increasing riboflavin intake did not improve performance.

Foods rich in riboflavin include dairy products, poultry, fish, grains, and enriched and fortified cereals. A daily multivitamin containing 100 percent of the DRI, or up to 1.3 milligrams, of riboflavin will help prevent a shortfall.

Niacin

Like the previously mentioned B-complex vitamins, niacin is involved in releasing energy from foods. Supplementing with too much extra niacin is not a good idea and may be harmful, according to a great deal of research. For example, supplementation with extra niacin may block the release of fat from fat tissue, causing a premature reliance on the use of stored carbohydrate and depletion of muscle glycogen. It may also impair aerobic performance. Excessive amounts of niacin could also contribute to liver damage.

The amount of niacin you need each day is linked to your caloric intake. For every 1,000 calories you eat daily, you need 6.6 milligrams of niacin, or 13 milligrams for every 2,000 calories. If you are using a carbohydrate formula that contains no niacin, make sure you take 6.6 milligrams of niacin for every 1,000 calories that you supplement. The best food sources of niacin are lean meats, poultry, fish, and wheat germ. Taking a multivitamin every day will help you guard against deficiencies.

Vitamin B_{12}

Vital to healthy blood and a normal nervous system, vitamin B_{12} is the only vitamin found primarily in animal products. It works in partnership with folic acid to form red blood cells in the bone marrow.

If you are a vegetarian who eats no animal foods, you must be sure to get enough vitamin B_{12}. Fermented and cultured foods such as tempeh and miso contain some

B_{12}, as do vegetarian foods fortified with the nutrient. The safest approach is to supplement with a multivitamin containing 3 to 10 micrograms of vitamin B_{12}.

If you are over 50 years old, your ability to absorb vitamin B_{12} from food may be limited. The Institute of Medicine recommends that you consume foods fortified with B_{12} or take a vitamin B_{12} supplement.

Folic Acid

Folic acid is the vitamin that, with B_{12}, helps produce red blood cells in the bone marrow. Found in green leafy vegetables, legumes, and whole grains, it also helps reproducing cells to synthesize proteins and nucleic acids.

Folic acid first attracted attention for its role in pregnancy. During pregnancy, folic acid helps create red blood cells for the increased blood volume required by the mother, fetus, and placenta. Because of folic acid's role in the production of genetic material and red blood cells, a deficiency can have far-reaching consequences for fetal development. If the fetus is deprived of folic acid, birth defects can result. Folic acid intake is so important to women in their childbearing years that foods are now being fortified with it. The most recent findings is that pregnant women should take a multivitamin supplement to ensure that they get enough folic acid.

Female athletes also need to be aware their folic acid intake. Those with low energy availability (LEA) may be at risk of low folic acid intakes, as well as low intakes of other essential vitamins and minerals. It is critical to examine the total dietary intake of female athletes to maintain adequate intakes of essential nutrients and energy.

There is renewed excitement about folic acid because of its protective role against heart disease and cancer. It reduces homocysteine, a protein-like substance, in the tissues and blood. High homocysteine levels have been linked to heart disease. Scientists predict that as many as 50,000 premature deaths a year from heart disease can be prevented if we eat more folic acid.

Recent scientific experiments have revealed that folic acid deficiencies cause DNA damage resembling the DNA damage in cancer cells. This finding has led scientists to suggest that cancer could be initiated by DNA damage caused by a deficiency in this B-complex vitamin. Other studies show that folic acid suppresses cell growth in colorectal cancer. It also prevents the formation of precancerous lesions that could lead to cervical cancer, a discovery that may explain why women who don't eat many vegetables and fruits (good sources of folic acid) have high rates of this form of cancer.

Stress, disease, and alcohol consumption all increase your need for folic acid. You should make sure that you're getting 400 micrograms a day of this vitamin, a level that is found in most multivitamins.

Pyridoxine

Pyridoxine, also known as vitamin B_6, is required for the metabolism of protein. It's also vital in the formation of red blood cells and the healthy functioning of the brain through its role in the synthesis of all neurotransmitters. The best food sources of pyridoxine are protein foods such as chicken, fish, and eggs. Other good sources are brown rice, soybeans, oats, and whole wheat.

Ever feel anxious before an athletic competition? If so, try supplementing with a cocktail of pyridoxine, thiamin, and vitamin B_{12}. By increasing levels of serotonin—a mood-elevating chemical in the brain—this trio has been found to reduce anxiety and thus improve competitive performance.

The DRI for pyridoxine ranges from 1.3 to 2.0 milligrams (see table 9.2 for details). If you're wondering whether your own intake of pyridoxine falls within safe bounds, rest assured that it probably does. A training diet that contains moderate amounts of protein will give you all the pyridoxine you need. In other words, there's no need to supplement. Besides, large doses (in excess of 50 milligrams a day) can cause nerve damage.

Pantothenic Acid

Pantothenic acid participates in the release of energy from carbohydrate, fat, and protein. Because this vitamin is so widely distributed in foods (particularly meats, whole grains, and legumes), it is rare to find a deficiency without a drop in other B-complex vitamins. They all work as a team.

The safe range of intake for pantothenic acid is 4 to 7 milligrams a day. Exercise does affect pantothenic acid metabolism but only to a slight degree. By following my strength-training nutrition plan in chapters 15 to 19, you'll take in plenty of this vitamin, enough to cover any extra needs you might have as a result of exercise.

Biotin

Biotin is involved in fat and carbohydrate metabolism. Without it, the body can't burn fat. Biotin is also a component of various enzymes that carry out essential biochemical reactions in the body. Some good sources of biotin are egg yolks, soy flour, and cereals. Even if you don't get the 30 to 100 micrograms you need daily from food, your body can synthesize biotin from intestinal bacteria. So there's no reason to supplement with extra biotin.

Together with choline and inositol, two other B-complex members, biotin is often found in lipotropic (prevents or reduces fat accumulation in the liver) supplements promoted as fat burners. However, there is no credible evidence that biotin or any other supplemental nutrient burns fat.

Some research shows that biotin levels are low in active people. No one is sure why, but one explanation is that it may have to do with exercise. Exercise causes lactic acid, a waste product, to build up in working muscles, and biotin is involved in the process that breaks down lactic acid. The more lactic acid that accumulates in muscles, the more biotin is needed to break it down. But don't rush out to buy a bottle of biotin. There is no need to supplement with this vitamin, because your body can make up for any marginal deficiencies on its own.

Although not so popular anymore, there are still strength trainers who are in the habit of concocting raw-egg milkshakes. Raw egg white contains avidin, a protein that binds with biotin in the intestine and prevents its absorption. Eating raw eggs (this includes pasteurized egg whites) on a consistent basis can thus lead to a biotin deficiency. But once eggs are cooked, the avidin is destroyed, and there is no danger of blocking biotin absorption.

Choline

Present in all living cells, choline is another B-complex vitamin. It is synthesized from two amino acids, methionine and serine, with help from vitamin B_{12} and folic acid. Choline works with inositol, another lipotropic dietary factor, to prevent fat from building up in the liver and to shuttle fat into cells to be burned for energy.

Choline is involved in the formation of the neurotransmitter acetylcholine in the body, as I explained in chapter 8. If acetylcholine is reduced in the nervous system, fatigue may set in. Because acetylcholine is the most abundant neurotransmitter in the body, acting every time we think or move, it's not surprising that low levels would lead to fatigue. Additionally, choline plays a central role in many other physiological pathways, including the cell membrane signaling involved in brain function and the methyl-group metabolism involved in hormone and energy metabolism.

Researchers at MIT studied runners before and after the Boston Marathon and found a 40 percent drop in their plasma choline concentrations. They don't know why this happened; however, they speculated that choline is used up during exercise to produce acetylcholine. Once choline is depleted, there's a corresponding drop in acetylcholine production, and when production falls off, the ability to do muscular work falls off.

A 2008 review published in the *International Journal of Sport Nutrition and Exercise Metabolism* pointed out that strenuous and prolonged physical activity may decrease circulating choline stores. Supplementing with choline prevents this, and may even improve endurance. The longer and harder you train, the more choline you use, and possibly use up.

Choline is best absorbed when taken as phosphatidylcholine (PC), which is the body's natural reservoir of choline and is also available as a supplement. PC is the major building block for all cell membranes, and it supports cell, tissue, and organ functions. Supplementing with PC helps maintain sufficient choline reserves for good health.

You can also boost absorption by taking PC with phosphatidylserine (PS), another key building block for cell membranes. PS dietary supplements also may help you improve your athletic performance by suppressing cortisol, a potent, catabolic (breakdown) stress hormone. Too much cortisol in the body, which can result from intense workouts, may have negative effects on your training, performance, and physique. Research has shown that short-term oral supplementation of 750 milligrams per day of phosphatidylserine for 10 days improves exercise capacity during high-intensity cycling and increases running performance. Supplementing with PS is a natural, drug-free choice for athletes who want to overcome the effects of exercise-induced stress.

Most vitamin supplements contain choline, and you should make sure to consume at least the DRI for choline daily. The effective dosage in sport studies is 0.2

gram of phosphatidylcholine per kilogram of body mass. This does not need to be any kind of loading strategy but can just be a maintenance program. The effective dosages for phosphatidylserine in exercise studies range from 300 to 800 milligrams per day for 10 to 15 days.

Other Vitamins

The fat-soluble vitamins A, D, and K are rarely promoted as exercise aids, most likely because they're toxic in large doses. Vitamin A, or retinol, is found primarily in animal sources such as liver, fish, liver oils, margarine, milk, butter, and eggs. Vitamin A is involved in the growth and repair of tissues, the maintenance of proper vision, and resistance against infection. It also helps maintain the health of the skin and mucous membranes. Massive doses in excess of the DRI can cause nausea, vomiting, diarrhea, skin problems, and bone fragility, among other serious problems.

Including beta-carotene, also known as previtamin A, is a safe way to ensure good vitamin A status and boost your antioxidant consumption. You have a natural governor in your body controlling vitamin A production: You will manufacture vitamin A from beta-carotene only if your body needs it. The best food sources of beta-carotene are orange, red, yellow, and dark green vegetables and fruits.

Vitamin D

Contrary to what most people believe, vitamin D is not a vitamin but a steroid hormone. It is produced in various parts of the body but exerts its influence elsewhere in the body—which is what hormones do. Your body can manufacture vitamin D on its own when your skin is exposed to sunlight. Just 15 minutes a day with your legs and face exposed to the sun without sunscreen several days a week usually supplies sufficient amounts of vitamin D. If you can't get out in the sun, live in northern climates where there is not too much sunlight, or frequently wear sunscreen, you may need to take supplements. The form of vitamin D manufactured by the liver and measured in the bloodstream is called calcidiol, or 25 hydroxyvitamin D-2. The activated vitamin D steroid hormone is processed by the kidneys and is known as calcitriol, or 25 hydroxyvitamin D-3. Calcitriol circulates as a hormone in your body regulating the amounts of calcium and phosphate in your bloodstream and maintaining the health of your bones.

As a steroid hormone, vitamin D regulates more than 1,000 vitamin D–responsive human genes and may influence athletic performance, particularly if you are deficient in this nutrient. Numerous studies over many decades have revealed that physical and athletic performance peaks when 25 hydroxyvitamin D-2 levels peak in the summertime and declines as the steroid hormone declines in the body in the wintertime. Athletes tend to have low vitamin D levels in winter, according to a number of studies. Several studies also document low vitamin D levels in athletes that participate in indoor sports. If you're an older athlete, make sure you get enough vitamin D from food and supplements, because elderly people are typically deficient in this nutrient. Supplements with vitamin D have been shown in numerous studies to boost performance in both younger and older adults with low blood levels of vitamin D.

Studies show that vitamin D reduces the risk for sport-related conditions such as stress fractures, total body inflammation, infections, and muscular function. Thus, raising your levels of vitamin D can reduce inflammation, pain, muscle weakness, and muscle-loss myopathy, while increasing muscle protein synthesis, ATP concentration, strength, jump height, jump velocity, jump power, exercise capacity, and physical performance. Vitamin D levels above 40 nanograms per milliliter of blood are required for fracture prevention, including stress fractures. Optimal musculoskeletal benefits occur when vitamin D is higher than 30 nanograms per milliliter of blood but not higher than 50 nanograms per milliliter.

In 2015, medical researchers went to the NFL and collected blood to study the vitamin D levels of 214 athletes among the athletes in attendance. Interestingly, inadequate vitamin D was present in 59 percent of the athletes, including 10 percent with deficient levels. Lower extremity muscle strain or core muscle injury was present in 50 percent of athletes, which was significantly associated with lower vitamin D levels. Athletes who had suffered numerous injuries also showed significantly lower vitamin D levels as compared with uninjured athletes. Even though football players practice outside during the heat of the day in the sunny summer months, they are typically somewhat covered up, blocking the sun's rays from reaching their skin and raising levels of vitamin D.

There is also a connection between vitamin D and weight management. Vitamin D helps your body better absorb calcium, which has a fat-burning effect. So for calcium to assist in fat burning, your body requires sufficient vitamin D. On the other hand, if the calcium levels in your body are low, a hormone called parathyroid hormone (PTH) and vitamin D increase in response to the shortage and trick your body into thinking it is starving. Consequently, you may pack away more calories in the form of fat and put on extra weight when this imbalance occurs.

Eight Reasons to Pump Up Your Vitamin D

1. Supports bone health
2. Bolsters immunity
3. Boosts mood when taken with the omega-3 fatty acid DHA
4. Assists in neuromuscular control
5. Helps regulate body weight
6. Helps prevent aging-related inflammation
7. Lengthens telomeres (a factor in longevity)
8. Decreases the risk of many chronic and degenerative diseases

To obtain enough vitamin D, don't rely on supplements alone. Instead, get at least 10 to 15 minutes of sun exposure daily during the summer months, and all year long if you live south of the 37th latitude. Also, include vitamin D-rich foods in your diet: fatty fish and fortified milk products. And, include vitamin D supplements as part of your daily routine. Each of us absorbs vitamin D differently, but the current recommendation for supplementation is 600 to 2,000 IU of the nutrient daily.

Vitamin K

The primary function of vitamin K is to assist in the process of normal blood clotting. It is also required for the formation of other kinds of body protein found in the blood, bone, and kidneys. However, research has revealed another side to vitamin K that most people were not aware of: It is vital for building healthy bones, which is why a number of calcium supplements are now being formulated with vitamin K. With a shortfall of vitamin K, bone can become weakened because of insufficient levels of osteocalcin, a protein involved in bone hardening. In one study with female athletes, 10 milligrams daily of vitamin K decreased the process of bone breakdown and increased bone formation. These improvements were measured by looking at the amount of osteocalcin (an indicator of bone formation), as well as at by-products of bone breakdown in the bloodstream and urine.

A vitamin K deficiency is extremely rare, and there's usually no need for supplementation unless recommended by your physician. The best food sources are dairy products, meats, eggs, cereals, fruits, and vegetables. The functions of vitamins A, D, and K and their possible roles in exercise performance are summarized in table 9.3.

Minerals and Performance

Minerals found naturally in food are particularly important to exercisers and athletes because of their involvement in muscle contraction, normal heart rhythm, oxygen transport, transmission of nerve impulses, immune function, and bone health. If you are not adequately nourished with minerals, a deficiency could harm your health, and this in turn could adversely affect your performance. What follows is a look at various minerals that can have a bearing on your performance. The functions of major and trace minerals are summarized in table 9.4.

Electrolytes

The tissues in your body contain fluids both inside cells (intracellular fluid) and in the spaces between cells (extracellular fluid). Dissolved in both fluids are electrolytes, which are electrically charged minerals or ions. The electrolytes work in concert, regulating water balance on either side of the cell membranes. Electrolytes also help make muscles contract by promoting the transmission of messages across nerve cell membranes. Electrolyte balance is critical to optimal performance and overall health. The two chief electrolytes are sodium and potassium. Sodium regulates fluid balance outside cells, whereas potassium regulates fluids inside cells.

TABLE 9.3   Vitamins A, D, and K

Vitamin A	
Exercise-related function	Growth and repair of tissues, including muscles; building of body structures.
Best food sources	Liver, egg yolks, whole milk, and orange and yellow vegetables.
Side effects and toxicity	Digestive system upset, damage to bones and certain organs.
DRIs for adults	Women, 700 mcg; pregnant women, 770 mcg; lactating women, 1,300 mcg; men, 900 mcg.
UL for adults	3,000 mcg.
Vitamin D	
Exercise-related function	Normal bone growth and development.
Best food sources	Sunlight, fortified dairy products, and fish oils.
Side effects and toxicity	Nausea, vomiting, hardening of soft tissues, kidney damage.
DRIs for adults	Women aged 19-70, 15 mcg; women aged 71+, 20 mcg; pregnant women, 15 mcg; lactating women, 15 mcg; men aged 19-70, 15 mcg; men aged 70+, 20 mcg.
UL for adults	100 mcg or 4,000 IU.
Vitamin K	
Exercise-related function	Involved in glycogen formation, blood clotting, and bone formation.
Best food sources	Vegetables, milk, and yogurt.
Side effects and toxicity	Allergic reactions, breakdown of red blood cells.
DRIs for adults (AI)	Women, 90 mcg; men, 120 mcg.

Sodium is obtained mostly from salt and processed foods. On average, Americans eat 2 to 3 teaspoons (12-18 g) of salt every day—far too much for good health. A healthier sodium target is 500 milligrams (the minimum requirement) to 2,400 milligrams per day, or no more than 1/4 teaspoon (1.6 g) of table salt each day.

Although some sodium can be lost from sweat during exercise, you don't have to worry about replacing it with supplements. Your usual diet contains enough sodium to replace what was lost. What's more, the body does a good job of conserving sodium on its own.

Severe sodium depletion, however, can occur during ultraendurance events such as triathlons that last more than four hours. Consuming 1/2 to 3/4 of a cup (120-180 ml) of sport drink every 10 to 20 minutes, along with adding salty foods to the diet, is enough to replenish most endurance athletes' needs for sodium. Thus, during an endurance event lasting longer than three hours, you want to have a

TABLE 9.4 Major Minerals and Trace Minerals

Major	
Calcium	
Exercise-related function	A constituent of body structures; plays a part in muscle growth, muscle contraction, and nerve transmission.
Best food sources	Dairy products and green leafy vegetables.
Side effects and toxicity	Excessive calcification of some tissues, constipation, mineral absorption problems.
DRIs for adults	Women aged 19-50, 1,000 mg; women aged 51+, 1,200 mg; pregnant women, 1,000 mg; lactating women, 1,000 mg; men aged 19-70, 1,000 mg; men aged 71+, 1,200 mg.
UL for adults	2,500 mg.
Phosphorus	
Exercise-related function	Metabolism of carbohydrate, protein, and fat; growth, repair, and maintenance of cells; energy production; stimulation of muscular contractions.
Best food sources	Meats, fish, poultry, eggs, whole grains, seeds, and nuts.
Side effects and toxicity	None known.
DRIs for adults	700 mg.
UL for adults	Women and men aged 19-70, 4,000 mg; aged 71+, 3,000 mg.
Potassium	
Exercise-related function	Maintenance of normal fluid balance on either side of cell walls; normal growth; stimulation of nerve impulses for muscular contractions; conversion of glucose to glycogen; synthesis of muscle protein from amino acids.
Best food sources	Potatoes, bananas, fruits, and vegetables.
Side effects and toxicity	Heart disturbances.
DRIs for adults (AI)	4.7 g; lactating women, 5.1 g.
Sodium	
Exercise-related function	Maintenance of normal fluid balance on either side of cell walls; muscular contraction and nerve transmission; keeps other blood minerals soluble.
Best food sources	Found in virtually all foods.
Side effects and toxicity	Water retention, high blood pressure.
DRIs for adults (AI)*	Women and men aged 19-50, 1.5 g; women and men aged 51-70, 1.3 g; women and men aged 71+, 1.2 g; pregnant and lactating women, 1.5 g.

Chloride

Exercise-related function	Helps regulate the pressure that causes fluids to flow in and out of cell membranes.
Best food sources	Table salt (sodium chloride), kelp, and rye flour.
Side effects and toxicity	None known.
DRIs for adults (AI)	Women and men aged 19-50, 2.3 g; women and men aged 51-70, 2.0 g; women and men aged 71+, 1.8 g; pregnant and lactating women, 2.3 g.

Magnesium

Exercise-related function	Metabolism of carbohydrate and protein; assists in muscular contractions.
Best food sources	Green vegetables, legumes, whole grains, and seafood.
Side effects and toxicity	Large amounts are toxic.
DRIs for adults	Women aged 19-30, 310 mg; women aged 31+, 320 mg; pregnant women aged 19-30, 350 mg; pregnant women aged 31+, 360 mg; lactating women aged 19-30, 310 mg; lactating women aged 31+, 320 mg; men aged 19-30, 400 mg; men aged 31+, 420 mg.
UL for adults	350 mg from supplements alone.

Trace

Iron

Exercise-related function	Oxygen transport to cells for energy; formation of oxygen-carrying red blood cells.
Best food sources	Liver, oysters, lean meats, and green leafy vegetables.
Side effects and toxicity	Large amounts are toxic.
DRIs for adults	Women aged 19-50, 18 mg; women aged 51+, 8 mg; pregnant women, 27 mg; lactating women, 9 mg; men, 8 mg.
UL for adults	45 mg.

Iodine

Exercise-related function	Energy production; growth and development; metabolism.
Best food sources	Iodized salt, seafood, and mushrooms.
Side effects and toxicity	Thyroid enlargement.
DRIs for adults	150 mcg; pregnant women, 220 mcg; lactating women, 290 mcg.
UL for adults	1,000 mcg.

Chromium

Exercise-related function	Normal blood sugar; fat metabolism.
Best food sources	Corn oil, brewer's yeast, whole grains, and meats.
Side effects and toxicity	Liver and kidney damage.

> *continued*

TABLE 9.4 > *continued*

Trace	
Chromium (continued)	
DRIs for adults (AI)	Women aged 19-50, 25 mcg; women aged 51+, 20 mcg; pregnant women, 30 mcg; lactating women, 45 mcg; men aged 19-50, 35 mcg; men aged 51+, 30 mcg.
Fluoride	
Exercise-related function	None known.
Best food sources	Fluoridated water supplies.
Side effects and toxicity	Large amounts are toxic and can cause mottling of teeth.
DRIs for adults (AI)	Women, 3 mg; men, 4 mg.
UL for adults	10 mg.
Molybdenum	
Exercise-related function	Involved in the metabolism of fat.
Best food sources	Milk, beans, breads, and cereals.
Side effects and toxicity	Diarrhea, anemia, and depressed growth rate.
DRIs for adults	45 mcg; pregnant and lactating women, 50 mcg.
UL for adults	2,000 mcg.
Boron	
Exercise-related function	No clear biological function in humans has been identified.
Best food sources	Fruit-based beverages and products, potatoes, legumes, milk, avocados, peanut butter, and peanuts.
Side effects and toxicity	Reproductive and developmental effects as observed in animals.
DRIs for adults	None established.
UL for adults	20 mg.
Vanadium	
Exercise-related function	No clear biological function in humans has been identified.
Best food sources	Mushrooms, shellfish, black pepper, parsley, and dill seed.
Side effects and toxicity	Large doses are extremely toxic and may cause excessive fatigue.
DRIs for adults	None established.

Note: Other important minerals that can affect your performance include zinc and selenium, which are included in table 9.1.

sport drink containing 200 to 300 milligrams of sodium per 8 ounces (240 ml). To restore fluid balance during recovery after endurance exercise, you need sodium in your beverage because it lets water enter your cells.

Drinking too much plain water (overhydration), however, can cause sodium and other electrolytes to become overly diluted. This imbalance can negatively affect performance.

Potassium works inside cells to regulate fluid balance. Potassium is also involved in maintaining a regular heartbeat, helping muscles contract, regulating blood pressure, and transferring nutrients to cells.

In contrast to sodium, potassium is not as well conserved by the body, so you should be sure to eat plenty of potassium-rich foods such as bananas, oranges, and potatoes. You need between 1,600 and 2,000 milligrams of potassium a day, which can be easily obtained from a diet plentiful in fruits and vegetables.

To get cut, some competitive bodybuilders use diuretics, drugs that increase the formation and excretion of urine in the body. This is a dangerous practice because diuretics can flush potassium and other electrolytes from the body. Life-threatening mineral imbalances can occur, and some professional bodybuilders have died during competition as a result of diuretic abuse. I can see no rational reason for taking diuretics for competitive purposes. The potential damage just isn't worth it.

Other Vital Minerals

Several other minerals could be low in your diet, particularly if you're a competitor and you frequently follow restrictive cutting diets.

Calcium

Ninety-nine percent of the calcium in the body is stored in the skeleton and teeth. The other 1 percent is found in blood and soft tissues. Calcium is responsible for building healthy bones, conducting nerve impulses, helping muscles contract, and moving nutrients into and out of cells. Exercise helps your body better absorb calcium. At the same time, high-intensity endurance exercise may cause your body to excrete calcium.

The chief sources of calcium in the diet are milk and other dairy products. However, almost every strength trainer and bodybuilder I have ever counseled has avoided dairy products like the plague during precompetition dieting. They believe that these foods are high in sodium, but I say that's nonsense. One cup (240 ml) of nonfat milk contains 126 milligrams of sodium and 302 milligrams of calcium. Two egg whites, a popular food in the diet of strength trainers and bodybuilders, contain 212 milligrams of sodium and only 12 milligrams of calcium. Sodium hardly seems to be a problem here, and there is no better low-fat source of calcium than nonfat milk.

So are milk and dairy products really your enemy? Absolutely not. As I pointed out earlier, milk in particular contains two proteins (whey and casein) that are involved in muscle building, fat burning, and recovery. (See chapter 2 for more information on these important milk proteins and how to use them.)

There's more to this story, however, and it has to do with the calcium in milk and dairy products. A number of studies show that this mineral may help you manage your weight. How? Calcium may assist the body in the breakdown of body fat. It appears that the more calcium a fat cell contains, the more fat the cell will burn.

In one widely publicized study, 32 obese adults were randomly assigned to one of the following diets for 24 weeks: (1) a standard diet containing 400 to

500 milligrams per day of calcium plus a placebo supplement; (2) a standard diet supplemented with 800 milligrams per day of calcium; or (3) a diet containing three servings per day of dairy products, providing 1,200 to 1,300 milligrams per day of calcium, plus a placebo supplement. Each diet cut calories by 500 calories a day. By the end of the experimental period, the average weight loss was 14.5 pounds (6.6 kg) with the standard diet, 19 pounds (8.6 kg) with the calcium-supplemented diet, and about 24.5 pounds (11 kg) with the high-dairy diet. Fat loss from the trunk region represented 19 percent of total fat loss on the standard diet, 50 percent of total fat loss on the calcium-supplemented diet, and 66.2 percent of total fat loss on the high-dairy diet.

In sum, dietary calcium intake clearly enhanced weight loss and fat loss in obese subjects who followed a reduced-calorie diet. Interestingly, higher calcium intake increased the percentage of fat lost from the trunk region. Finally, consuming calcium in the form of dairy products was significantly more effective than taking calcium supplements. I have to add here, however, that the last finding, though significant, should be interpreted cautiously, because the study was funded by the National Dairy Council.

But the story doesn't end with dairy calcium alone. In a study of mother-daughter pairs in Poland, different dietary patterns that included dairy, and it's contribution to total dietary calcium, were investigated relative to the influence on obesity, waist circumference, weight-to-height ratio, BMI, and body composition. Despite having a calcium intake that was generally lower than the estimated adequate requirement (EAR) for calcium, mothers who included regular dairy foods in the dietary patterns had a significantly decreased incidence of obesity, and daughters had a significantly increased incidence of thinness. High-fat dairy foods and beverages contributed to even better outcomes of decreased waist circumference and central adiposity, dispelling the idea that high-fat dairy will lead to overconsumption of calories and fat gain. The authors theorize that specific dairy fats may reduce oxidation and chronic inflammation, enhancing calcium absorption. Other factors such as dairy casein and lactose also increase calcium bioavailability, as well as the ability of calcium to bind unconjugated bile acids and free fatty acids from the gastrointestinal tract and prevent fat absorption.

No one knows yet whether calcium from other foods such as leafy greens has the same effect. Additional research needs to be conducted to ascertain similar benefits. The take-home message is that if you're trying to drop weight, don't drop dairy products, and be sure to select low-fat products.

Overall, the calcium in dairy foods is essential to maintaining good health. With plenty of high-calcium foods, your diet provides the calcium needed to maintain healthy blood calcium levels. If you don't have enough in your diet, your body will draw calcium from bones to maintain blood calcium levels. As more and more calcium is removed from bones, they become brittle and break. The most susceptible areas are the spine, hips, and wrists. An exit of calcium from the bones can lead to the bone-weakening disease osteoporosis.

It is vital to obtain calcium by eating calcium-rich foods—namely, nonfat milk and dairy products. If for some reason you cannot or will not drink milk, try nonfat yogurts. They are equally high in calcium, and they often do not cause the intestinal problems that some people experience from milk. You can also obtain calcium from alternative sources if you are on a milk-free diet. Table 9.5 lists those sources.

Some people are lactose intolerant and can't digest milk. They lack sufficient lactase, the enzyme required to digest lactose, a sugar in milk that helps you absorb calcium from the intestine. If you are lactose intolerant, try taking an enzyme-replacement product such as Lactaid. These products replace the lactase you are

TABLE 9.5   Alternative Sources of Calcium for Milk-Free Diets

Food	Amount	Calcium (mg)	Calories
Collards, frozen, cooked*	1/2 cup (95 g)	179	31
Soy milk (fortified)	1 cup (240 ml)	150	79
Mackerel, canned	2 oz (56 g)	137	88
Dandelion greens, raw, cooked*	1/2 cup (53 g)	74	17
Turnip greens, frozen, cooked*	1/2 cup (72 g)	125	25
Mustard greens, frozen, cooked*	1/2 cup (75 g)	76	14
Kale, frozen, cooked*	1/2 cup (65 g)	90	20
Tortillas, corn	2	80	95
Molasses, blackstrap	1 tbsp (21 g)	176	48
Orange	1 large	74	87
Sockeye salmon, canned, with bone, drained	2 oz (60 g)	136	87
Sardines, canned, with bone, drained	2 medium	92	50
Boston baked beans (navy or pea bean), vegetarian, canned	1/2 cup (127 g)	64	118
Pickled herring	2 oz (60 g)	44	149
Soybeans, cooked	1/2 cup (90 g)	88	149
Broccoli, cooked	1/2 cup (78 g)	36	22
Rutabaga (Swedish or yellow turnip), cooked, mashed	1/2 cup (120 g)	58	47
Artichoke, cooked	1 medium	54	60
White beans, cooked	1/2 cup (90 g)	81	124
Almonds, blanched, whole	1/4 cup (36 g)	94	222
Tofu	2 oz (60 g)	60	44

*Frozen, cooked vegetable greens are higher in calcium than fresh, cooked greens. If you eat the fresh variety, you need to double your portion to get the same amount of calcium.

TABLE 9.6   A Day's Worth of Calcium

Food	Amount	Calcium (mg)	Calories
Orange juice, calcium fortified	1 cup (240 ml)	300	112
Nonfat milk	1 cup (240 ml)	301	86
Tofu	4 oz (120 g)	120	88
Low-fat yogurt, fruit	8 oz (230 g)	372	250
Mozzarella cheese, part-skim	1 oz (30 g)	229	73
Turnip greens cooked, chopped	1 cup (72 g)	250	60
Total		**1,572**	**669**

missing and will digest the lactose for you. Another option is Lactaid milk. Available at most supermarkets, Lactaid milk is pretreated with the lactase enzyme.

Calcium supplements may be in order, too. The most bioavailable source of calcium as a supplement is calcium citrate. Calcium supplements are best taken with all of the other bone-building minerals such as magnesium, boron, and vitamin D.

The DRIs for calcium from food and supplements are 1,000 milligrams for women and men aged 19 to 50, and 1,200 milligrams for women and men aged 51 and over (see table 9.4). The National Institutes of Health (NIH) recommends supplementation with calcium and vitamin D (which helps the body absorb calcium) by people not getting the DRIs, including women who develop the female athlete triad. If you have some calcium in your diet, don't take all 1,000 or 1,200 milligrams of calcium in a supplement. Too much calcium in the diet can cause kidney stones in some people.

For the prevention and treatment of osteoporosis in postmenopausal women, many physicians recommend 1,500 milligrams of calcium daily. Table 9.6 illustrates how to get a day's worth of calcium from food.

Iron

The major role of iron is to combine with protein to make hemoglobin, a special protein that gives red blood cells their color. Hemoglobin carries oxygen in the blood from the lungs to the tissues. Iron is also necessary for the formation of myoglobin, found only in muscle tissue. Myoglobin transports oxygen to muscle cells to be used in the chemical reaction that makes muscles contract.

As a strength trainer or bodybuilder, you are constantly tearing down and rebuilding muscle tissue. This process can create an additional need for iron, a mineral that is enormously essential to human health. What's more, there seems to be a common increase in iron losses from aerobic exercises or sports that involve pounding of the feet, such as jogging, aerobic dancing, and step aerobics. Also at risk for low iron are women who exercise more than three hours a week, have been pregnant within the past two years, or eat fewer than 2,200 calories a day.

Low iron can impair muscular performance. A shortfall of iron can lead to iron-deficiency anemia, the final stage of iron loss, characterized by a hemoglobin concentration below the normal level. Athletic training does tend to deplete iron stores for a number of reasons, including physical stress and muscle damage. Another reason for low iron and iron-deficiency anemia is an inadequate intake of iron. Studies of the diets of female athletes, who likely need to take in even more than the daily requirement (18 mg) to compensate for training-induced losses, indicate daily intakes of roughly 12 milligrams. Other possible reasons for low iron are losses that occur in the gastrointestinal tract, in sweat, and through menstruation.

The best sources of dietary iron are liver and other organ meats, lean meat, and oysters. Iron is found in green leafy vegetables, too, although iron from plant sources is not as well absorbed as iron from animal protein.

Strength trainers and other active people tend to shy away from iron-rich meats because of their high fat content. But you can increase the iron in your diet without adding a lot of beef or animal fat. If you don't eat any meat at all, you must pay careful attention to make sure that you get the iron you need. Here are some suggestions:

- Eat fruits, vegetables, and grains that are high in iron. You won't get as much iron as from animal foods, but the plant foods are the lowest in fat. Green leafy vegetables such as kale and collards, dried fruits such as raisins and apricots, and iron-enriched and fortified breads and cereals are all good plant sources of iron.

- Enhance your body's absorption of iron by combining foods high in iron with a rich source of vitamin C, which improves iron absorption. For example, drink some orange juice with your iron-fortified cereal with raisins for breakfast. Or sprinkle some lemon juice on your kale or collards.

- Avoid eating very high-fiber foods at the same meal with foods high in iron. The fiber inhibits the absorption of iron and many other minerals. Avoid drinking tea and taking antacids with high-iron foods; they also inhibit the absorption of iron.

- Try to keep some meat in or add some meat to your diet. Lean red meat and the dark meat of chicken and turkey are highest in iron. Eating 3 to 4 ounces (90-120 g) of meat three times a week will give your iron levels a real boost. And if you combine your meat with a vegetable source of iron, you will absorb more of the iron from the vegetables.

- You might need an iron supplement. Eight milligrams for men and 18 milligrams for women 19 to 50 years old, or 100 percent of the DRI for iron, may be a big help. Don't pop huge doses of iron, though. The more iron you take at one time, the less your body will absorb. Also, excess iron can lead to hemochromatosis, a disorder that causes iron buildup in major organs and the eventual deterioration of liver function.

Zinc

Zinc, one of the antioxidant minerals, is important for hundreds of body processes, including maintaining normal taste and smell, regulating growth, and promoting wound healing.

My research has revealed that female bodybuilders, in particular, don't get enough zinc in their diets. Zinc is an important mineral for people who work out. As you exercise, zinc helps clear lactic acid buildup in the blood. In addition, zinc supplementation (25 mg a day) has been shown to protect immunity during periods of intense training.

There is not much research on zinc supplementation and exercise performance. Interestingly, though, one study shows that if you're an endurance athlete who follows a diet that is rich in carbohydrate but low in protein and fat, you could be setting yourself up for a zinc deficiency, resulting in a loss of too much body weight, greater fatigue, and poor endurance.

Too much zinc might be a bad thing, however. It has been associated with lower levels of good cholesterol (HDL) and thus may increase your risk of cardiovascular disease. What's more, excess zinc over time may create mineral imbalances and produce undesirable changes in two substances involved in calcium metabolism: calcitonin, a hormone that boosts calcium in bones by drawing it from soft tissue, and osteocalcin, the key noncollagen protein needed to help harden bone.

By eating zinc-rich foods, you can get just the right amount, which is 8 milligrams a day for women and 11 milligrams a day for men. The best sources of zinc are meat, eggs, seafood (especially oysters), and whole grains. If you restrict your intake of meat, taking a multivitamin-multimineral each day will help fill in the nutritional blanks.

Magnesium

Magnesium, a mineral that is in charge of more than 400 metabolic reactions in the body, has been touted as an exercise aid. One study hints at a link between magnesium and muscle strength. Men in a test group were given 500 milligrams of magnesium a day, an increase of 100 milligrams over the DRI of 400 milligrams. Those in a control group took 250 milligrams a day, significantly less than the DRI. After both groups weight trained for eight weeks, their leg strength was measured. The supplemented men got stronger, whereas those in the control group stayed the same. But many researchers are not yet convinced that magnesium is a strength builder. They caution that the magnesium status of the subjects before the study was unknown. Generally, magnesium consumption is a bit below recommended levels, and may be even lower in the diets of athletes who restrict their energy, carbohydrate, or fat consumption. Therefore, moderately low magnesium status may be common among strength trainers. That's an important point, because supplementing with any nutrient in which you are deficient is likely to produce some positive changes in performance and health. Basically, the current train of scientific thought on magnesium supplementation is that it does not affect aerobic power or muscle strength.

Magnesium promotes calcium absorption and helps in the function of nerves and muscles, including heartbeat regulation. The DRI for magnesium for men ranges from 400 to 420 milligrams, and for women, 310 to 360 milligrams (see table 9.4). The best dietary sources of magnesium are nuts, legumes, whole grains, dark green

Food First

Always count on food first. Food is your body's best source of vitamins and minerals. Take the time to plan a healthy, well-balanced diet full of fruits, vegetables, grains, beans, lean meats, and dairy foods, and use the diet-planning guidelines in chapter 13. Along with dedicated training, a good diet with the correct balance of protein, the right kinds of carbohydrate, and the right kinds of fat is your best ticket to building a better body.

---

vegetables, and seafood. These foods should be plentiful in your diet. You can also supplement these foods with a daily multivitamin-multimineral formulated with 100 percent of the DRI for magnesium.

Selenium

An antioxidant mineral, selenium works in partnership with vitamin E to fight damaging free radicals. Selenium is vital for a healthy immune system, boosting your defenses against bacteria and viruses, and it may reduce the risk of certain cancers, particularly in the prostate, colon, and lungs. As for performance, some studies have shown that selenium reduces lipid peroxidation after prolonged aerobic exercise, but this effect did not enhance athletic endurance in people who supplemented with selenium.

Selenium is found naturally in fish, meat, wheat germ, nuts (particularly brazil nuts), eggs, oatmeal, whole-wheat bread, and brown rice. Most people have to make sure they eat foods rich in selenium to get enough. You can supplement but do so carefully. There is a narrow margin between the DRI of 55 micrograms and the UL of 400 micrograms.

10

Muscle-Building Products

You train hard. You're building body-hard muscle. Still, you want to know if there isn't something else—besides intense workouts and healthy food—that can help you gain a little faster, something that will give you a muscle-building edge with less effort.

Yes, there definitely is. In fact, there are several things you can do to pack on lean muscle. Unfortunately, not all of them are safe—or legal. Anabolic steroids, although approved for medical use and available by prescription only, are among the most abused drugs among athletes. *Anabolic* means "to build," and anabolic steroids tend to make the body grow in certain ways. They do have muscle-building effects, but they're also dangerous. Once practiced mainly by elite athletes, abuse of anabolic steroids has spread to recreational and teen athletes and is now a national health concern. The 2010 Monitoring the Future study funded by the National Institute on Drug Abuse showed that 0.5 percent of 8th-graders, 1.0 percent of 10th-graders, and 1.5 percent of 12th-graders had abused anabolic steroids at least once in the year prior to being surveyed. Table 10.1 lists some of the dangers associated with these drugs.

A trend related to anabolic steroid abuse is the use of androstenedione and androstenediol, prohormones or precursors to testosterone. Testosterone is the male hormone responsible for building muscle and revving up the sex drive. Legally considered a controlled substance in the same category as anabolic steroids, androstenedione is not without side effects, including acne, hair loss in genetically susceptible people, abnormal growth of breast tissue (gynecomastia), negative blood cholesterol profiles that can lead to the increased risk of heart disease, and potentially reduced testosterone output. Use of this family of compounds may also result in a positive drug test.

TABLE 10.1 Health Dangers of Anabolic Steroids

Liver disease	Masculinization in women
High blood pressure	Muscle spasms
Increased LDL cholesterol	Headache
Decreased HDL cholesterol	Nervous tension
Fluid retention	Nausea
Suppressed immunity	Rash
Decreased testosterone	Irritability
Testicular atrophy	Mood swings
Acne	Heightened or suppressed sex drive
Gynecomastia	Aggressiveness
Lowered sperm count	Drug dependence

Another class of banned or illegal substances, nonsteroidal selective androgen receptor modulators (SARMs) seem to have a more favorable anabolic/androgenic ratio than steroids and produce fewer side effects. Often referred to as prohormones by those trying to sell them to you, make no mistake—these are anabolic steroids; they just appear a little earlier in the biochemical production chain. Their chemical composition is slightly different from anabolic steroids, and therefore they may fall under the wire of substance control in the nutritional supplement category. However, the FDA has issued warning letters to manufacturers and told consumers to stop using products that contain them. According to the FDA, among the dangers associated with SARMs are liver toxicity and increased risk of heart disease and stroke. As an athlete, you must be aware that these are banned substances equal to anabolic steroids. Several dietary supplement products, including a carbohydrate–electrolyte replacement product, are on the high-risk list for SARM contamination. Regardless of whether the presence of SARMs is intentional or accidental on the part of the manufacturer, you are the one who will be held responsible if supplements you use cause a positive drug test result.

Prohibited and Banned Substances: What You Must Know

The most important information for you to know is that any product can be contaminated with a prohibited or banned substance. Perhaps even more important these days is the knowledge that prohibited and banned substances can occur naturally in foods, herbs, and botanical preparations at a level that will give you a positive blood doping test. The onus is on you, the athlete, to do the research and make informed decisions.

To keep up to date on what substances are banned, the best resource is the World Anti-Doping Agency (WADA) Prohibited List, found on the website of the U.S. Anti-Doping Agency (USADA): www.usada.org/substances/prohibited-list. (In addition to the Prohibited List, the USADA website has a plethora of information and guidelines as well as real stories of athletes who have been sanctioned for doping violations.) Broken down by categories, the WADA Prohibited List identifies which substances and methods are prohibited in competition versus outside of competition and, in some cases, which substances and methods are banned for a specific sport. For athletes who are required to test at any time, prohibited substances are *always* prohibited, regardless of whether it is competition season.

To be well-informed about what you are ingesting, you must do more than just read ingredient labels or the manufacturers' claims. There are controversies over some ingredients, such as peptide hormones and growth factors. Colostrum, the first milk produced by a mammal after birthing, is known to be very high in immune factors and bioactive proteins, such as IGF-1. Cow milk colostrum, sold as a nutritional supplement, is not on the prohibited list; however, the IGF-1 that it contains is banned. If you end up with abnormally elevated IGF-1 blood levels, you can be prosecuted for doping. The research data on colostrum supplementation has not shown abnormally elevated IGF-1 levels from recommended doses, but that is not an absolute protection for you. If you are a drug-tested athlete and choose to use these types of products, you should do your own blood tests to see how your body responds to the doses you are using.

Supplement manufacturers sometimes advertise their products in a different category than where it appears in the WADA Prohibited List. The supplement industry often defines stimulants differently from USADA. Higenamine, derived

When Is a Substance Considered for Inclusion in the WADA Prohibited List?

To answer this question, I had an enlightening conversation with Dr. Amy Eichner, special advisor on drugs and supplements for USADA. According to Dr. Eichner, a substance or method will typically be considered for the WADA Prohibited List if the substance or method meets any two of the following three criteria:

1. It enhances, or has the potential to enhance, sport performance.
2. It represents an actual or potential health risk to the athlete.
3. It violates the spirit of sport.

Take note of those last two criteria: Something that does not enhance performance could still be a banned substance. In other words, if you use a substance with the intention of cheating and it is discovered, it is cheating even if what you used does not have the potential to help you win. Additionally, an individual can be sanctioned by USADA for possession of a prohibited substance or for intention to give a prohibited substance to an athlete. So coaches, beware!

Categories of Substances Prohibited and Banned by WADA

Anabolic agents

Peptide hormones, growth factors, related substances, and mimetics

Beta-2 agonists

Hormone and metabolic modulators

Diuretics and masking agents

Manipulation of blood and blood components

Chemical and physical manipulation

Gene doping

Stimulants

Narcotics

Cannabinoids

Glucocorticoids

Beta-blockers

Other nonapproved substances

---

from a variety of fruits and plants, is often sold as a fat burner and a preworkout supplement. But it is classified as a beta-2 agonist by WADA and is therefore on the WADA Prohibited List. You risk a doping ban if you use this supplement. Other danger zones include general self-care and alternative medicine products, particularly those from compounding pharmacies. Several recent positive drug tests have been traced to compounding pharmacy preparations.

Now we enter the realm of sport nutrition supplements that are uniquely positioned to promote exercise performance, or at least claim to do so. While we need vitamins and minerals whether or not we exercise, supplements like creatine and beet root juice are not considered essential nutrients.

This next section covers the evidence-based ingredients that definitely work or that have promise based on the current level of research. Again, there just isn't room to list all the products that don't have any research evidence to support their claims, or that the evidence shows don't work, or that frankly may even be dangerous. Trust that if the product isn't listed here, it's not worth it.

Products That Meet and Possibly Meet Marketing Claims

The products in this category have numerous research studies that back up the marketing claims (table 10.2), or they are accumulating an early body of evidence that looks promising. In the right setting, these products can work or may work.

TABLE 10.2 Rating of the Supplements

Supplement	Meets marketing claims	Possibly meets marketing claims
Caffeine	✔	
Carbohydrate–protein sport drinks	✔	
Protein supplements	✔	
Creatine	✔	
Carbohydrate and carbohydrate–electrolyte solutions	✔	
Beta-alanine		✔
Beta-hydroxy-beta-methylbutyrate (HMB)		✔
Branched-chain amino acids (BCAAs)		✔
Gelatin/collagen and vitamin C		✔
Sulfur (methylsulfonylmethane)		✔
Glucosamine chondroitin		✔
L-carnitine		✔
Sodium bicarbonate		✔
DHA and EPA	✔	
Coenzyme Q10 (CoQ10)		✔
Glycerol		✔
Probiotics/prebiotics	+	+
*Phosphatidylcholine (PC)		✔
*Phosphatidylserine (PS)		✔
*Taurine		✔
*Theacrine		✔
*Tart cherry juice		✔
**Guarana	✔	
**Maté	✔	
**Ginseng		✔
**Green tea		✔
**Ginger		✔
**Turmeric (curcumin)		✔

*These are covered in chapter 11 on products for boosting the brain and nervous system.

**These are covered in chapter 12 on botanicals.

+Some do and some do not meet marketing claims. Consumers need to read about different cultures and products and understand the target issue.

When I say that the supplements meet their marketing claims, it doesn't mean that I recommend that you use them. It just tells you that what is claimed on the label is substantiated by research. Also in this section are those products that possibly meet their marketing claims as supporting by fairly new but good science. You should choose to use or not use supplements based on your exercise goals, lifestyle, and attention to all the factors that support the enhancement of strength and power. Supplements will not help you if you don't have your diet, training, and recovery dialed in.

Caffeine

Caffeine, a drug found in coffee, tea, soda, and over-the-counter pharmaceutical preparations, can have a wide range of effects depending on your sensitivity to it. You might feel alert and wide awake, or you might get the jitters. Your heart might race, or you might race to the bathroom (caffeine in large amounts is a diuretic).

Caffeine lingers in the body, so even small amounts can accumulate over time. It has a half-life of four to six hours, meaning that it takes that long for the body to metabolize half the amount consumed. Because of its half-life, caffeine can become counterproductive. If you drink small amounts during the day, they add up, and you eventually reach a point at which your body has more caffeine than it can handle. By increasing anxiety or restlessness, caffeine reduces the body's ability to function. Other unwanted side effects are upset stomach, irritability, and diarrhea.

Caffeine also inhibits the absorption of thiamin (a vitamin important for carbohydrate metabolism) and several minerals, including calcium and iron. Women who consume caffeine regularly (4 or more cups [1 or more L] of coffee a day or 330 mg of caffeine) and have a low intake of calcium in their diet (fewer than 700 mg a day) may run a greater risk of developing osteoporosis, or brittle bone disease.

How It Works

Most research on caffeine has focused on endurance sports. The main finding is that for many endurance athletes, caffeine may extend performance. Caffeine influences many biochemical pathways in the body, but the most relevant research on extension of endurance performance focuses on why caffeine makes you perceive that you are doing less work than you really are during exercise. It states that caffeine, because of its direct effect on the central nervous system, might have the psychological effect of making athletes feel they are not working as hard, or it may somehow maximize the force of muscular contractions. We now know that caffeine can cross the blood–brain barrier and antagonize the effects of adenosine, the neurotransmitter that causes drowsiness by slowing down nerve cell activity. In the brain, caffeine looks like adenosine and can bind to adenosine receptors on brain cells. But caffeine doesn't have the same action as adenosine, so it doesn't slow down nerve cell activity. Instead, it stimulates brain chemicals to secrete epinephrine, the flight-or-fight hormone that makes you feel better while working out. Currently, this is the prevailing theory most supported by the research.

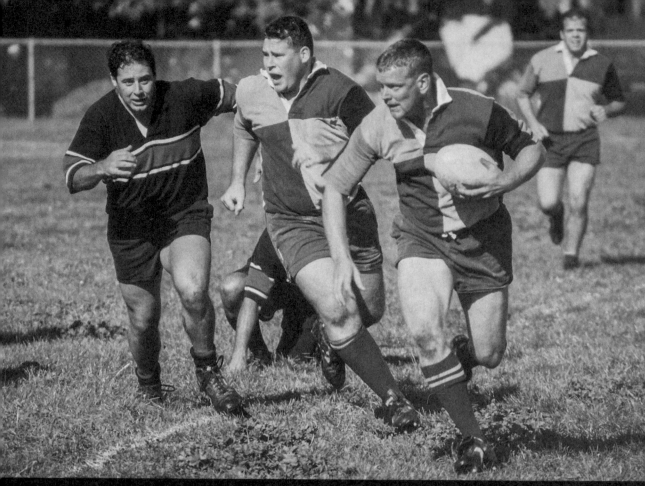

High-intensity sports require the right kinds of fuel to keep muscles strong and energy levels high.

Photodisc/Getty Images

Caffeine Use in Power Sports

Does caffeine supplementation help with power sports? Yes, according to a mound of research. A 2010 review report looked at 29 studies that tested caffeine's ability to enhance performance during power exercise, such as sprinting team sports and resistance training. Eleven of the 17 studies showed significant improvements in team sport exercise and power-based sports with caffeine ingestion, but the greatest improvements were shown in elite athletes who were not regular caffeine users. Six of the eleven studies showed benefits of caffeine ingestion with resistance training.

The reason caffeine works in power sports probably has to do with its ability to trigger the release of epinephrine from the adrenal glands. This results in improved muscle contraction. When this happens, perceived exertion is reduced, letting you push more weight without making a conscious decision to work harder. Basically, it seems that caffeine can improve strength over time, which of course leads to greater muscle mass. Caffeine is a bona fide ergogenic aid: A large collection of studies shows that it can improve exercise performance by 22 percent. More good news: The amount of coffee it takes to enhance performance—about 16 ounces (480 ml), or 2 cups—does not have a dehydrating effect on the body.

The Caffeine–Carbohydrate Duo

Some of the most breakthrough research on caffeine has to do with its interaction with carbohydrate. Basically, caffeine taken with carbohydrate boosts sport performance. Case in point: British scientists investigated the effects of the simultaneous consumption of carbohydrate and caffeine on athletic performance. Soccer players who drank a beverage with carbohydrate (6.4 percent) plus caffeine (160 mg) during a game simulation performed with higher intensity than they did when they drank a carbohydrate drink without caffeine or a placebo.

Well-Trained Athletes Do Best

Studies also show that caffeine works best as a power booster if you're well-conditioned. Proof of this comes from experiments with swimmers, whose sport is anaerobic as well as aerobic. Highly trained swimmers improved their swimming velocity significantly after consuming 250 milligrams of caffeine and then swimming at maximal speed. Untrained, occasional swimmers didn't fare as well. The same group of researchers had previously conducted experiments with untrained subjects who cycled against resistance after supplementing with caffeine. Again, caffeine didn't provide much of a performance boost in untrained people.

Whether or not caffeine supplementation works best in nonhabitual users of caffeine is really not clear. While we used to think that habitual use minimized the impact of caffeine around exercise, a number of recent studies have shown, at least in those studies, to be incorrect. Habitual users benefited just as much from caffeine supplementation prior to exercise when compared to the nonhabitual users. So this may be another time when personalization is the key. However, don't wait until game day to try using caffeine. Test out your reaction to caffeine long before it's going to really count. Lastly, a new study of the genetics of caffeine metabolism shows that whether caffeine enhances or hinders your performance may be dictated by your genes.

The Final Word on Caffeine

The International Society of Sports Nutrition has taken the following position on caffeine and performance:

1. Caffeine is effective for enhancing sport performance in trained athletes when consumed in doses between approximately 3 to 6 milligrams per kilogram of body weight. Higher doses do not result in greater enhancements in performance.

2. Caffeine exerts a greater ergogenic effect when consumed in a dry state (mixed with liquid) as compared to coffee.

3. Caffeine can enhance vigilance during bouts of extended exhaustive exercise.

4. Caffeine is ergogenic for sustained maximal endurance exercise and has been shown to be highly effective for time trial performance.

5. Caffeine supplementation is beneficial for high-intensity exercise, including team sports such as soccer and rugby, both of which are categorized by intermittent activity within a period of prolonged duration.

6. Caffeine improves strength and power performance.

7. Caffeine can act as a diuretic in high doses, but athletes should not use it to trigger fluid losses.

One of the main reasons I like caffeine as a sport supplement is that it enhances certain aspects of mental performance, particularly vigilance, even if you're rested, and it has even more generalized effects if you're sleep deprived. By that, I mean that it improves cognitive (thinking) functions that are compromised by lack of sleep. Ultimately, this means that you can more easily push through those final reps, extra sets, or endurance laps or legs if you're feeling a little less fatigue.

Keep in mind, though, that caffeine may aggravate certain health problems, such as ulcers, heart disease, high blood pressure, and anemia, to name just a few. Stick to your doctor's advice. Above all, don't substitute caffeine for sound, commonsense nutritional practices for extending energy, and don't use it regularly to make up for getting a good night's sleep.

Carbohydrate–Protein Sport Drinks

Unimaginable as it may seem, it is within your control to retool your body for more lean muscle and less fat—and do it naturally—all with a simple formula and routine. Here's how: Immediately after your workout, drink a liquid carbohydrate supplement that contains protein. This routine will jump-start the muscle-building process, plus boost your energy levels.

The simple formula is 12 ounces (360 ml) of carbohydrate and protein in liquid form taken immediately after your strength-training regimen. This is the time your body is best able to use these nutrients for muscle firming and fat burning. The supplement I use with my clients is my Kleiner's Muscle-Building formulas, featured in chapter 20. For a long time, I've used these formulas with many of my bodybuilding clients, and soon after they begin drinking the formulas, we observe a major shift in their body composition from less fat to more muscle.

How It Works

How does this formula help muscles get stronger and firmer? Exercise, of course, is the initial stimulus. You challenge your muscles by working out, and they respond with growth. But for muscle building to take place, muscles need protein and carbohydrate in combination to create the right hormonal climate for muscle growth.

What happens is this: Protein and carbohydrate trigger the release of insulin and growth hormone (GH) in your body. Insulin is a powerful factor in building muscle. It helps ferry glucose and amino acids into cells, reassembles those amino acids into body tissue, and prevents muscle wasting and tissue loss. GH increases the rate of protein production by the body, spurring muscle-building activity, and it also promotes fat burning. Both hormones are directly involved in muscle growth. Your body is primed for growth thanks to this simple muscle-gain formula.

Scientific Proof

Research into the effect of carbohydrate–protein supplements on athletes and exercisers supports what I've observed for years. Here are some examples:

- In one scientific study, 14 normal-weight men and women ate test meals containing various amounts of protein: none (a protein-free meal), 15.8 grams, 21.5 grams, 33.6 grams, and 49.9 grams. All subjects combined their protein intake with 58 grams of carbohydrate. Blood samples were taken at intervals after the meal. The protein-containing meals produced the greatest rise in insulin compared with the protein-free meal. This study points out that protein has an insulin-boosting effect.

- In another study, nine experienced male strength trainers were given water (which served as the control), a carbohydrate supplement, a protein supplement, or a carbohydrate–protein supplement. They took their designated supplement immediately after working out and again two hours later. Right after exercise and throughout the next eight hours, the researchers drew blood samples to determine the levels of various hormones in the blood, including insulin, testosterone, and GH.

  The most significant finding was that the carbohydrate–protein supplement triggered the greatest elevations in insulin and GH. The protein works hand in hand with postexercise carbohydrate to create a hormonal climate that's highly conducive to muscle growth.

- If you've started strength training later in life, consuming protein after your workout is very important. Researchers in Denmark instructed a group of men (aged 74 and older) to have a protein drink consisting of 10 grams of protein, 7 grams of carbohydrate, and 3 grams of fat either immediately after or two hours after each training session. The study lasted 12 weeks. By the end of the study, the best gains in muscular growth occurred when the subjects consumed liquid protein immediately after their workouts. The point here seems to be that the sooner you replenish with protein, the better results you can obtain.

More Energy

If you supplement with a carbohydrate–protein beverage after your workout, you'll notice something else: higher energy levels. Not only does this nutrient combination stimulate hormone activity, but also it starts replenishing muscle glycogen, which means more muscle energy. The harder you work out, the greater your muscular gains will be.

When protein is added to the supplement mix, your body's glycogen-making process accelerates faster than if you just consumed carbohydrate alone. Some intriguing research proves this point. In one study, nine men cycled for two full hours during three different sessions to deplete their muscle glycogen stores. Immediately after each exercise bout and again two hours later, the men drank a straight carbohydrate supplement, a straight protein supplement, or a carbohydrate–protein supplement. By looking at actual biopsy specimens of the muscles, the researchers observed that the rate of muscle glycogen storage was significantly faster in men who consumed the carbohydrate–protein mixture.

Why such speed? It's well known that eating carbohydrate after prolonged endurance exercise helps restore muscle glycogen. When protein is consumed along with carbohydrate, there's a surge in insulin. Biochemically, insulin is like an acceleration pedal. It races the body's glycogen-making motor in two ways. First, it speeds up the movement of glucose and amino acids into cells, and second, it activates a special enzyme crucial to glycogen synthesis.

In another study, a group of athletes performed enough exercise to deplete their glycogen reserves. Afterward, part of the group consumed a carbohydrate–protein supplement; the other consumed a 6 percent glucose–electrolyte solution. Both groups exercised again. Endurance-wise, the carbohydrate–protein group outlasted the other group by 66 percent.

In a similar study, eight endurance-trained cyclists performed two 2-hour exercise bouts designed to deplete their glycogen stores. After exercise and again two hours later, they consumed either a carbohydrate–protein supplement or a carbohydrate-only formula. The carbohydrate–protein formula contained 53 grams of carbohydrate and 14 grams of protein, whereas the carbohydrate formula contained 20 grams of carbohydrate. The effects of the carbohydrate–protein supplement were quite remarkable: Glucose levels rose by 17 percent, and insulin levels increased by 92 percent. Furthermore, there was 128 percent greater storage of muscle glycogen when athletes took the carbohydrate–protein supplement compared with when they took the carbohydrate-only formula.

Scientific research indicates that for hard trainers, the optimal combination of protein and carbohydrate after exercise is 0.5 gram per kilogram body weight protein to 1.0 to 1.2 grams per kilogram body weight carbohydrate, to fully replenish muscle glycogen, stimulate muscle protein synthesis, and begin to tamp down muscle protein breakdown. This formula is based on the needs of hard training; total carbohydrate consumption can be lower if you are training at lower intensity or for a short duration. Also, if you want an effective protein dose but no extra, 20 to 25 grams of whey protein should be a good target.

A question often arises as to whether you should eat your postexercise meal or drink it in the form of a carbohydrate–protein supplement. Let's turn to some scientific data for the answer. Researchers at Ithaca College in New York tested whether a whole-foods meal, a supplemental drink of protein and carbohydrate, a carbohydrate-only beverage, or a placebo would have any effect on insulin, testosterone, or cortisol levels following resistance training. The study revealed that the supplemental drink of protein and carbohydrate had the most effect but mostly in terms of increasing insulin levels. As noted before, insulin is essential for driving the manufacture of glycogen, so it looks as though your best meal after a workout is one that is in liquid form. That's why my clients love my smoothies! You can find a variety of smoothie recipes in chapter 20.

However, as I've said throughout *The New Power Eating*, I always put food first. So here's what I tell my clients: I like smoothies and shakes for exactly the research reason stated above. Furthermore, because of my clients' busy lives, if they don't drink something right away after training or practice, they may not get any food for many hours afterward. So a liquid supplement is also a very important convenience that they can take with them in their gym bags. Oftentimes they freeze them the night before, and by the time they need to drink them they have defrosted. Or for the most convenience, they use powdered supplements and just add water after practice. If you can go right home or to a restaurant after training and eat plenty of nutrient-dense whole food, that is also an excellent choice. The key here is timing. While you don't have to eat or drink your supplement immediately after training, the sooner the better. If hours are going to pass before you eat, then drink a shake that will start your recovery, and save enough protein and carbohydrate to have a good selection of foods for your next meal.

Protein Supplements

Protein supplements are a convenient way to consume high-quality, fat-free, lactose-free animal- or plant-based protein after workouts or between meals. A variety of these supplements are on the market. Each has unique benefits to exercisers, strength trainers, and other athletes.

Table 10.3 guides you through the differences in processing. Here's a rundown of the different protein sources.

Bovine Colostrum

A clear premilk fluid and life's first food for every newborn mammal, colostrum is loaded with growth factors, amino acids, and bioactive protein that help the newborn develop in its first week of life. Several brands are on the market.

Colostrum is similar to whey protein in both protein efficiency ratio (PER) (3.0) and protein digestibility score (PDCAAS) (1.0). What's more, it is low in fat and free of lactose. Because of its naturally high content of insulin-like growth factors, colostrum is banned by the National Collegiate Athletic Association (NCAA) and the USOC. If you are not affected by these organizations, you might try colostrum

TABLE 10.3 Supplemental Protein: What's the Difference?

Forms of protein	Characteristics
Hydrolysates	Hydrolysates are proteins that have been partially broken down. This makes them taste more bitter, but taste has fortunately improved with newer products. Hydrolysates are extremely well absorbed and virtually free of any potential allergens.
Isolates	Isolates have the highest protein concentration (90%-95%) and contain very little (if any) fat, lactose, and minerals. These have been removed to "isolate" the protein.
Concentrates	Concentrates have a protein concentration ranging from 25 to 89%. Concentrates are less processed than the other forms of protein and contain some lactose, fat, and minerals.

Protein Supplements and Weight Loss

In addition to being used in muscle-building diets, protein supplements are frequently used in weight-loss diets. Increasing dietary protein has been shown to be a successful weight-loss strategy, and protein supplements are an easy way to increase protein without increasing carbohydrate and fat.

One reason whey protein is so effective for weight loss is that it is high in leucine, an amino acid that regulates muscle mass, but also helps you reduce body fat during weight loss. Research shows that 2.5 grams is the ideal dose of leucine for fat loss, that whey protein contains 10 percent leucine, and that other proteins contain slightly less. So a dose of 25 grams of whey protein will contain the ideal dose of leucine.

Although recent research shows that very high levels of dietary protein (3.4 grams per kilogram of body weight per day) can be safe in healthy subjects and continue to support advanced lean mass gains, such high levels of protein intake have not been studied in terms of the impact from minimizing other foods in the diet. The question remains whether a very high protein diet that lacks a wide variety of foods, and thus lacks the consumption of all nutrients and food factors, will enhance muscle recovery, growth, and, moreover, sport performance.

---

for its easy digestibility if you are looking for any possible strength-building edge. It is probably the most expensive of all protein supplements.

Egg Protein

The protein obtained from egg whites (ovalbumin) is considered the reference standard against which to compare types of protein. Egg protein was traditionally the protein of choice for supplements but is rather expensive. The PER of egg protein is 2.8; the PDCAAS is 1.0. If you like variety in your protein supplements, this one has value.

Soy Protein

Despite being low in the amino acid methionine, soy is an excellent source of quality protein. Soy protein concentrate (70 percent protein) and isolate (90 percent protein) are particularly good protein sources for vegetarians. Soy protein isolate also contains isoflavone glucosides, which have a number of potential health benefits. The PER of soy protein is 1.8 to 2.3; the PDCAAS is 1.0. The downside of soy protein is that it is not as effective at muscle building as whey protein. On the other hand, if you are a vegetarian or you don't consume milk protein, soy protein is an excellent alternative for boosting protein intake, especially immediately after exercise.

Whey Protein

Whey is a component of milk that is separated off to make cheese and other dairy products. It is high in B-complex vitamins, selenium, and calcium. In addition, whey appears to boost the levels of the antioxidant glutathione in the body.

Along with colostrum, whey protein represents the highest-quality protein available in supplements. It is digested rapidly, allowing for fast uptake of amino acids. Also available are whey protein hydrolysate, ion exchange whey protein isolate, and cross-flow microfiltration whey protein isolate. These differ slightly in their amino acid profiles, fat content, lactose content, and ability to preserve glutamine. It is unclear whether these small differences would have any impact on exercise performance. Using the isolated form of whey is a good idea if you want to reduce the amount of carbohydrate you consume. However, you will get less calcium and other minerals from this form of whey.

Casein Protein

Casein comprises 80 percent of the protein found in cow's milk. It is a major component of cheese and is also found as a food additive. Calcium and phosphorus are major components of casein. The opposite of rapidly digested whey protein, casein forms a gel-like compound in the stomach that creates a timed-release effect—a slow, steady release of amino acids into the bloodstream.

Creatine

Creatine is one of the most important natural fuel-enhancing supplements discovered thus far for strength trainers. Unlike a lot of supplements, creatine has been extensively researched. The results of a PubMed.gov scientific research literature search using the key words "creatine," "human," and "exercise" found 4,253 relevant citations. Among those studies that have focused on the performance-enhancing value of creatine, about 70 percent report positive effects. These exciting experiments show that creatine produces significant performance improvements in sports that require high levels of strength and power, including strength training, rowing, and cycling sprints. Another big plus for creatine: Many studies have shown gains in body mass averaging 2 to 5 pounds (0.9-2.3 kg) during 4 to 12 weeks of training. Also, creatine improves overall performance, which means that you can train harder while supplementing with creatine. That translates into greater muscle gains. Thus, supplementing with creatine seems to be a safe and effective method to increase muscle mass.

Studies of the influence of creatine supplementation on performance have been conducted in both male and female athletes, but the results have been more consistently positive with male athletes. The research suggests that females may not receive the same level of strength and muscle mass enhancement as males.

Creatine received a major thumbs-up in a 2010 review article published in the *Journal of the International Society of Sports Nutrition*, and in 2017 the ISSN Journal reinforced that position with an updated position paper and added more information from many new studies. In addition, recent position stands by the American Dietetic Association, Dietitians of Canada, and the American College of Sports Medicine on nutrition for athletic performance all drew similar conclusions. The authors continue to state that creatine is the most effective nutritional supplement available to athletes to increase high-intensity exercise capacity and muscle mass during training. In addition, creatine seems to have many medical applications that make it a particularly important supplement for brain and central nervous system conditions.

Sound good? You bet. Who wouldn't prefer a bona fide natural supplement such as creatine over synthetic, dangerous compounds such as steroids? Creatine is the ticket to greater strength and improved muscularity.

How It Works

Creatine is produced in the liver and kidneys at a rate of about 2 grams a day from arginine, glycine, and methionine, three nonessential amino acids. About 95 percent of the body's creatine travels by the blood to be stored in the muscles, heart, and other body cells. Inside muscle cells, it's turned into creatine phosphate (CP), a compound that serves as a tiny energy supply, enough for several seconds of action. CP thus works best over the short haul in activities such as strength training that require short, fast bursts of activity. CP also replenishes your cellular reserves of ATP, the molecular fuel that provides the power for muscular contractions. With more ATP around, your muscles can do more work.

Although there are several different forms of creatine, the greatest number of studies have evaluated creatine monohydrate as the test factor. Manufacturers eager to separate their product from the rest of the market make extravagant claims about the solubility, the absorption, or the reliability of their products. This is what the scientists from ISSN have to say:

> Claims that different forms of creatine are degraded to a lesser degree than creatine monohydrate in vivo or result in a greater uptake to muscle are currently unfounded. Clinical evidence has not demonstrated that different forms of creatine such as creatine citrate, creatine serum, creatine ethyl ester, buffered forms of creatine, or creatine nitrate promote greater creatine retention than creatine monohydrate.

Vegetarians May Benefit Most

Since the greatest dietary source of creatine is from meat, vegans and vegetarians typically have low levels of muscle creatine. By supplementing with creatine, lacto-ovo vegetarians (who typically have lower stores of creatine in their bodies) can increase their muscular stores of creatine to levels similar to those of people who eat meat and experience better synthesis of ATP.

Supplementing with creatine has been shown to increase bone mineral content and bone density in older men who engage in strength training. This benefit may be related to enhanced muscle mass and strength due to taking the creatine. Men tend to lose both muscle mass and bone mass as they age, so this finding is quite promising in terms of quality of life for older men.

As a strength trainer, you load creatine into your muscles just as endurance athletes do with carbohydrate. Consequently, you can push harder and longer in your workouts because creatine boosts the pace of energy production in your muscle cells. Creatine supplementation doesn't build muscle directly. But it does have an indirect effect: You can work out more intensely, and this translates into muscle gains. Once in the muscles, creatine appears to induce intramuscular fluid retention, or volumization, which in turn may influence carbohydrate and protein metabolism.

The Latest Word on Creatine

More than one thousand articles have been written on the influence of creatine supplementation on strength, power, and athletic performance. A new area of creatine research, how creatine may influence medical conditions involving the brain and nervous system, has greatly increased the number of publications addressing the possible benefits of creatine supplements. This is discussed further in chapter 11.

How Much?

Creatine supplements swell the ranks of creatine in your muscles, giving the working muscles another fuel source in addition to glycogen from carbohydrate. The question is, how much creatine do you need? You do get creatine from food—roughly 1 gram a day. But that's not enough to enhance strength-training performance.

Creatine usually comes in a powdered form. The latest scientific research shows that the most rapid method of increasing muscle creatine stores is to consume approximately 5 grams of creatine, four times a day for five to seven days, or alternatively based on your body weight: 0.3 gram per kilogram of body weight of creatine, four times per day for five to seven days. Follow this loading dose with 3 to 5 grams of creatine per day thereafter (perhaps 5-10 g/day for larger athletes) to maintain elevated stores. Ingesting smaller amounts of creatine, 2 to 3 grams per day, will increase muscle creatine stores over a three- to four-week period. It will take a little longer to reach saturation levels compared to the loading dose, but the results are virtually the same once you reach saturation. You will not see benefits prior to reaching saturation.

Because creatine levels will be maintained in your muscles for about four to six weeks, another strategy is to cycle on and off creatine rather than using the loading maintenance phases. Start with a dose of 5 grams per day for about six weeks. Cycle off the creatine for about four to six weeks, and then go back on it again. Your muscle levels and training results will remain high during the off period. This strategy will lighten the strain on your wallet, while still giving you competitive results. The choice is completely yours, but the fastest route to muscle creatine saturation is the loading dose for five to seven days.

The question of when to supplement with creatine seems to be answered by research that shows nonsignificant differences. A Canadian study conducted over a six-week period found that supplementing with creatine after working out can increase muscle size. This particular study focused on arm muscle, and the effect was more pronounced in men than in women. On the other hand, taking creatine before intense aerobic exercise improved energy production during exercise. Creatine is so well absorbed that it doesn't seem to matter when you take it, so just add it to your regimen when it fits.

Here's an important fact about creatine supplementation: Although it doesn't matter when you take creatine, what you take with it can make a difference. Even though creatine is highly absorbed, combining creatine with carbohydrate or carbohydrate plus protein may increase muscle creatine retention levels.

Creatine is nontoxic, and studies have been unable to find any negative side effects to its use when dosage recommendations are followed, other than weight gain. It does not interfere with normal body fluid shifts that occur when exercising or competing in the heat—good news to endurance athletes who often train or compete in hot weather. Creatine has actually been shown to enhance cellular hydration in athletes training outdoors in the heat of the summer. But if you take too much at once, you can experience an upset stomach.

My stand has always been that you must have your nutrition, your training, and your rest dialed in before you add creatine to your program, so that you can really evaluate if it is making a difference for you. Of course, always check with your physician before supplementing with anything new.

Carbohydrate and Carbohydrate–Electrolyte Solutions

Carbohydrate supplements and carbohydrate–electrolyte solutions are beneficial for athletes competing in high-intensity sports lasting less than one hour or events that last an hour or longer. These solutions do two things: supply an exogenous source of carbohydrate to the working muscles, decreasing the use of muscle and liver glycogen stores, and replace water and electrolytes lost through sweat. During competition, athletes can thus run, bike, or swim longer because the supplemental carbohydrate has spared stored glycogen.

Most drinks are about 6 to 8 percent carbohydrate. The carbohydrate may be one or more of a selection of low-molecular-weight carbohydrates: a monosaccharide simple sugarlike glucose or fructose; a disaccharide such as sucrose, ordinary table sugar (a complex of glucose and fructose); maltodextrin, an oligosaccharide complex carbohydrate derived from corn; or a combination of these. Low-molecular-weight carbohydrates create high osmolality in the gastrointestinal tract, which attracts water toward the carbohydrate molecules and into the gut lumen. If too much of these carbohydrates are consumed within too short a period of time, this leads to bloating, gastric upset, cramping, and potentially diarrhea. This is why recommendations for carbohydrate consumption during exercise has always been limited to 40 to 60 grams of carbohydrate per hour, despite the higher amounts of carbohydrate utilization during high-intensity exercise and competition events.

One incomplete solution to this problem has been to combine several different carbohydrates into one formula, referred to as multitransport carbohydrate formulas. When maltodextrin is combined with glucose and fructose, they are emptied from the stomach and transported across the intestinal membrane into the bloodstream at different rates, lessening the buildup in the gut and decreasing gastric discomfort. This allows more carbohydrate, possibly up to 90 grams per hour, to be consumed and utilized during exercise. Athletes have found that they need to train the gut to get used to this mix of higher levels of low-molecular-weight carbohydrate, and they need to start lower and raise their intake over time to avoid gastric upset. Individuals report a range of comfort (or discomfort) levels with the slightly higher doses per hour.

A more complete strategy may be to try a high-molecular-weight (HMW) complex carbohydrate–starch supplement. The high molecular weight leads to lower osmolality, significantly faster stomach emptying, markedly less gastric distress, and generally a greater capacity to consume much more carbohydrate per hour of exercise. Several published research studies on a HMW fractionated starch amylopectin (Vitargo) has supported this data. Studies also report very rapid glycogen recovery after exercise, nearly two times that seen from maltodextrin plus sugars two hours postexercise, as well as enhanced endurance and resistance exercise performance.

There's no evidence that electrolytes improve exercise performance for general workouts. For events lasting less than three hours, they're not required unless you have a mineral deficiency diagnosed by your physician or your daily sweat losses total more than 3 percent of your body weight, or 4.5 pounds (2 kg) in a 150-pound (68 kg) athlete. Endurance and ultraendurance athletes exercising more than three hours are among those who do need to replace electrolytes. Unless you count yourself in this elite class of athlete, if you are eating a diet rich in whole foods, you are getting enough of these minerals.

In addition to the ability of carbohydrate–electrolyte solutions to replenish fluids, electrolytes, and carbohydrate, they may strengthen your immune system. This amazing news comes from Appalachian State University, where researchers put two groups of marathoners through high-intensity treadmill exercises for two and a half hours. One group drank 25 ounces (750 ml) of a carbohydrate–electrolyte solution (Gatorade) 30 minutes before exercise, 8 ounces (240 ml) every 15 minutes during exercise, and a final 25 ounces (750 ml) over a 6-hour recovery period. The other group replenished fluids on the same schedule but with a noncarbohydrate placebo solution.

The researchers took blood samples from the marathoners and found that the carbohydrate–electrolyte solution drinkers had lower levels of cortisol in their blood than the other exercisers did. Cortisol is a hormone that suppresses immune response. So apparently when the body is well fed, stress is reduced and cortisol levels remain at normal levels, helping to maintain more optimal immune function. Because this is just one study, obviously it offers no final and complete answers on the carbohydrate–immunity connection. This research is intriguing, nonetheless.

Other research has found that consuming a sport drink during aerobic exercise can enhance feelings of pleasure, meaning that you may not notice feelings of discomfort while working out. For people who don't like to exercise, sipping a sport drink, or perhaps even a flavored noncaloric drink, may spark motivation simply because it makes them feel better.

What About Carbohydrate Gels?

Carbohydrate gels are highly concentrated sources of carbohydrate with a pudding-like consistency and are usually packaged in single-serve pouches. Designed as a convenient package for athletes and exercisers participating in endurance activity, these products are usually a mixture of simple carbohydrate with flavoring, and some are formulated with protein as well. These gels are quickly absorbed into the bloodstream and thus are a good source of immediate energy, particularly during extended exercise. Research has found that carbohydrate gels that contain protein extend performance longer than plain carbohydrate gels and may be a better choice. However, a significant proportion of people get stomach upset and nausea from protein during exercise. When using these gels, make sure to take in sufficient water to process the carbohydrate and protein and to prevent dehydration. Reminder: These are low-molecular-weight carbohydrates, so too much too fast will lead to gastric upset, especially if you neglect to drink water.

Carbohydrate–electrolyte solutions are designed primarily for endurance athletes. But they also have application for strength trainers in two important ways. First, if you train aerobically—particularly in the heat—these supplements prevent electrolyte and fluid depletion. Second, if you're training intensely and lifting heavy for 45 minutes or more, extra fluid and fuel mean more energy.

There has also been speculation on whether these drinks have any influence on oxidative damage in the aftermath of exercise. In strength trainers who were given a sport drink or a placebo, researchers could find no difference in oxidative stress. Sport drinks apparently don't help heal muscle damage following exercise. Adding protein to a sport drink in the form of amino acids has been shown to help with muscle recovery and muscle protein synthesis, however, particularly in novice strength trainers who drank a sport drink spiked with six additional grams of amino acids. The mixture significantly elevated insulin concentrations for an anabolic effect and decreased levels of the stress hormone cortisol, decreasing the stress effects of exercise on the body. Adding protein to these drinks has been shown to reduce the mental fatigue involved in exercise as well.

Beta-Alanine

This is a naturally occurring nonessential amino acid found in the muscle portion of animal protein, such as in beef, chicken, pork, fish, lamb, and others. It is a component of carnosine, a protein-like compound that is concentrated in actively contracting muscles. Carnosine is a buffering agent, meaning that it prevents certain enzymatic reactions within the muscle cell that increase acid buildup, dampening the burn in your muscles when you are working all out. Beta-alanine increases muscle carnosine, allowing for high-intensity exercise to proceed longer.

Scientists became interested in beta-alanine when they discovered a naturally occurring, unusually high level of carnosine in the muscles of a significant number of championship strength and power athletes. By controlling the natural rise in lactic acid that results from high-intensity exercise, these athletes could likely perform extra reps or perform a greater number of multiple sprints before muscle burn forced them to quit. To help those who are not naturally able to produce high levels of muscle carnosine, initial studies tried supplementing the diet with carnosine. It was found that carnosine is metabolized during digestion and does not raise muscle carnosine levels. So the researchers turned to supplementing with beta-alanine, an essential ingredient for carnosine production, and saw that it could raise muscle carnosine levels. The next step was to show that the more beta-alanine you have in your muscles, the better you can perform.

The research with beta-alanine has been methodical and primarily positive, although all studies are not in agreement. Supplementation with beta-alanine has been shown to increase muscle carnosine content and therefore total muscle buffering capacity, with the potential to elicit improvements in physical performance during high-intensity exercise. Studies of beta-alanine supplementation and exercise performance have demonstrated improvements in performance during multiple bouts of high-intensity exercise and in single bouts of exercise lasting more than 60 seconds. Similarly, beta-alanine supplementation has been shown to delay the onset of neuromuscular fatigue. Although beta-alanine does not improve maximal strength or aerobic capacity, some aspects of endurance performance, such as anaerobic threshold and time to exhaustion, can be enhanced.

Although most of the studies have used male subjects, two investigations from the University of Oklahoma studied women and resulted in different outcomes. In 2006, Dr. Jeff Stout and colleagues examined the effects of 28 days of beta-alanine supplementation on several parameters associated with intense exercise performance in 22 women. The subjects were supplemented with either beta-alanine or a placebo and performed an incremental exercise test on a cycle ergometer to exhaustion. The beta-alanine group significantly outperformed the placebo group in anaerobic, but not aerobic, metabolic, and performance measurements.

In 2010, University of Oklahoma researchers again investigated the effect of beta-alanine supplementation, this time on 44 women performing high-intensity interval training (HIIT) for six weeks. The subjects were split into three test groups: beta-alanine, placebo, or control (no supplement at all). The training consisted of riding a cycle ergometer three times per week with five 2-minute work intervals separated by 1 minute of passive recovery at varying intensities of workload ranging from 90 to 110 percent of their maximum workload (recorded during an initial measure of peak aerobic capacity). All groups improved their cardiorespiratory fitness, but there was no difference in the measurements among the three groups. The scientists concluded that HIIT was an effective and time-efficient method to improve maximal oxygen uptake. No benefit from beta-alanine was shown.

So what's the bottom line? I can tell you that in my practice I have clients who wouldn't train without beta-alanine, and those who haven't seen any difference in their training or race results. Most likely, clients in this second set are not different from the original elite athlete subjects studied for their naturally high levels of muscle carnosine. Perhaps they have reached the stratosphere of athletic performance partly as a result of a natural ability to produce more muscle carnosine, so supplementation does not lead to any noticeable or statistically measurable effect. For those less capable of producing carnosine, supplementation may work seemingly like magic to decrease muscle burn and fatigue, thereby enhancing high-intensity training and conditioning, leading to improved performance.

My take on beta-alanine is that if you participate in high-intensity training, competition, or both, it's worth a try. Use it in the following way: The loading phase for beta-alanine appears to be 28 days (4 weeks). Dosages in research studies range from 3.2 to 6.4 grams per day, separated into four or more doses per day. Single dosage amounts greater than 800 milligrams can lead to a transient tingling and paresthesia in the extremities, which can be eliminated by using timed-release formulas and smaller doses. Beta-alanine is available in a number of supplement formulas, even mixed with creatine. Already, one study has shown that beta-alanine combined with creatine delayed the onset of muscular fatigue better than beta alanine or creatine alone.

Beta-Hydroxy-Beta-Methylbutyrate (HMB)

Found in grapefruit, catfish, and other foods, beta-hydroxy-beta-methylbutyrate (HMB) is a breakdown product of leucine, a branched-chain amino acid. The body produces it naturally from proteins containing leucine.

Studies show that HMB may be anticatabolic; that is, it inhibits the degradation of muscle and protein in the body, so you can possibly train harder on successive days. Preliminary research on HMB indicates that 1.5 to 3 grams a day can assist with increasing muscle mass, decreasing body fat, and boosting strength levels if you are just beginning a strength-training program. There is some indication, although little evidence so far, that HMB may be protective of lean body mass in the elderly and after injury with immobilization.

Branched-Chain Amino Acids (BCAAs)

The BCAAs are leucine, isoleucine, and valine. During endurance exercise, levels of these amino acids fall, which may contribute to fatigue during competition. Emerging but limited research suggests that supplementation with BCAAs may enhance performance, particularly if you compete in endurance events. One study found that marathoners who consumed a sport drink containing BCAAs increased their performance by as much as 4 percent. Not all studies have shown a positive effect, however. In addition, some proportion of exercisers report gastric upset and nausea from protein during exercise.

Here are some guidelines based on what is currently known about BCAA supplementation: Dosages of 4 to 21 grams daily during training and 2 to 4 grams per hour with a 6 to 8 percent carbohydrate–electrolyte solution before and during prolonged exercise have been shown to improve physiological and psychological responses to training. In other words, athletes felt better mentally and physically during exercise. Theoretically, BCAA supplementation during hard training may help reduce fatigue, too, as well as prevent protein degradation in your muscles.

BCAAs are also part of some strength trainers' supplement arsenal. Leucine is the primary signal for muscle protein synthesis (MPS), but leucine does not act alone. All essential amino acids must be available for MPS to continue. However, it appears that once MPS has been stimulated and the building blocks from whole proteins are present, adding additional BCAAs may support continued MPS.

You can buy BCAAs in a bottle, but you can also find them in dairy products and in whey protein powder. Refer to chapter 2 for more information on BCAAs in food.

Collagen and Vitamin C

Another possibly useful supplement regime to watch for more evidence on, collagen is the primary structural component of connective tissues such as bone, tendon, ligament, and cartilage. All athletes, and especially weightlifters, put high demands on their connective tissues, and injury is not uncommon. The supplement combination of gelatin or hydrolyzed collagen plus vitamin C offers the building blocks for potential repair and renewal of connective tissues. Both the pathways and the mechanism of enhanced tissue synthesis from gelatin or hydrolyzed collagen in humans have been demonstrated in short-term studies, with longer-term studies showing improvement in cartilage function in patients with osteoarthritis. A 24-week randomized clinical trial in athletes showed that 10 grams of collagen hydrolysate significantly decreased knee pain. More research is needed to confirm these findings, determine the proper dosing, and answer many more questions regarding impact on healing after injury, prevention of damage from strength training, and whether supplementation enhances performance.

Glucosamine Chondroitin

There are so many claims about glucosamine chondroitin that many people are confused about which, if any, claims are backed by reliable published literature. Therefore, I am pleased that a recently published position paper has been endorsed by the European Society for Clinical and Economic Aspects of Osteoporosis, Osteoarthritis and Musculoskeletal Diseases (ESCEO). The authors of the paper confirm that there is evidence of efficacy of decreasing symptoms of osteoarthritis with the supplementation of glucosamine and chondroitin. However, the authors caution that,

> *while all preparations may claim to deliver a therapeutic level of glucosamine or chondroitin not all are supported by clinical evidence. Only patented crystalline glucosamine sulfate (pCGS) is shown to deliver consistently high glucosamine bioavailability and plasma concentration in humans, which corresponds to demonstrated clinical efficacy. Similarly, clinical evidence supports only the pharmaceutical-grade chondroitin sulfate. (Bruyère et al. 2018, p. 111)*

Sulfur (methylsulfonylmethane)

Hard training often results in extra inflammation, pain, and soreness after exercise, especially 24 to 72 hours following exercise. Throughout *The New Power Eating*, I recommend a number of foods and supplements to lessen the unchecked inflammation and discomfort, including a protein-carbohydrate recovery shake, a plant-rich diet, EPA and DHA, vitamin D, and creatine. Let's now add methylsulfonylmethane (MSM) to the mix.

Also known as dimethyl sulfone or $DMSO_2$, MSM is a form of dimethyl sulfoxide (DMSO), an organic sulfur compound from lignan. It has been used to improve immune function, reduce inflammation, and help repair bodily tissue. It is also a popular joint health supplement. The reason for these benefits is because MSM provides biologically active sulfur, the fourth most plentiful mineral in the body and needed for many different critical bodily functions every single day.

Studies have shown that MSM reduces postexercise inflammation, tissue damage, and discomfort, with some additional data on reduction of immunosuppression postexercise. Effective doses in studies have been 3 grams a day of MSM (OptiMSM brand) without any timing specificity for supplementation.

L-Carnitine

Recent research from the United Kingdom has shown that increasing total muscle carnitine content reduces muscle carbohydrate use during low-intensity exercise, consistent with an increase in the use of fat by the muscle. However, during high-intensity exercise, muscle carnitine loading results in more efficient energy metabolism, reducing energy use during anaerobic exercise. Together, these metabolic effects result in a reduced perception of effort and increased work output during a validated exercise performance test.

The other exciting finding from this study was simply that it was the first time scientists had been able to load carnitine into the muscle. The scientists discovered that when 2 grams of L-carnitine is consumed with 80 grams of very fast, high- molecular-weight carbohydrate (Vitargo), leading to a rapid rise in insulin levels, carnitine loaded into the muscle cells. The subjects followed the loading regimen twice daily for 24 weeks. Ultimately, the L-carnitine–loaded subjects had enhanced exercise performance. We don't have much more data on this protocol, but it might be worth a try if you are at elite levels of performance and looking for every edge you can get.

Soda Loading

For many years, a handful of strength trainers and other athletes have put their faith in the alkaline power of sodium bicarbonate (better known as baking soda) and have practiced soda loading. Extracellular metabolic acidosis, a by-product of intense work effort, eventually leads to the point of fatigue. Soda loading may offset fatigue by negating the build-up of extracellular acidic metabolic by-products.

POWER PROFILE: A Champion With Type 1 Diabetes

Leanne Stanley has won multiple championships: Canadian and World Outrigger Canoe Champion, Canadian Surfski Champion, Gorge Downwind Champion, World Dragon Boat Champion, among others.

I first met this champion at a strength and conditioning conference in Kelowna, British Columbia, where I was giving a presentation. Afterwards, she came up front to ask a few questions, introducing herself as someone who "paddles a little bit." At dinner that evening, I learned from the conference organizer that Leanne was a Canadian national champion outrigger canoeist. It sells Leanne short to call her an outrigger canoeist, because she competes at just about every sport on a platform in the water: SUP, surf ski, Dragon Boat, and more. I also learned that she has type 1 diabetes and wears an insulin pump and continuous glucose monitor.

Leanne was searching for two things: A better way to fuel her performance, and a diet to help her drop about 10 pounds of fat but gain strength and power. Leanne knew how to manage her diabetes fairly well. We worked together to dial in her fueling around training; specifically, how we could borrow from her carbohydrate intake during the day to add it to her fueling for training. Her calories were on target but not their distribution. By controlling her carbohydrate intake during the day, we made room for about 60 extra grams of protein, which her strong, nearly 5-foot-10-inch body really needed for recovery every day.

She had a 300-calorie daily energy deficit from her diet. We allowed 100 grams of carbohydrate in meals and snacks, and a minimum of 135 grams of carbohydrate spread out before, during, and after (with whey protein) her high-intensity training sessions. As her training sessions elevated, she increased her carbohydrate supplementation. On her low-intensity days, she reduced to 105 grams of carbohydrate around training. Leanne finds her proper dosage of carbohydrate based on the feedback from her body and her continuous glucose monitor.

When I started working with Leanne, she shared the story with me that she was known as the "burp girl" on the competition circuit, because the witch's brew of carbohydrate supplements she was using to keep herself semifueled on the race course and during training gave her horrible GI discomfort. We discovered that Vitargo, a high-molecular-weight, pure-starch supplement, worked beautifully for her, fully fueling her training yet keeping her comfortable throughout her sessions and competitions. The powder also allowed her to perfectly match her carbohydrate intake to her physiological needs.

The combination of the diet adjustments in food and supplements made an enormous difference for Leanne. She dropped her weight, upped her power, and went on to win more national titles in outrigger canoe and surf ski competitions, along with a win at Queen Lili, a fourth at Na Wahine O Ke Kai, a fourth at the 2017 inaugural World Va'a Distance Championships with Team Canada, and a fourth in the V1—all prestigious competitions in her sport.

Research data support the theory that a more alkaline, plant-rich diet is favorable for exercise and recovery, especially as we age. Research has also found that alkaline diets may

- preserve muscle mass in older men and women and in younger, unhealthy patients;
- correct growth hormone secretion to improve bone health;
- decrease your risk of cardiovascular disease;
- improve body composition, memory, and cognition; and
- decrease chronic low back pain.

Foods that promote alkalinity are vegetables, fruits, legumes, and most plant foods and are an excellent basis for a health-promoting, high-performance diet. Caution: Although much research is being done on soda loading (discussed below), I still feel that adding baking soda to your diet is definitely not the way to create a more alkaline diet on a daily basis. But I am all for a plant-rich diet.

Soda loading has been researched somewhat under the radar for decades but recently has begun to come into its own. Although several products have been studied, sodium bicarbonate appears to be the most effective in improving high intensity exercise lasting from 1 to 7 minutes at a dosage of 0.3 g/kg body weight, with a peak blood level at 60 to 180 minutes after consumption, although these levels can be highly variable. Higher dosages do not improve performance. The evidence supporting sodium citrate and calcium lactate are much weaker. Several studies have strong evidence supporting improvements in single high intensity bouts of exercise, but the evidence is not as clear with repeated bouts of exercise. Also, while the evidence is very appealing, do not ignore the fact that effective doses of soda loading come with side effects, most prominently mild to severe gastrointestinal distress such as stomach pain and diarrhea. When sodium bicarbonate is taken with a meal that contains carbohydrate and fluid, symptoms may be lessened. You must practice with this strategy. It is definitely not something to try first on race or competition day.

A buffering option that works within the cell is beta-alanine, discussed above. Studies are being done on the tactic of combining sodium bicarbonate with beta-alanine to enhance work performance, but so far the results are equivocal. This strategy may be worthwhile to experiment with during training, but the data on supplementing with beta-alanine alone are probably the most convincing once the potential negative side effects of soda loading are considered.

11

Products for Boosting the Brain and Nervous Systems

I began to understand the full potential of the impact of food and supplements on the brain and central nervous system (CNS) when I worked with a clinically depressed all-star NBA player in the 1990s. At that time, there wasn't anything in the nutrition science literature about the impact of food or ingredients on the brain, but I was certain that the restricted diet that he was following was causing harm to his mood, mental focus, sense of mental energy, and ability to cope with stress.

It was well known that certain essential nutrients play important roles in the health and function of the brain and CNS, but I knew he wasn't deficient in those. I dove into the science of neurobiology, and I was fortunate to find, among others, the writings and research of Dr. Eric Kandel, a Nobel prize–winning neurobiologist from Columbia University. Putting nutritional biochemistry together with the science of learning and memory led to my new approach to the timing and combining of food and nutrients in the diets of my clients. It was a step beyond sport nutrition, adding nutrition for the brain and CNS to feeding muscles for training and performance.

Honestly, the impact was magical. Every client felt it: better mood, better focus, more sustained mental energy, improvements in ability to cope with stress, as well as noticeably better rest, relaxation, and sleep. And unexpectedly, their body composition goals were achieved faster. Everything in their bodies just worked better. The last two editions of *Power Eating* contained a lot of this information, both quietly woven into the programs as well as frankly discussed. I didn't want to distract from the major topic of physical performance, strength, and power. To focus only on the concept of nutrition for the brain and CNS, I wrote a book in 2007 called *The Good Mood Diet*.

Today, there is a lot of attention on brain health and performance, and athletes and coaches are well aware of the impact of the mental game. That's why this edition has made nutrition and the brain a priority. I have added this chapter on specialized products (as opposed to food, which I discuss in chapter 8) that boost the brain and nervous system. This up-to-date list will guide you to the truth about the current products and the evidence that supports their claims.

Protein–Carbohydrate Partnership

Chapter 8 goes into the detail of how protein and carbohydrate together are an ideal feel-great food combination, by working in partnership to affect the neurotransmitters in your brain. This combo ideally comes in from whole foods, but many busy fitness enthusiasts and athletes depend on a meal replacement shake for an occasional snack. If that's you, then look for carbohydrate as well as protein in your shake formula to help you stay feeling good all day.

In particular, whey protein is high in the bioactive protein lactalbumin, known to help stress-prone individuals cope with stress and anxiety. So if you're wondering what ingredients will matter, look for the most natural formulation you can find that includes whey protein and some carbohydrate.

Caffeine

The previous chapter covered caffeine in detail, but aside from drinking it in your coffee or tea, you should know that the data support better performance enhancement when you use a powder, capsule, or pill. These supplements will provide a controlled and consistent dose of caffeine for a more reliable result.

For performance enhancement, most studies recommend 3 to 6 milligrams per kilogram of body weight, taken about an hour prior to exercise. The effects last for approximately four to six hours. Some studies have shown effects with dosages of 2 milligrams per kilogram of body weight. I have found that many of my clients can get a consistently reliable and measurable effect from as little as 70 to 80 milligrams of caffeine, but the effects wear off sooner. Oftentimes for a standard one- to two-hour workout, this is a desirable effect.

Theacrine

Consumed for centuries as a natural constituent of teas and coffees, theacrine is found naturally in plant foods including kucha tea (*Camellia assamica var. kucha*), Cupuacu fruit (*Theobroma grandiflorum*) and various coffee (*Coffea*) species and is grown in wild woodland at moderate altitude (1,370 m) in various parts of China. In early animal and human studies, theacrine is reported to enhance mental energy, focus, concentration, and attention without the negative side effects of jitteriness, nausea, and habituation often reported from caffeine.

A recent, two-part human study of 200 milligram and 400 milligram doses of theacrine (Teacrine) showed the following:

1. Theacrine is safe and well tolerated at these doses over a period of seven days, without a sign of habituation.
2. In comparison to placebo under double-blind conditions, theacrine administration at 200 milligrams resulted in more energy, less fatigue, better concentration, and better mood.
3. Under a less-desirable, open-label study design, the 200 milligram dose resulted in improvements in willingness to exercise, motivation to train, and libido, whereas the 400 milligram dose did not show any of these outcomes.

This fairly new-to-the-market product has some good early science behind it. If you want a caffeine-like boost without any of the negative side effects, theacrine might be worth a try. In addition, there is research showing the safety of combining caffeine and theacrine, and the manufacturer of Teacrine does make a product that contains both.

I have recommended this product in particular to my clients who participate in shooting sports and other competitions where a steady hand is equally as important as energy, mental clarity, and focus. The anecdotal reports have been generally positive, but are certainly not research-quality data.

Taurine

One of the most abundant amino acids in the body, taurine is found in the central nervous system and skeletal muscle and is very concentrated in the brain and heart. It is manufactured from the amino acids methionine and cysteine, with help from vitamin B_6. Animal protein is a good source; taurine is not found in vegetable protein.

Taurine appears to act on neurotransmitters in the brain. There have been reports on the benefits of taurine supplementation in treating epilepsy to control motor tics such as facial twitches. The effectiveness of taurine in treating epilepsy is limited, however, because it does not easily cross the blood–brain barrier.

Taurine is also an effective cellular protector against exercise-induced DNA damage. It appears to reduce muscle damage caused by exercise, thereby accelerating recovery between workouts. Other research indicates that supplemental taurine may improve exercise performance by increasing the muscles' force of contraction (strength). In addition, taurine may exert an insulin-like effect. Research hints that it might improve insulin resistance and help the body better use glucose. It also appears to reduce triglycerides and blood levels of harmful cholesterol.

With high-intensity exercise, blood levels of taurine increase, possibly as a result of its release from muscle fibers. Because of its association with neurotransmitters in the brain, taurine has recently been advocated as a supplement to enhance attention, cognitive performance, and feelings of well-being. One study investigated these possibilities with a supplement containing caffeine, taurine, and glucuronolactone (a natural detoxifier derived from carbohydrate metabolism) and found that these ingredients had positive effects on human mental performance and mood. But because a combination of ingredients was tested, there's no way of knowing how much of the effect was the result of taurine alone.

Research into taurine in athletes is very limited and is mostly conducted either in animals or in combination with other ingredients in energy drinks. Many more studies need to be done to verify its benefits. However, because of the possible effectiveness of supplemental taurine in other populations, it is a supplement to watch.

Creatine

Creatine has many benefits and is discussed in several places throughout *The New Power Eating*, but what may end up being creatine's most important function is its role within the brain. Research into how creatine may influence medical conditions involving the nervous system has greatly increased the number of publications addressing the possible benefits of creatine supplements. In addition to research on injury prevention and rehabilitation and enhanced tolerance to exercise in the heat, creatine is under heavy investigation for potential brain and spinal cord neuroprotective capacity.

Traumatic brain injuries, spinal cord injuries and concussions during contact sports, military exercises, and work-related accidents and other accidents are all topics of immense discussion and research. A number of studies have examined the effects of creatine supplementation on traumatic brain injury (TBI), cerebral ischemia, and spinal cord injuries (SCI). In summary, the findings of many of these studies provide strong evidence that creatine supplementation may limit damage from concussions, TBI, or SCI.

Research is also under way to examine the impact of creatine on various metabolic and synthesis disorders, neurodegenerative diseases, ischemic heart disease, memory and the aging brain, and its involvement in certain complications of pregnancy.

The evidence on creatine and the brain is so abundant and convincing that it is the position of the International Society of Sports Nutrition that

> *Given all the known benefits and favorable safety profile of creatine supplementation reported in the scientific and medical literature, it is the view of ISSN that government legislatures and sport organizations who restrict and/or discourage use of creatine may be placing athletes at greater risk—particularly in contact sports that have risk of head trauma and/or neurological injury thereby opening themselves up to legal liability. This includes children and adolescent athletes engaged in sport events that place them at risk for head and/or spinal cord injury. (Kreider et al., 2017, 13)*

I recommend that all my masters-level clients, women and men, supplement with 1 teaspoon (5 g) of creatine daily for brain health. I give the same recommendation to all my youth athlete clients who participate in sports with any risk of head injury, from football to skiing.

EPA and DHA

Both EPA and DHA are important for healthy brain function and your entire central nervous system. They appear to help prevent chronic degenerative diseases of the brain and memory loss. DHA, in particular, is a mood booster.

It is a good idea to supplement your diet with fish oil. Enough research justifies its use; however, you need to choose wisely. The product you choose should be a good source of EPA and DHA, with at least 1,000 milligrams combined of DHA and EPA. The recommended dose for supplementation or through diet is 1,000 milligrams per day of a combination of DHA and EPA. Under certain circumstances DHA or EPA are recommended alone, but in general the combination works quite well.

If you cannot consume fish oil, I highly recommend supplementation from a vegan algae-based product. Always tell your physician or health care provider before taking supplements if you also take prescription medications or need any kind of medical intervention or surgery.

Youth athletes and masters athletes, in addition to the traditional young adult athlete users of creatine, may find that creatine supplements provide brain and spinal cord benefits, particularly when participating in contact sports.

iStockphoto/Grafissimo

Phosphatidylcholine (PC) and Phosphatidylserine (PS)

PS and PC have both been shown to play an important role in brain cell health and memory function. These two phospholipids are required to create the channels in brain cell membranes that allow nutrients to pass into the cells and toxins to pass out. Research from the National Institutes of Mental Health has shown that supplementing with PS and PC may slow the rate of progression of degenerative diseases of the brain. These are critical compounds to have in our diets.

Phosphatidylserine (PS) is a fat-soluble nutrient that is most concentrated in the brain, where it supports many crucial nerve cell functions, including mood and brain health. It is available as a supplement (extracted from soybeans), and it has been well studied.

Here's what some of the research shows:

- Taking 300 milligrams daily of PS for a month helped young adults better cope with stress (from taking a mental arithmetic test).

- Male soccer players who supplemented with 850 milligrams of PS for 10 days increased their running time to exhaustion. This benefit probably has to do more with the ability of PS to reduce anxiety and improve mood than anything else, because the nutrient had no real effect on preventing muscle damage, oxidative stress, or lipid peroxidation. A study with cyclists looked at similar parameters and also found that PS has a positive effect on performance. Again, this may have occurred because of the ability of PS to improve mood. If your mood is good, you're naturally going to feel like exercising because you have better mental energy.

- Most vitamin supplements contain choline, and you should make sure to consume at least the DRI for choline daily. The effective dosage in sport studies is 0.2 gram of phosphatidylcholine per kilogram of body mass. This does not need to be any kind of loading strategy but can just be a maintenance program. The effective dosages for phosphatidylserine in exercise studies range from 300 to 800 milligrams per day for 10 to 15 days. Studies that investigated cognitive function and memory, and support during periods of mental stress associated with physical stress, suggested a range from 100 to 300 milligrams of phosphatidylserine per day. In the soccer study above, 850 mg was given safely for 10 days, but we do not have long-term data on that level.

Citicoline

A form of choline getting a lot of attention is citicoline, or CDP-choline. It has been found in a number of studies to

- have a positive effect on memory and behavior in elderly patients with chronic cerebrovascular disorders;
- be helpful in the management of neurodegenerative conditions such as senile dementia, Alzheimer's disease, and Parkinson's disease;
- slow the progression of Alzheimer's disease;
- increase blood flow to the brain;
- increase levels of two neurotransmitters, noradrenaline and dopamine, in the central nervous system;
- inhibit brain inflammation; and
- help accelerate recovery in head trauma patients, including possibly athletes who have suffered concussions.

The common dose is 1,000 milligrams, and studies show it is well tolerated with no adverse effects.

Another form of choline delivery, alpha glycerylphosphorylcholine, or Alpha-GPC, has been shown in very early studies possibly to have an impact on certain types of physical performance. There are minimal data despite the fact that products with such claims are already on the market. So, I am only including this because of the gaining marketing momentum and not because I think it is worth trying yet.

Probiotics

I have talked about foods containing probiotics, but it is also a good idea to supplement with them because of their effect on the gut-brain axis. The science and our understanding of specific types of probiotic cultures are changing and updating so rapidly that it's hard to make a specific recommendation here, but I can make some general recommendations.

Species of *Bifidobacterium* and *Lactobacillus* are most commonly studied as cultures for a healthy daily regimen. While the exact species matters, I can only give you the general family because the target on species just changes too fast. I recommend that you do a little of your own research on the cultures included in products that you consider, asking the manufacturer for published data on their product or on that specific culture species and the number of live culture cells required for efficacy.

Prebiotics

As you feed your body, you also have to feed your microbiota with prebiotics, which are the food for the probiotic bacteria in your gut. As I mentioned earlier, a variety of fibers will feed your microbiota, such as whole grains, onions, apple skins, bananas, garlic, honey, leeks, and artichokes. Or you can consciously create a daily prebiotic regimen of 1 to 2 tablespoons of flaxseed meal. I grind flaxseeds fresh daily, but preground flaxseed meal is just as effective.

Tart Cherry Juice

There have been a number of studies investigating the anti-inflammatory impact of Montmorency tart cherries and tart cherry juice on exercise-induced inflammation, with mixed results on the clinical impact on pain and muscle soreness. However, one very interesting area not commonly discussed is the naturally high melatonin content of tart cherries, and the potential to enhance sleep, especially as we age.

One study gave subjects 8 ounces (240 ml) of tart cherry juice in the morning and nighttime for two weeks. The supplementation was associated with a significant reduction in insomnia severity and wake-after-sleep-onset in adults with chronic insomnia. A later study replicated the study but in a population of young, healthy adults. One week of tart cherry juice supplementation increased urinary melatonin concentrations, total sleep time, and sleep efficiency (the amount of time in bed spent asleep) compared with a placebo juice. Bottom line, early clinical evidence supports the possible sleep-promoting effect of tart cherries.

Mood-Boosting Herbs

Among the most popular of self-prescribed medications, many herbs are promoted as brain and mood boosters. But keep in mind that certain brain-boosting herbs, particularly *Ginkgo biloba* and ginseng, interfere with normal blood clotting and can lead to excessive blood loss during surgery. Mood-boosting herbs such as St. John's wort and kava kava dangerously heighten the sedative effects of anesthesia.

Several botanicals do influence mood. They are typically not as potent as drugs and take longer to show an effect. Although side effects may also not be as potent as the negative side effects from drugs, they do exist, so dosages should always be according to label directions. Here's a rundown of these mood boosters:

- Passion flower helps with calming, anxiety reduction, and better sleep.
- Chamomile helps with calming, anxiety reduction, and better sleep.
- *Ginkgo biloba* improves blood flow to the brain for clearer thinking.
- Kava kava elevates mood and well-being, induces relaxation, and may lower anxiety. (I don't recommend it, though, because there are serious and dangerous side effects, including liver damage.)
- St. John's wort relieves mild depression. (Caution: This herb can interfere with other drugs and should be used only under the care of a physician.)

If you're still curious and want to try an herbal supplement as a brain or mood booster, do so with care by following a few precautions:

- Choose good-quality supplements by reputable manufacturers.
- Keep in mind that cost is not always a reliable gauge of quality.
- Do not exceed recommended dosages.
- Get advice from a trained health care professional.
- In general, supplement with simpler rather than more complicated formulas.
- Liquid forms may be easier during active treatment (easier to swallow and more easily absorbed).
- Consider taste and ease of swallowing in choosing the form of a supplement.
- Disclose any use of botanicals and herbal supplements to your health care team.

Products Marketed as Nootropics

Nootropics is a marketing term used to encompass the category of drugs and supplements presumed to enhance cognition. When searched on Google, there are nearly as many articles warning of scams as ads promoting products claiming to have nootropic properties. This chapter has included only the compounds that have a substantial or significant amount of research evidence behind such claims, and clear data on safety. Any other products on the market are fairly untested in both safety and efficacy. This does not mean they will never have data, but the evidence does not yet support inclusion.

For information on herbal supplements outside their effects on mood, see chapter 12.

12

Botanicals for Performance

Herbs are the most popular self-prescribed medication. They now come in capsules, tablets, liquids, and powders. Of the $20 billion spent on dietary supplements in the United States, more than $5 billion is spent on herbal supplements alone. Those sales figures increase by 3 to 5 percent each year. Herbs are heavily promoted as bodybuilding supplements with little evidence that they work (although we have more data now than ever before). Also, herbs can even do harm.

An herb is a plant or part of a plant valued for its medicinal qualities, its aroma, or its taste. Herbs and herbal remedies have been around for centuries. Even Neanderthal people used plants for healing purposes. About 30 percent of all modern drugs are derived from herbs. Cooking with herbs and botanicals is a very powerful way to influence your mind–body health. I encourage you to enhance the healing properties of your foods by adding more herbs and botanicals to your diet. In this chapter, however, I'll be focusing more on supplements. The information in this chapter can help guide you through the often-confusing maze of herbs and lead you to those that can be helpful.

Natural but Not Always Safe

It's a common but dangerous notion to think that because herbs are natural, they are safe. What separates plant-derived drugs from herbal supplements is careful scientific study. Makers of herbal supplements in the United States are not required to submit their products to the FDA, so there is no regulation of product quality or safety. Without the enforcement of standards, there is only a meager chance that the contents and potency described on labels are accurate. Some eye-opening proof of this was found in a study conducted at the UCLA Center for Human Nutrition. Researchers analyzed commercial formulations of saw palmetto, kava kava, echinacea, ginseng, and St. John's wort. They purchased six bottles each of two lots of supplements from nine manufacturers and analyzed their contents. There were differences in what was actually in the product versus what was stated on the labels, particularly with echinacea and ginseng. Even the product labels varied in the information provided. Dosage recommendations and information about the herbs often varied.

This study reflects an important problem with herbal products. When products that are not standardized are tested for effectiveness, conclusive evidence on what works and what doesn't is hard to come by, no matter how well the study is designed. What you are taking may not be the same in any way as the extract that was tested.

Many herbal supplements can be contaminated, too, although this is usually not the case with well-known mainstream store brands. For this reason, try to purchase herbal supplements from reputable manufacturers. Also, make sure the product lists all ingredients on the label and that it is certified by a good laboratory.

Because there's no universal quality-control regulation of the industry, the danger of chemical contamination of herbal supplements is real. Were the plants sprayed with any chemicals before harvesting or processing? Other toxic contaminants or banned or illegal substances may enter the product during processing as well. For instance, a study testing herbal products for prohibited anabolic androgen steroids and growth hormone (GH) found that 15 percent contained prohormones (variants of hormones) that were not declared on the label. Most of these substances were manufactured in the United States but were sold in European countries. Products that are purchased by mail order from other countries are even more questionable than those purchased in the United States.

Herbs are classified as food supplements by the FDA. Labeling them as medicines would require stringent testing to prove their safety and effectiveness. This costs millions of dollars per herb, an investment few manufacturers are willing to make. Fortunately for consumers, supplements can no longer be labeled with unsubstantiated claims. The latest government regulations require that the supplement industry abide by the same labeling laws that govern packaged foods. This means that any supplement bearing a health claim must support the claim with scientific evidence that meets government approval. Any product marketed as a way to cure, modify, treat, or prevent disease is regulated as a drug by the FDA.

What you see on supplement labels now are structure and function claims. This means that manufacturers are allowed to make claims about the impact of dietary supplements on the structure or function of the body, but these claims must be truthful. An example of such a claim is, "Vitamin C is involved in immune function."

Besides quality control, there are other concerns with herbal supplementation. It's not uncommon to have an allergic reaction to drugs, even those that have been tested and manufactured with strict safeguards. Therefore, it is even more likely that untested herbs, which are consumed in large amounts, may also produce allergic reactions. These reactions can sometimes be fatal. Herbs can interact with prescribed medications, too. If you're taking any medications, you should consult your physician, pharmacist, or dietitian before using any herbal supplement.

In addition, if you're scheduled for surgery and are taking herbal supplements, let your physician know well in advance of your operation. Certain herbs, particularly *Ginkgo biloba*, garlic, ginger, and ginseng, interfere with normal blood clotting and can lead to excessive blood loss during surgery. Mood-boosting herbs such as St. John's wort and kava kava dangerously heighten the sedative effects of anesthesia.

Pregnant and nursing mothers should avoid all herbal preparations. If you are pregnant or nursing, ask your physician or dietitian about specific herbal teas, because even these can cause harmful reactions in a developing baby or nursing infant. Don't give herbal supplements or remedies to children, either. There is virtually no medical information about the safety of herbs for children. Your best intentions could result in serious harm.

Being better informed about the benefits, limitations, and risks of herbal supplementation will help you decide which herbs to try. The following is a rundown of well-known herbs that may help enhance performance.

Herbal Supplements That Meet Marketing Claims

Much of the research on herbal supplements has been conducted outside the United States, but experts agree that the products listed here have been well tested for efficacy. Even so, herbs can act as powerful drugs. Approach them with the same respect as you would any prescription medication.

Buchu

Culled from a shrub native to South Africa, the leaves of this herb are usually made into a tea and other supplement forms. Buchu is a mild diuretic, and in that regard it may help rid your body of excess water weight. It is also an antiseptic that fights germs in the urinary tract.

Buchu is generally considered safe, although herbalists recommend taking no more than 2 grams two or three times a day.

Fo-Ti

Ancient Chinese herbalists swore that this member of the buckwheat family is one of the best longevity promoters ever grown. According to herbalists, fo-ti exhibits different properties depending on the size and age of its root. A fist-sized 50-year-old plant, for example, keeps your hair from turning gray. A 100-year-old root the size of a bowl preserves your cheerfulness. At 150 years old and as large as a sink, fo-ti makes your teeth fall out so that new ones can grow in. And a 200-year-old plant restores youth and vitality. Or so the folk tales go.

Fo-ti has a reputation as a good cardiovascular herb. Supposedly, it lowers cholesterol, protects blood vessels, and increases blood flow to the heart. Fo-ti does act as a natural laxative, however, and in this regard it's probably a safe herb.

Guarana

Guarana is a red berry from a plant grown in the Amazon valley. It contains seven times the caffeine as coffee beans and is widely sold in health food stores as a supplement to increase energy. It is also found in energy drinks and energy waters. The supplement is made from the seeds of the berry.

Guarana is used in a number of natural weight-loss supplements. It is believed to increase thermogenesis (body heat) and thus stimulate the metabolism. In large doses, guarana may also cause the body to lose water because the caffeine it contains is a diuretic. As for a possible performance benefit, guarana has been shown to increase blood glucose in animals. Whether that holds true for humans, however, remains to be seen. A note of caution: If you're sensitive to caffeine, it's best to leave guarana alone.

Maté

Another caffeinated herb is maté. Touted as a natural upper, it has a caffeine content of 2 percent. Maté is found in some natural weight-loss supplements because it is believed to help control appetite. Like guarana, it is found in energy drinks and energy waters. It also has a mild diuretic effect and thus may produce temporary water weight loss. Medical experts say the herb is relatively safe when taken in small quantities for short periods of time.

Please keep in mind that both guarana and maté contain caffeine. I've had clients come to me thrilled that they are off caffeine, only to find out that they've been drinking energy waters containing one of these herbs! They haven't quit caffeine at all; they went from caffeine in their coffee to caffeine in their herbal water. Read labels to watch for these herbs. You do have to be well informed about herbs that naturally contain caffeine; the label will not list caffeine unless caffeine itself is an additive ingredient.

Herbal Supplements That Possibly Meet Marketing Claims

Research is still not clear on whether the claims made about the herbs in this category are true—maybe they are; maybe they aren't. If you try these herbs, remember that you are being the guinea pig. It may be preferable to wait to see how the research pans out before trying them yourself.

Beetroot Juice

Beetroot juice, with its active ingredient nitrate, appears to help prolong time to exhaustion by reducing oxygen intake and making exercise less tiring. This is called greater energy efficiency and is seen to work in studies predominantly with recreational and nonelite athlete subjects. Studies with beetroot juice show that subjects who took this botanical needed less oxygen and had lower blood pressure than those who did not take it. Other benefits found in research included better performance and heart function while exercising.

Nitrates are compounds found naturally in various foods, including beetroots, green leafy vegetables, cured meats, and tea. Nitrates are converted in the body to various other compounds, including sodium nitrite, and part of this process involves bacteria found in the mouth and digestive tract.

Dietary nitrates used to be forbidden for fear of increased cancer risk from the converted nitrites, but new science tells us that they aren't necessarily bad for our health and can even jack up blood flow and energy during exercise. Nitrates are the active natural compound in beetroot juice. They are also found abundantly in celery, spinach, and collard greens.

How exactly does beetroot juice work? Basically, it doubles the amount of nitrate in the blood and reduces the rate at which muscles use their source of energy, ATP. But I must emphasize that the subjects who appear to receive the greatest benefits are not elite athletes. Recreational and subelite athlete subjects have received the greatest benefit from supplementation.

See chapter 20 for my Banana Beet Orange antioxidant smoothie that includes beets in its ingredient list. This recipe does not give the efficacious dose of beetroot juice, but certainly adds to your total nitrate intake for the day.

Using beetroot juice supplements may be the easiest way to ingest adequate amounts of dietary nitrate, but a side effect of this strategy may be red urine and stools. There are other great sources of nitrates, including spinach, collard greens, raw leaf lettuce, and vegetable juice. The beneficial amount of dietary nitrate consumed in most studies ranges from 300 to 500 milligrams.

Cayenne

Cayenne pepper, that spice you use to make foods taste hot, may be a bona fide fat burner. It contains a compound called capsaicin, which has been shown in studies to enhance energy expenditure and increase fat burning.

A lot of athletes have trouble using this supplement, however. It tends to create a burning sensation in the stomach. Fortunately, a less-hot form of capsaicin, the capsinoid dihydrocapsiate, has been developed from sweet peppers. Supplementing with this new nonspicy formulation is an exciting alternative option for this fat burner. Available data suggest that it's best to take 3 milligrams daily to obtain the fat-burning benefit without the burning sensation in the stomach.

Echinacea

Echinacea is a member of the sunflower family. There are three species used medicinally—*purpurea, angustifolia,* and *pallida.* The German Commission E, Germany's equivalent to the U.S. FDA, has approved *Echinacea purpurea* as supportive therapy for colds and chronic infections of the respiratory tract. The Commission's monograph, a publication describing scores of herbs and their therapeutic applications, notes that echinacea preparations increase the number of white blood cells in the body. White blood cells destroy invading organisms, including cold viruses.

A stringent scientific review study of echinacea conducted in 2006 analyzed 16 trials of the herb. It concluded that some evidence has found that the aerial parts of *Echinacea purpurea* are effective for the early treatment of colds in adults, but that these results are not fully consistent.

Weakened immunity is often seen in athletes and highly active people—which is why many sport scientists recommend supplementing with echinacea. However, I am not one of them. One reason is that if you suffer from hay fever, taking echinacea puts you at risk for a severe reaction, even anaphylactic shock, a life-threatening allergic reaction. Allergies in general appear to be on the rise, so I believe that taking an herb such as this is not worth the risk.

Don't supplement with echinacea if you have an autoimmune disease such as lupus or a progressive illness such as multiple sclerosis, because the herb may over-stimulate your immune system and do further damage. Also, don't take echinacea orally for longer than eight weeks.

Ginseng

Used for thousands of years in the Far East as a tonic to strengthen and restore health, ginseng has more recently been touted as a performance-boosting herb for exercisers and athletes. For background, ginseng comes from the root of a medicinal plant in the ginseng family (*Araliaceae*). There are various types of ginseng, including those in the *Panax* classification and a botanical cousin called Siberian ginseng, also known as eleuthero or ciwujia, its Chinese name, for short.

Panax ginseng and eleuthero are approved medicines in Germany. In fact, the German Commission E states in its monographs that these ginsengs can be used "as a tonic for invigoration and fortification in times of fatigue and debility, for declining capacity for work and concentration, also during convalescence" (Blumenthal, 2000, 174).

In the United States, the FDA considers ginseng a food. According to one nutritional analysis, 100 grams of *Panax* ginseng root contain 338 calories; 70 grams of carbohydrate; appreciable amounts of vitamins A, B_1 (thiamin), B_2 (riboflavin), B_{12}, C, and E; as well as the minerals niacin, calcium, iron, and phosphorus.

The main active constituents of the *Panax* species are plant steroids called ginsenosides. Eleuthero's active constituents are plant steroids known as eleutherosides, which differ in chemical structure from ginsenosides but have similar properties. The mechanisms of action of these chemical components are complex, but scientists theorize that they increase the size of the mitochondria (the energy factories of cells), stimulate the production of adrenal hormones, and enhance the transmission of brain chemicals called neurotransmitters, among other functions.

In herbal medicine, all ginsengs are considered to be "adaptogens." Coined by a Soviet scientist in 1947, the term refers to a class of agents that build resistance to physical stress, enhance performance, extend endurance, and stimulate the body's recovery power after exercise.

Summarizing much of the research that's been done, Dr. Luke Bucci in a review paper noted that *Panax* ginseng supplements may enhance physical and mental performance if taken long enough and in sufficient enough doses. Further, he stated that ginseng is more effective in untrained subjects or subjects older than age 40. There are no acute or immediate effects from ginseng supplementation, either. It is a supplement that acts over at least an eight-week period of time.

In other research, when doses are at least 2 grams of the standardized extract for longer than eight weeks, significant improvements in physical or psychomotor performance are almost always seen. Siberian ginseng, different from *Panax* ginseng, has not shown any influence on physical performance. Further studies and better studies are needed on both Siberian ginseng and *Panax* ginseng.

Clearly, there is conflicting research on ginseng. How do we make sense of the data? The most valid explanation is the wide variability among commercial ginseng products. An analysis of 24 roots and products (including softgels, tablets, dry-filled capsules, and teas) showed great variations in the concentrations of ginsenosides. Another study revealed that ginseng products vary in content even across lots of the same brand, and that some products contain no ginsenosides at all. In addition, the chemical composition of commercial ginseng products varies according to the age of the root, its cultivation, the part of the root used, and manufacturing methods.

When it comes to ginseng, knowing what you're buying can be difficult. And taking ginseng is a questionable practice. There are known side effects of large doses and long-term use: high blood pressure, nervousness, insomnia, low blood pressure, sedation, painful breasts, breast nodules, and vaginal bleeding. In addition, ginseng reacts with many drugs. Ginseng is contraindicated for use with stimulants, including excessive use of caffeine. Talk to your physician and pharmacist about potential interactions with any medications you're taking.

Green Tea

Derived from the leaves and leaf buds of an evergreen plant native to Asia, green tea is of interest to fitness-minded people because it may help encourage weight loss. Certain natural chemicals called catechins are abundant in green tea; animal and human studies show that these chemicals appear to increase fat burning and stimulate thermogenesis, the calorie-burning process that occurs as a result of digesting and metabolizing food. Green tea is also an excellent anti-inflammatory.

A study by Japanese researchers in 2001 reported that tea catechins (600 mg/day) taken with the diet for 12 weeks in men promoted weight loss, a decrease in body mass index (BMI), and a decrease in waist circumference compared to subjects consuming a placebo with a small amount of catechins.

Green tea used in conjunction with caffeine has also been widely studied. In 2011, researchers published a review of the mechanisms contributing to the anti-obesity effects of green tea and reported their findings in the *Journal of Nutritional Biochemistry*. They stated that the predominant hypothesis is that the green tea catechins influence the sympathetic nervous system, increasing energy expenditure and promoting fat oxidation. Caffeine also influences sympathetic nervous system activity, acting synergistically to increase the antiobesity effects. The researchers speculate that other potential mechanisms are involved, too, including appetite suppression, an increase in fat-burning enzymes, and less absorption of calories.

Does green tea help boost exercise performance? Studies looking into this have found no effect. I believe more research is needed in this area.

Even the amount that you need to consume for weight loss isn't yet clear. A 1999 study in Maryland resulted in weight loss when using 6 1/4 cups (1.5 L) of tea per day for four days. The more recent Japanese study on men (mentioned earlier) found successful results from 2 1/2 cups (600 ml) every day for 12 weeks. If you are caffeine sensitive, you might want to start with the lower dose, and definitely don't drink the tea in the evening before bed.

Whether or not green tea pans out as a true antiobesity agent, it's worth drinking for other reasons. Research has found that the natural chemicals in green tea may protect against periodontal disease, some cancers, and heart disease. Unless you're sensitive to caffeine, green tea or extracts containing it are very safe and probably beneficial to health.

Anti-Inflammatory Botanicals

A big part of Power Eating is including anti-inflammatory foods in your diet. One way to do this is to use botanicals that fight inflammation. Here are my top picks for anti-inflammatory botanicals.

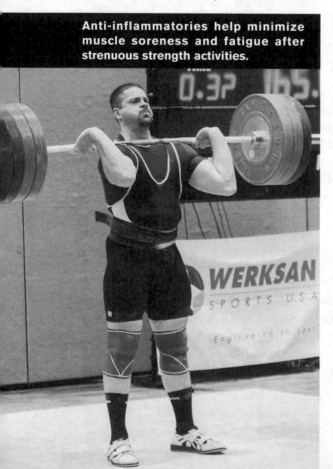

Anti-inflammatories help minimize muscle soreness and fatigue after strenuous strength activities.

Ginger

This popular herb helps relieve symptoms of mild muscle pain and works like non-steroidal anti-inflammatory drugs but without the negative side effects on your digestive tract. The recommended dose is between 2 and 7 grams daily. Ginger is also helpful for mild nausea; I recommend it to my clients who get nervous prior to competing in an event or race. Ginger comes in capsules and lozenges.

Turmeric

This spice is used widely in Indian cooking. It contains a potent anti-inflammatory and antioxidant called curcumin. Curcumin works through several well-established pathways. As an antioxidant, it boosts levels of glutathione, one of the body's chief antioxidants. It also blocks

Sport Nutrition Fact Versus Fiction: Are Functional Foods the New Training Staple?

If you've ever taken a bite of a sport bar, swilled a glass of calcium-fortified orange juice, or slurped a soup beefed up with herbs such as St. John's wort or echinacea, you've feasted on a functional food.

Technically, the term *functional food* refers to a food product that enhances performance or is beneficial to health. In its position paper on functional foods, the Academy of Nutrition and Dietetics defines these products as "any modified food or food ingredient that may provide a health benefit beyond the traditional nutrients it contains" (American Dietetic Association, 2009, 735-746).

Products that fit this definition include the following:

- ***Foods in which sugar, fat, sodium, or cholesterol have been reduced or eliminated.*** Fat-free cheese, reduced-sugar jam, or low-sodium soup are all examples. Functional foods such as these are beneficial to people on restricted diets and may be helpful in preventing or controlling obesity, cardiovascular disease, diabetes, and high blood pressure.

- ***Foods in which naturally occurring ingredients have been increased.*** Breakfast cereal and pasta that have been enriched with additional fiber or vitamins are good examples. Foods modified in this way can play an important role in preventing disease.

- ***Foods enhanced with nutrients not normally present.*** Folic acid–enriched bread and soups or soft drinks spruced up with therapeutic herbs are good examples. Enriched foods help people take in higher levels of health-protective nutrients and can be important in maintaining general wellness.

- ***Probiotic yogurt and other dairy products to which special healthy bacteria have been added as a part of the fermentation process.*** These foods are believed to enhance the growth of healthy flora in the intestines, which improve digestion and prevent disease.

- ***Sport foods targeting the nutrient and energy needs of athletes and exercisers.*** These include sport drinks with added electrolytes; protein powders formulated with creatine, amino acids, and other nutrients; and sport bars packed with vitamins, minerals, or herbs. Functional foods such as these are designed to provide energy, enhance muscle growth, and replenish nutrients lost during exercise.

Should you incorporate these foods into your diet if you're not already doing so? The answer is yes, particularly if convenience is important and you're trying to enhance muscle health, strength, and growth. Sport foods, in particular, can help you achieve those goals. However, think of functional foods as supplements to your diet rather than as substitutes for real food. Ultimately, the best way to fuel your body is always to eat a varied, nutrient-rich diet of lean protein and dairy products, fruits, whole grains, vegetables, and the right kinds of fat.

the formation of prostaglandin E2, a compound that promotes inflammation within the body. You can reap the benefits of curcumin by spicing your foods with turmeric.

Flavonols

These phytochemicals are strong antioxidants and anti-inflammatories. They include quercetin, kaempferol, and myricetin, as well as the citrus bioflavonoids that include naringenin, hesperetin, and others. Green tea also contains flavonols. These beneficial compounds are easy to obtain from food. Foods rich in quercetin include capers, the green leafy vegetable lovage, apples, and chamomile tea. Kaempferol is found in tea, broccoli, cabbage, kale, beans, endives, leeks, tomatoes, strawberries and grapes, and in botanical supplements including *Ginkgo biloba* and propolis. Myricetin is found in grapes, berries, onions, tea, and walnuts. Flavonols are found most abundantly in citrus fruits, dark chocolate, and all types of teas.

Other important and potent anti-inflammatory and antioxidant botanicals with good supporting evidence include grape seed extract, elderberry, pomegranate, nettles, devil's claw, frankincense, flaxseed, milk thistle, and white willow bark.

Plans and Menus

This part of the book is where you put your knowledge to work. You have the foundation, the information, and hopefully, the inspiration. Now let's put it all into practice, designing your own personalized Power Eating plan. To begin, determine your goals: Do you want to maintain weight, build muscle, lose weight, or cut fat? Are you in your off-season trying to gain, or approaching a championship and planning for a peak? Are you new to strength training, or have you been training for years? Chapter 13 will walk you through the steps I take when I design a client's customized nutrition plan. With the information here, you can figure your calories and map out your protein, carbohydrate, and fat needs based on your personal goals, just as I would if you came to my office. Chapter 13 also provides the information you need to customize all of the menu plans presented in later chapters. Chapter 14 gives you the ultimate competitive nutrition strategies for preparing your body to peak for competition. I've kept no top-level professional secrets from these pages—it's all here.

Each of the five diet strategies (maintaining weight, building muscle, cross-training, losing weight, and cutting fat) in chapters 15 through 19 offers a menu plan designed especially for novice strength trainers, or those who work out three or four times per week, and one for highly muscled, experienced strength trainers who work out five or more times per week. The menu plans are also divided into plans geared for women and those geared for men. The plans begin with the mathematical models I designed to create the menus. By plugging in your weight, you can create your own personalized diet plan. The menus in this section are examples based on the needs of a 180-pound (82 kg) man and a 130-pound (59 kg) woman. If your weight is different, just plug it into the formulas and you can create a personalized plan.

The menus are similar in food choices so you can easily move from one strategy to the next as your training goals change. Some menus place exercise in the morning and others place it in the late afternoon so you can see how to customize a menu to your training schedule. Always make sure to have a preworkout snack and a postworkout snack or meal. Menu planning takes some time and effort, but the results are worth it!

To experiment with periodizing your carbs with your training, make sure to prefuel with carbs on high intensity, heavy training days. If your next training session is lower intensity, you don't need heavy recovery carbs or prefueling carbs for that workout. Then the night before a heavy workout, have carbs, and again prefuel with carbs. That's a cycle that has had promise with some athletes.

Once you've designed your diet, have some fun with the recipes in chapter 20. This chapter includes the special power drinks I created for the clients and teams I've worked with over the years. These drinks can be used in place of commercially-produced liquid supplements. Enjoy experimenting with added greens, either fresh or frozen, for vitamin, mineral, and anti-inflammatory potency. You won't even know the veggies are there. Add liquid or powdered supplements to your drinks for an extra boost. My family and I particularly enjoy the smoothies, and we make them daily. They're a great way to sneak in extra protein, fruit, and vegetable servings. Don't miss the power breakfasts, either—they will give your day a tasty and energy-charged start. And I am very proud to again include recipes designed by Shar Sault, two-time consecutive winner of the drug-tested World Figure Title of Ms. Natural Olympia. Shar is an awesome role model and a dear friend.

Most of all, train hard and Power Eat!

13

Developing a
Power Eating Plan

There are different schools of thought regarding the ideal way to help people change their dietary behaviors. One school has a less defined approach, giving guidelines and strategies for menu selection, but no specific menu plans. I have found that this method works best with people who don't have highly specific goals or those who are doing just about everything right but need a tweak here and there. For most people this approach leaves too much room for error and results in their never quite accomplishing their performance and physique goals. People with very idealized goals need a targeted plan so that they make strategic choices. That is why I offer specific plans that outline exactly how to eat to achieve your goals. You undertake rigorous training and need a diet to support that training.

The Power Eating plan begins with determining the proper calorie level and then the right distribution of protein, fat, and carbohydrate to meet your goal. Menu development is based on a food group exchange plan that I have tweaked just a bit based on state-of-the-art nutrition science. Food group exchanges force you to have variety in your diet and at the same time allow you to personalize your program through food choices and exchanges or swapping among groups. Use the sample diets as a starting point, and then add or subtract servings to meet your personalized protein, carbohydrate, and fat needs based on the goal-oriented formulas that I include with each menu plan.

I provide a lot of examples of fat servings to give you the freedom to customize your plan. Lower-fat and nonfat milk and very lean and lean protein sources are the primary choices in the meal plans. The one exception is a whole egg, which is a medium-fat protein. There is also space in your diet for healthier, high-performance fats from sources such as vegetable oils, olive oils, nuts, and seeds in place of animal fat that is higher in saturated fat. Consider any low-fat or fat-free protein supplements as very lean protein servings.

To use more medium-fat protein sources such as soy products, as well as the occasional high-fat protein source, just exchange, or swap, one very lean protein serving plus one fat serving for one medium-fat protein serving. Exchange one lean protein serving plus one fat serving for one high-fat protein serving. Refer to the Nutrients per Food Group Serving table to become proficient at food group exchanges. Remember that you can easily determine your fat grams once you have calculated your total calories and your protein and carbohydrate needs. In most cases, all the leftover calories are fat calories. Divide fat calories by 9 to get your total fat grams per day. Or you can directly calculate your recommended fat grams per day by using the formula for grams per kilogram or pound of body weight per day. Then multiply your fat grams by 9 to get your total fat calories per day.

You will also be able to use your recommended added teaspoons of carbohydrate or sugar mostly as sport fuel, and learn how to use these to your advantage. Engineered sports-specific nutrition can assist you in muscle fuel during exercise and recovery and work best around exercise.

A note on alcohol: Too much alcohol on a regular basis will slow your training, halt your fat loss, and even impair your health and safety. Thus, alcohol is not part of the Power Eating plan.

Creating Your Diet Plan

Once you have calculated your daily nutrient and calorie needs, use the Nutrients per Food Group Serving table that follows to design your diet. This table shows the amount of nutrients in one serving from each food group. Make sure that you include choices from all of the food groups to ensure a well-balanced diet. Add liquid supplements to meet additional carbohydrate, protein, and calorie needs. To simplify periodizing your diet to align with your training program, put your exercise-specific fueling into snacks before, during, and after exercise. These snacks

Nutrients per Food Group Serving

Food groups	Carbohydrate (g)	Protein (g)	Fat (g)	Calories
Bread and starch	15	3	1 or less	72-81
Fruit	15	-	-	60
Nonfat milk	12	8	0-1	80-89
Low-fat milk	12	8	3	107
Added carbohydrate or sugar (1 tsp, 4 g)	4	-	-	16
Vegetables	5	2	-	25
Very lean protein	-	7	0-1	35
Lean protein	-	7	3	55
Medium-fat protein	-	7	5	75
Fat	-	-	5	45

Adapted from American Diabetes Association and American Dietetic Association, Exchange Lists for Meal Planning (Alexandria, VA: American Diabetes Association, 1995).

can be eliminated on rest days and low-volume training days. Refer to the serving size charts in the next section to learn about serving sizes for each food group.

Knowing Your Portions

A portion is the amount of food used to determine the numbers of servings for each food group; it is the physical measurement of one serving. The amount of food that makes up a portion is not usually what you would think of as a serving, however. For example, one portion of cooked pasta is just 1/2 cup (70 g). If you have pasta for dinner, you would likely eat at least 1 cup (140 g), but since one serving is 1/2 cup, one cup of pasta equals two servings from the bread and starch group.

Learning the portion sizes for servings is the foundation of success. It is the method by which calorie control is built into the Power Eating plan. If you are eating portions that are too large or too small, the plan will not work. The following charts list portion sizes (for one serving) for foods in each food group. In the beginning, you should refer to this chart frequently, as well as weigh and measure foods to get a handle on portion sizes. After a few weeks, you will be able judge the size on your own.

Milk and Yogurt Group

Each portion contains 90 to 110 calories.

Food	Size of one portion
Nonfat or low-fat milk	1 cup (240 ml)
Evaporated nonfat milk	1 cup (240 ml)
Nonfat dry milk powder	1/3 cup (22 g)
Plain nonfat yogurt	1 cup (230 g)
Plain nonfat Greek yogurt	6 ounces (173 g)
Nonfat or low-fat soy or rice milk, fortified with calcium and vitamins A and D	1 cup (240 ml)

	Calories	Protein (g)	Carbohydrate (g)	Fat (g)	Calcium (mg)	Vitamin D (IU)
Cow's milk (2% fat)*	120	8	12	5	300	101
Almond, unsweetened*	29	1	1	2.5	451 mg	101
Cashew, unsweetened*	36	0	1	3.5	101	139
Coconut, unsweetened*	420	3	9	42	0	0
Hemp, unsweetened*	110	3.5	11.6	5.6	10	0
Rice*	113	0.7	22	2.3	283	2.4
Soy**	80	7	4	4	300	180

Comparison of 1 cup (240 ml) of cow's milk to 1 cup of other common calcium and vitamin D-fortified beverages (when available) used as substitutes.

*United States Department of Agriculture Agricultural Research Service USDA Food Composition Databases, https://ndb.nal.usda.gov.

**Manufacturer's data (Silk) for fortified product.

Vegetable Group

Each portion contains approximately 25 calories.

Food	Size of one portion
Most cooked vegetables	1/2 cup (81 g)
Most raw vegetables	1 cup (30-100 g)
Raw lettuce	2 cups (56 g)
Sprouts	1 cup (30 g)
Vegetable juice	6 oz (180 ml)
Vegetable soup	1 cup (240 ml)
Tomato sauce	1/2 cup (120 ml)
Salsa (made without oil)	3 tbsp (45 g)

Fruit Group

Each portion contains about 60 calories.

Food	Size of one portion
Most fruits, whole	1 medium
Most fruits, chopped or canned in own juice	1/2 cup (120 g)
Melon, diced	1 cup (156 g)
Berries, cherries, grapes (whole)	3/4 cup (80 g)
Fruit juice	1/2 cup (120 ml)
Banana	1 small
Grapefruit, mango	1/2
Plums	2 each
Apricots	4 each
Strawberries, whole	1 1/4 cup (180 g)
Kiwi	1 each
Prunes, dried	3 each
Figs	2 each
Raisins	2 tbsp (28 g)
Juice: cranberry, grape, fruit blends (100% juice)	1/3 cup (80 ml)
Cranberry juice cocktail (reduced calorie)	1 cup (240 ml)

Bread and Starch Group

Each portion contains 60 to 100 calories.

Food	Size of one portion
Bread	1 slice
Pita	1 small (1 oz)
Bagel, English muffin, bun	1/2 small (1 oz)
Roll	1 small
Cooked rice, cooked pasta	1/2 cup (97 g)
Tortilla	6 in. round (15 cm)
Crackers, large	2, or 3-4 small
Croutons	1/3 cup (13 g)
Pretzels, baked chips	1 oz (30 g)
Rice cakes	2 each
Cooked cereal	1/2 cup (119 g)
Cold cereal, unsweetened	1/2-1 cup (15-30 g)
Granola	1/2 cup (30 g)
Corn, green peas, mashed potato	1/2 cup (105 g)
Corn on the cob	1 medium
White or sweet potato baked, with skin	1 small
Plantain, slices and cooked	1/3 cup

Protein

Each protein portion contains about 35 to 75 calories. Very lean servings contain 35 calories and 0 to 1 gram of fat; lean, 55 calories and 3 grams of fat; and medium-fat, 75 calories and 5 grams of fat.

Food	Size of one portion
Very lean	
White meat skinless poultry	1 oz (30 g)
White fish	1 oz (30 g)
Fresh or canned tuna in water	1 oz (30 g)
All shellfish	1 oz (30 g)
Beans, peas, lentils*	1/2 cup (100 g)
Cheeses and processed sandwich meat with 1 g of fat	1 oz (30 g)
Egg whites	2 each

> continued

Food	Size of one portion
Lean	
Select or choice grades of lean beef, pork, lamb, or veal trimmed of fat	1 oz (30 g)
Dark-meat skinless poultry or white-meat chicken with skin	1 oz (30 g)
Oysters, salmon, catfish, sardines, tuna canned in oil	1 oz (30 g)
Cheese and deli sandwich meat with 3 g of fat	1 oz (30 g)
Parmesan cheese	1 oz (30 g)
Medium-fat	
Most styles of beef, pork, lamb, veal trimmed of fat, dark-meat poultry with skin	1 oz (30 g)
Ground turkey or chicken	1 oz (30 g)
Cheese with 5 g of fat	1 oz (30 g)
Cottage cheese, 4.5% fat	1/4 cup (56 g)
Whole egg	1 each
Tempeh	4 oz or 1/2 cup (120 g)
Tofu	4 oz or 1/2 cup (120 g)

*One portion counts as one very lean protein and one starch.

Fats and Oils

Each portion contains about 45 calories.

Food	Size of one portion
Butter (stick) and oils	1 tsp (5 g)
Cream cheese and heavy cream	1 tbsp (15 g)
Half and half, whipped cream, sour cream	2 tbsp (30 g)
Salad dressing, full fat	1 tbsp (15 g)
Avocado	1/8 medium (2 tbsp, or 30 g)
Olives, black	8 large
Nuts	6-10
Seeds	1 tbsp (9 g)
Peanut butter and other nut butters	1/2 tbsp (8 g)

Added Carbohydrate or Sugar

I use this category not only to help you understand where sugar is added in foods but also to set a placeholder for sports fuel. The best place for added carbohydrate of sugar in your diet is around exercise, to fuel your training and recovery. Sometimes you have extra calories leftover in your diet to add some extra carbs, even extra sugar, as part of desserts or treats. The best way to do that is to be informed about your choices.

There is no way that I could give you an exhaustive list of all the added sugar in foods. By July 2018 food manufacturers will begin to put that information on the label. You can also figure it out yourself, just as I do, by following these basic guidelines. Every 1 teaspoon, or serving, of sugar contains 4 grams of carbohydrate and 16 calories (no protein or fat).

Cereals and grains

Grains do not contain any sugar. By looking at the Nutrition Facts label on the side of a box of cereal such as Shredded Wheat, you'll see 0 grams of sugar in a serving. Therefore, the manufacturer adds any sugar contained in a cereal. Most sweetened cereals contain 8 grams of sugar per serving, which is the equivalent of 2 teaspoons of added sugar, and many contain much more. The exception is cereals with added fruit. Some of the sugar in these cereals comes from the fruit. Look at the ingredient label. If any kind of sugar is listed ahead of the fruit, you know that the greatest proportion of the added sugar is not from the fruit. The same concept goes for breads, crackers, and other grain products. Any sugar on the label is added in processing.

Milk and yogurt

One cup (8 ounces, or 240 ml) of milk contains 12 grams of natural milk sugar, or lactose. If you look at the Nutrition Facts label on a carton of milk, you will see that one serving (1 cup) contains 12 grams of sugar. Any amount of sugar above that is added, as in chocolate milk and other flavored milks.

Yogurt cartons are generally 6 oz (180 g). A carton of plain yogurt will contain about 12 grams of natural milk sugar. Anything above that is added sugar. Most yogurts are sweetened with at least 4 teaspoons of added sugar, and many use 6 teaspoons or more.

Fruit and fruit juices

A medium-sized piece of fruit contains about 15 grams of carbohydrate. Some of that is fiber, often 2 to 3 grams, and the rest is natural fruit sugar. When purchasing canned or frozen fruits and fruit juices, you must read the ingredients label to check for added sugar. Any amount of sugar above 15 grams for 1/2 cup (120 g) of canned or frozen fruit or 1/2 cup (120 ml) of fruit juice is added to the product.

Vegetables, vegetable juices, and soups

A medium-sized vegetable contains 5 grams of carbohydrate and no sugar. Any sugar listed on the Nutrition Facts label is added to the product.

Beverages

Obviously, water has no amount of natural sugar. So if you're looking at the Nutrition Facts label on the side of a soft drink can, all the sugar is added, and it usually amounts to about 10 teaspoons (50 g) per 12-ounce (360 ml) can. Typical sport drinks contain about 12 grams of sugar per cup, equivalent to 3 teaspoons (15 g) of added sugar per serving. Some sport drinks report dosing in grams of carbohydrate or sugar on the label. To determine your allowance for training, refer to the menu plans in chapters 15 through 19. This same principle can be applied to most bottled beverages that do not contain any milk or fruit juice. When it comes to fruit juice concentrates added as sweeteners to beverages and foods, the juice is highly refined in the processing and is little more than sugar syrup. Ingredients such as white grape juice concentrate are virtually the same as added sugar.

Personalizing the Plan

To achieve the greatest strength and muscle gain, follow these guidelines when designing your diet:

1. Assess Calorie Needs Based on Body Weight

As your weight changes, you must recalculate energy and nutrients. Chapters 15 through 19 outline the calorie needs for each phase of the plan to help you do this.

Training to Maintain Muscle

Men who train five or more times per week need 42 calories per kilogram of body weight a day (3,444 calories a day for a 180 lb [82 kg] man). Women who train five or more times per week may be able to increase muscle at 44 to 50 calories per kilogram of body weight a day (2,950 calories for a 130 lb [59 kg] woman) and maintain at about 38 to 40 calories per kilogram of body weight a day (2,360 calories). The larger and more muscular a woman is, the more calories she can handle for maintenance.

Smaller women may need fewer than 38 calories per kilogram of body weight per day to maintain weight. There is a lot of trial and error with women, because all the research has been done on men and because levels of activity vary widely. For the rest of the phases, women should generally choose the lower end of the calorie ranges. Always check your final calorie numbers against the energy availability calculations from chapter 7. Stay above 30 calories per kilogram of lean body mass (LBM) to support both health and performance. This diet is great for bodybuilders, powerlifters, and weightlifters, as well as for recreational strength trainers and multisport athletes. Novice trainers should follow the novice guidelines.

Building

This plan requires 44 to 52 or more calories per kilogram of body weight a day, depending on the intensity of training (4,264 or more calories for a 180 lb [82 kg] man; 2,596 to 2,950 calories for a 130 lb [59 kg] woman). Start low and add calories as needed. As stated earlier, women will likely be able to build at 44 calories per kilogram of body weight a day. Smaller women should try slightly fewer calories when beginning a building program and work up from there. This diet is good for all competitive and recreational strength trainers. Novice trainers should follow the novice guidelines.

Losing Fat

To lose fat and begin to sculpt (10 to 12 weeks of precontest dieting), you'll need 35 to 38 calories per kilogram of body weight a day (3,116 calories for a 180 lb [82 kg] man; 2,065 calories for a 130 lb [59 kg] woman). Because it's more difficult for women to lose fat than it is for men, women should choose the lower calorie range and increase aerobic exercise in order to burn 300 to 400 calories a day. Again, smaller women may need fewer calories. This recommendation is primarily for bodybuilders. Novice trainers should follow the novice guidelines.

Cutting

This plan requires 30 calories per kilogram of body weight a day (7 to 14 days maximum) for women (1,711 calories for a 130 lb [59 kg] woman) and 32 calories per kilogram of body weight a day for men (2,624 calories for a 180 lb [82 kg] man). If you are a smaller woman who has been losing fat at a lower calorie level, decrease recommended calories here as well. Use this approach only when absolutely necessary. This diet is only for bodybuilders or others trying to make a weight class—not for powerlifters or Olympic weightlifters.

Powerlifters and Weightlifters Trying to Make a Weight Class

After dieting to build muscle, go back to the maintenance diet ideally, or fat-loss diet if necessary, for two weeks before your meet and use your goal weight for the calculations. This will allow for loss of body fat without loss of muscle, strength, or power. This strategy is also a good basic diet for overweight strength trainers who want to lose body fat.

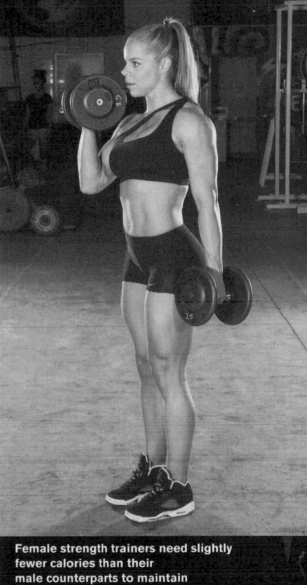

Female strength trainers need slightly fewer calories than their male counterparts to maintain muscle.

2. Calculate Your Protein Needs

Protein needs change with both energy intake and training goals. Although the menu plans in chapters 15 through 19 provide grams per pound of body weight, you can easily convert your weight from pounds to kilograms by dividing your weight by 2.2. Make sure to cover your protein needs during all four diet strategies. If you are a vegan, add 10 percent more protein to all of the plans.

Maintenance	1.5-1.8 grams per kilogram of body weight a day
Building	Women: 2.0-2.2 grams per kilogram of body weight a day
	Men: 2.2-2.5 grams per kilogram of body weight a day
Losing fat	2.2 grams per kilogram of body weight a day
Cutting	2.3-2.5 grams per kilogram of body weight a day; 2.5 grams per kilogram of body weight a day for those eating a mostly vegetarian or vegan diet

3. Calculate Your Carbohydrate Needs

Calculate your carbohydrate needs as 5 to 7 grams per kilogram of body weight a day. Strength trainers need closer to 5 to 6 grams per kilogram of body weight a day for maintenance and 6.5 to 7 grams per kilogram of body weight a day for building. Cross-trainers who do an intense, ultra-type sport such as an Ironman event need closer to 6 to 10 or more grams per kilogram of body weight a day. Novice athletes need less carbohydrate at all levels of training, but the amount will increase as they increase their training intensity.

During fat-loss and cutting phases, women and men need different amounts of carbohydrate. Here is the amount of carbohydrate needed per kilogram of body weight per day.

Losing fat	Women: 2.5 to 3.5 grams per kilogram
	Men: 3 to 4 grams per kilogram
Cutting	Women: 1.8 to 2.9 grams per kilogram
	Men: 2.3 to 3 grams per kilogram

4. Calculate Your Fat Needs

The rest of your calories will be 25 to 30 percent of the total. Fat sources should be predominantly monounsaturated and polyunsaturated, including omega-3 fat, with much less saturated fat.

To find the number of fat grams you need in your plan, first determine the calories of protein and carbohydrate that you have calculated for yourself (1 g protein = 4 calories; 1 g carbohydrate = 4 calories). Then subtract those calories from the total number of calories needed for your weight and training phase, and you have the number of fat calories you need. Fat contains 9 calories per gram, so if you divide the fat calories by 9, you have your grams of fat.

Here's an example of a maintenance diet for a novice 180-pound (82 kg) man:

Calories	33 calories per kilogram
	33×82 kg = 2,706 calories
Protein	1.5 grams per kilogram
	1.5×82 kg = 123 g protein
Carbohydrate	4.5 grams per kilogram
	4.5×82 kg = 369 g carbohydrate
Fat	The leftover calories, or 1 g per kilogram

Calculate the calories in the protein and carbohydrate grams:

$$123 \text{ g protein} \times 4 \text{ calories/g} = 492 \text{ protein calories}$$
$$369 \text{ g carbohydrate} \times 4 \text{ calories/g} = 1,476 \text{ carbohydrate calories}$$
$$492 + 1,476 = 1,968 \text{ protein and carbohydrate calories}$$

Then, calculate the fat calories and grams.

$$2{,}706 \text{ total calories} - 1{,}968 \text{ protein and carbohydrate calories} = 738 \text{ fat calories}$$
$$738 \text{ fat calories} / 9 \text{ calories} = 82 \text{ g of fat}$$

So, the diet consists of 2,706 calories, 123 grams of protein, 369 grams of carbohydrate, and 82 grams of fat. Then, by using the chart of the nutritional content of food groups, you can write your own diet. Use the menus that I have written as your guide. An easy solution is to add or subtract portions from the menus that I have already written for you. For instance, if you need to subtract carbohydrate grams, remove some servings of sugar; if you need to subtract fat grams, remove some servings of fat, and so on.

Genetics and Meal Planning

There are plenty of popular diets that do your meal planning for you. Atkins, for example, wants you to ramp up protein and fat and slash carbohydrates. Weight Watchers pushes nutrient-poor, high-sodium, reduced-calorie processed meals with lengthy ingredient lists, including added sugars, hydrogenated oils, and white flour. The Mediterranean diet advocates eating lots of complex carbohydrate, lean protein, and some healthy fat like olive oil. Paleo emphasizes lots of animal protein, veggies, and fruits but no dairy or grain foods.

Though all these diets are different, they still take a cookie-cutter approach to meal planning—meaning they are not based on our individual differences. Writing in the October 18, 2007, issue of *Nutrition Journal*, Colorado researchers said, "It has long been suspected that 'one size does not fit all' in terms of determining the optimal diet for an individual, and this has been demonstrated over the recent years in studies on gene-diet interactions and the emergence of nutrigenetics. The goal of nutrigenetics is to add a level of personalization to a prescribed diet, by adjusting it according to genetic variation" (2).

So here's where genetics meets nutrition (nutrigenetics) as they enter the picture together. Your genetics can affect how your body responds to protein, carbohydrate, and fat even to the point of whether you'll gain or lose weight from the same intake of these macronutrients. Here are a few examples of how your genetics could influence your predisposition for weight gain.

Let's say you decide to go on a high-fat diet such as the ketogenic diet or the Atkins diet. After all, your best friend lost a ton of weight on one of those, so why shouldn't you? Well, it's not that easy; again, due to individual, genetic differences. Genetically, many people will gain weight from high amounts of fat in their diets. It's just how they're wired. So, if you've been unsuccessful on those diets, you may need to cut back on dietary fat. It's that simple.

In a similar vein, paleo diets tend to be high in saturated fat. There are also diets that emphasize eating a lot of coconut oil, a saturated fat. Again, there are several genetic variants that, if you have them, will increase your odds of gaining weight from a diet high in saturated fat. My advice is to watch how your body responds to saturated fat, as well as all other types of fats. Are you trying to lose weight while

POWER PROFILE: Diet SOS!

This client was a 49-year-old, highly competitive, 70.3 Ironman competitor and bank executive from the Dominican Republic. His goals were to increase performance by increasing strength, power, and endurance, while maintaining his body weight.

One issue I noticed after analyzing his diet was that he had a wide fluctuation in energy intake from day to day:

1,862 to 3,500 calories

125 to 197 grams protein

192 to 509 grams carbohydrate

60 to 90 grams fat

His estimated resting metabolic rate (RMR) was 1,837 calories a day, and he usually expended 1,300 to 3,500 calories daily, depending on the day's training. This athlete needed to smooth out his energy intake to be more consistent day to day for better recovery and building, with only the energy around training adjusted as needed.

Because of time demands from work and travel, as well as family, this took some planning and preparation, but he was highly motivated to move up competitively. Here is what I recommended:

2,540 calories a day (30.5 calories per kg)

150 grams protein a day (1.8 g per kg)

300 grams carbohydrate a day (3.6 g per kg)

83 grams fat a day (1 g per kg)

His food intake needed some boosting, so we added one whole egg daily and more servings of fruits and vegetables, with a goal of at least five servings of fruits a day and nine servings of vegetables a day. We added up to 280 grams of carbohydrate in 35-gram scoops of Vitargo, depending on the day's training, for nutrition pre- and posttraining and during training, plus 20 grams of whey protein isolate for recovery. Other supplements that were added included creatine monohydrate, caffeine, beta-alanine, beet root juice, and electrolytes.

It took serious food planning and preparation to achieve daily consistency, but the extra effort to eat a consistent diet and fully fuel his training paid off. He very quickly felt stronger and had multiple age-category successes.

eating a lot of fat but gaining it instead? If so, you may be genetically predisposed to dietary fat–generated weight gain. So high-fat diets are not right for you.

Cutting carbohydrate is a popular way to try to lose weight; there's no doubt about it. For some people though, cutting carbohydrate will increase the likelihood of weight gain. In that case, you'll need to plan your meals so that you get more calories from good carbohydrate sources, such as whole grains, fruits, legumes, and starchy vegetables, rather than from junk carbohydrate sources like sodas, sweets, desserts, and so forth. For others, even a moderate-carbohydrate diet will pack on pounds, while a low-carbohydrate diet will take them off.

The same advice applies here: Be very aware of whether you gain or lose weight based on the distribution and amount of macronutrients in your diet. And know that any failure to take off pounds is not really a failure, and it's not your fault. It's your genetics.

Your genetics, however, is not your destiny. You can control your food–gene interactions by choosing the right foods for your body and designing the right meals to fuel your body, which is why the Power Eating plan is all about individualizing your nutrition. So let your body be your guide. If you are a big carbohydrate burner, you will feel uncomfortable, and may not get the best results, when carbohydrate calories drop too low. If that's you, then raise carbohydrate a little and drop fat calories to maintain the calorie recommendation. If your body is an easy fat burner and you're trying to cut weight, then you may do well with less carbohydrate and more fat but within the calorie target zone. Population data tell us that there are more people (at least more people who have been tested) that are carbohydrate burners than are easy fat burners. Take a saliva-based genetic test if you really want to know what's in your genes. There's power, and confidence, in information.

Adjusting the Plan for Competitive Bodybuilders and Physique Athletes

If you're preparing for a contest, begin the fat-loss phase 10 to 12 weeks before your contest. Decrease calories and increase your aerobic exercise. However, if you simply up the intensity and duration of your aerobic exercise, you'll lose some muscle, along with fat. The solution is to do high-intensity interval training (HIIT). It enables you to get extremely defined, without burning up precious muscle mass. HIIT involves performing intervals of high-intensity exercise at a rate near 90 percent of your maximum heart rate (MHR) interspersed with intervals of slower-paced activity. It is fine to do some aerobic work, but ramp up your HIIT training.

If you're not looking as ripped as you would like, follow the cutting program for one or two weeks prior to your contest. Consume 29 to 32 calories per kilogram of body weight a day for this phase. This will allow for a final loss of 3 to 4 pounds (1.4 to 1.8 kg), as long as you keep up your HIIT. Make sure to increase your protein intake to 2.3 to 2.5 grams per kilogram of body weight a day.

Sticking to Your Plan

For these strategies to work, you have to stick to your Power Eating plan. Design your diet with foods that you like. Use the sample diets in chapters 15 through 19 to help you design your personal plan. If you don't like the foods you're supposed to eat, you won't stick to the plan. If you're using liquid supplements, try different brands and flavors to find ones you like.

Sport Nutrition Fact Versus Fiction: Fast-Food Nutrition

If yours is an on-the-go lifestyle, I've included many fast and delicious recipes that you can prepare in under 10 minutes and take with you on the road. Alternatively, it's fine to eat at some of the alternative new slightly-less-than-fast-food restaurants on occasion. The key is to make the right choices—those that are low in fat and high in nutrition. Fortunately, this style of alternative fast-food restaurant today caters to the healthier preferences of consumers. So if you're really serious about your training, get serious about your eating, too (see appendix B for a guide to restaurant eating and healthy fast food).

When you get caught without the food you need, here are some fast-food tips to keep you on track.

- Always order the regular-sized (vs. large) sandwiches, because they are lower in unhealthy fat and calories.
- Instead of ordering a bigger sandwich, order a salad and low-fat milk.
- Stay away from fried foods.
- Don't eat the high-fat tortilla shells from taco salads.
- Request that sour cream and secret sauces be left off your order.
- Top your baked potato with chili instead of fatty cheese sauce.
- Drink water instead of soda.

Whatever you order, order just one!

Pay attention to your body and plan to eat when you're hungry. You might want to pick specific times of the day to eat rather than depending on the pace of each day. But also be aware of whether you are hungry or thirsty; sometimes we confuse thirst with hunger. Keep food and drink on hand wherever you go. The most successful strength trainers always have a backpack full of food and drink that goes with them everywhere. This way, they can stick to their timed eating patterns, and if they get hungry, they're not dependent on vending machines or other snack foods that are high in fat and sodium.

When you're trying to lose fat, you might find it difficult to eat at restaurants, and it might be especially difficult to travel. If you must do either, try to find restaurants that specialize in healthy fare. They should be able to easily adjust their menu to meet your personal needs. Don't forget to ask what's in the recipe. A menu description may be misleading. You can even ask for foods that aren't on the menu—restaurants may be able to accommodate your request.

Remember to always recalculate your requirements based on your present weight. If you have gained weight during a building or bulking phase and now want to lose weight, use your new weight rather than that of the prebulking phase.

Habits and Goals: Track Your Nutrition From the Inside

An essential way to stick with your plan is to focus on habit change and goal achievement, and you can do these through tracking your behavior, physically and emotionally. Tracking is simply a matter of logging what you do as you do it, including how you feel when you stay on track. The data you log reinforces positive actions, locks in your new habits for the long run, and gets you to your goals. Here are some guidelines and worksheets to help you.

TRACK YOUR NUTRITION FROM THE INSIDE

Planning ahead for how you will mindfully change an old habit into a new, healthier habit is a proven way to keep yourself on track. *Logging* what you do as you do it, and how you feel when you stay on track will reinforce your actions to lock in your new habits for the long run.

For the best results, *track yourself in real time*. It's often difficult to accurately remember activities that you did hours earlier. You will begin to see that what you eat, when you eat, and what you do can change the way you feel, which can drive the choices that you make in the following hours and days.

The choices that you make will change the way you feel on the inside, which will both drive and reinforce your food choices and habitual behaviors. *Review and save* your logs at the end of the day, the week, and the month to track your progress. Pay close attention to what you did and how you felt. *Celebrate* your accomplishments. You're on track to feeling great!

Feel Great Nutrition Guidance Goals

Group 1: Generally for women who would like to taper with a moderately active lifestyle (don't exercise as much as you'd like)

Group 2: Generally for men who would like to taper with a moderately active lifestyle (don't exercise as much as you'd like), or women who are exercising more rigorously (1-2 hr) and still would like to taper

Group 3: Generally for those who exercise regularly at higher intensities (1-2 hr), and would still like some body sculpting

If you exercise at high intensities for long duration, add more fueling around exercise to optimize workouts, maximize recovery, and increase muscle mass and strength.

Feel Great Exercise Guidance Goals

Exercise at least 30 minutes, 6 days/week. Include strength training, cardiovascular training, and flexibility/breathing routines throughout the week.

From S.M. Kleiner and M. Greenwood-Robinson, *The New Power Eating* (Champaign, IL: Human Kinetics, 2019).

Success Tracker

Get on track for success!

1. Target one of your performance or health goals.
2. Target one daily action that will get you moving toward your goal. The action can be about diet or training, but it can also be anything in your life that you want to change to support your goal.
3. Determine exactly when and where you will perform this action each day.
4. At the place and time that you have selected in step 3, you must accomplish the action.
5. Consistency is key! At first you must be very mindful that you perform your selected action, but over time your new action will become routine. It often takes about 10 weeks to get to that point.
6. SUCCESS! You are one step closer to your goal!!
7. Now build on your success by choosing the next daily action that will move you closer to one of your performance or health goals and plug it into the SUCCESS TRACKER.

My target goal *(Example: Take a 30 minute walk every day.)*:

My daily action *(Example: After dinner, when I finish my tea, I will get up and take a walk before I clean up the kitchen.)* • **I will** *(be specific, including when and where)*:

Your Success Track Sheet:

	WEEK 1	WEEK 2	WEEK 3	WEEK 4	WEEK 5	WEEK 6	WEEK 7	WEEK 8	WEEK 9	WEEK 10
Monday	○	○	○	○	○	○	○	○	○	○
Tuesday	○	○	○	○	○	○	○	○	○	○
Wednesday	○	○	○	○	○	○	○	○	○	○
Thursday	○	○	○	○	○	○	○	○	○	○
Friday	○	○	○	○	○	○	○	○	○	○
Saturday	○	○	○	○	○	○	○	○	○	○
Sunday	○	○	○	○	○	○	○	○	○	○

Done on 5 days or more?

How routine does it feel?
Rate from 1 (not at all routine) to 10 (completely routine)

Adapted from B. Gardner, P. Lally, and J. Wardle, "Making Health Habitual: The Psychology of 'Habit-Formation' and General Practice," *British Journal of General Practice* 62 no. 605 (2012): 664-666. From S.M. Kleiner and M. Greenwood-Robinson, *The New Power Eating* (Champaign, IL: Human Kinetics, 2019).

Feel Great Food Tracker Goals
(circle answer)

Did I respond to my hunger?	YES	NO
Did I recognize thirst?	YES	NO
Was I mindful when I was satisfied?	YES	NO
Did I combine carbohydrate, protein and fat?	YES	NO
Did I plan my eating times to meet my needs?	YES	NO

Feel Great Nutrition Suggested Daily Serving Goals

	Group 1	Group 2	Group 3
Whole grains and starchy vegetables	4	5	6
Fruits	3	3	4
Vegetables	5	6	6
Dairy or legumes	3	3	4
Proteins (1 oz)	9 + 1 egg	11 + 1 egg	14 + 1 egg
Fats	5	6	8
Water (8 oz)	5	5	5
(check off your group)	◯	◯	◯

Make a checkmark to track daily serving numbers for each food group:

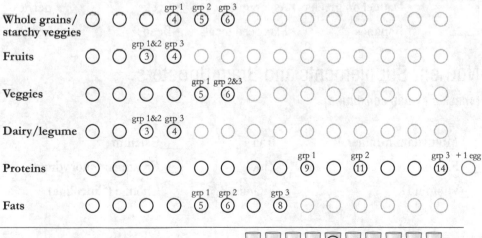

Whole grains/starchy veggies ◯ ◯ ◯ ④(grp 1) ⑤(grp 2) ⑥(grp 3) ◯ ◯ ◯ ◯ ◯ ◯ ◯

Fruits ◯ ◯ ③(grp 1&2) ④(grp 3) ◯ ◯ ◯ ◯ ◯ ◯ ◯ ◯ ◯

Veggies ◯ ◯ ◯ ◯ ⑤(grp 1) ⑥(grp 2&3) ◯ ◯ ◯ ◯ ◯ ◯ ◯

Dairy/legume ◯ ◯ ③(grp 1&2) ④(grp 3) ◯ ◯ ◯ ◯ ◯ ◯ ◯ ◯ ◯

Proteins ◯ ◯ ◯ ◯ ◯ ◯ ◯ ◯ ⑨(grp 1) ◯ ⑪(grp 2) ◯ ◯ ⑭(grp 3) ◯(+1 egg)

Fats ◯ ◯ ◯ ◯ ⑤(grp 1) ⑥(grp 2) ◯ ⑧(grp 3) ◯ ◯ ◯ ◯ ◯

Cross off at least 5 glasses of water/day: ▯ ▯ ▯ ▯ ⑤ ▯ ▯ ▯ ▯ ▯

From S.M. Kleiner and M. Greenwood-Robinson, *The New Power Eating* (Champaign, IL: Human Kinetics, 2019).

Diet Booster Goals

Daily Nutrition Nibble: Probiotic Foods for Gut Health

(check off when one is consumed daily)

- Yogurt
- Kombucha
- Miso

- Kefir
- Kimchi
- Buttermilk

- Sauerkraut
- Tempeh
- Natto

- Pickles
- Kvass
- Olives

Daily Nutrition Nibble: Prebiotic Foods for Gut Health

Prebiotics are a special form of nondigestible carbohydrate that feed the probiotics (aka, good bacteria). When prebiotics and probiotics are combined, they work together to create a healthy environment inside of your gut while promoting proper digestion. Here are some foods that contain prebiotics:

(check off when one is consumed daily)

- Artichokes
- Dandelion greens
- Bananas

- Onions
- Asparagus
- Flax seed meal

- Garlic
- Leeks
- Beans

- Chicory
- Berries
- Lentil

Nutrient Supplements and Brain Boosters:

(check off when consumed)

___Multivitamin-mineral

___Fish oil

___Vitamin D

___Iron

___Zinc

___Vitamin B$_{12}$

___Calcium

___Creatine monohydrate

___Choline (Citicoline)

From S.M. Kleiner and M. Greenwood-Robinson, *The New Power Eating* (Champaign, IL: Human Kinetics, 2019).

THE GOOD MOOD DIET©

The 10 Habit Commandments

1. Think about what you NEED to eat, not what you can't eat next.

2. Always combine starches with protein or healthy fat.

3. Nourish yourself before and after exercise, and every 2-1/2 to 3 hours all day long.

4. Dairy 3 times/day: AM, after exercise, PM.

5. Egg yolk or soy every day.

6. Nuts every day.

7. Fish 5 times/week.

8. 5 to 6 cups of water every day.

9. Eat a variety of vegetables, including a food from the carotene-rich, brassica and allium, families each day.

10. Eat a variety of fruits, including a food from the citrus, berries, and others categories each day.

From S.M. Kleiner and M. Greenwood-Robinson, *The New Power Eating* (Champaign, IL: Human Kinetics, 2019).

Did I exercise at least 30 minutes?
(check off the activity you did today)

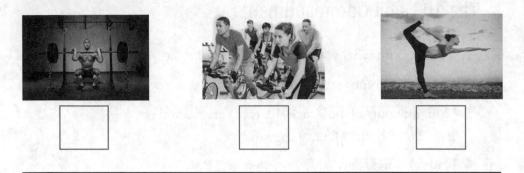

☐ ☐ ☐

Good Mood Bottom Line
How do I feel at the end of the day?

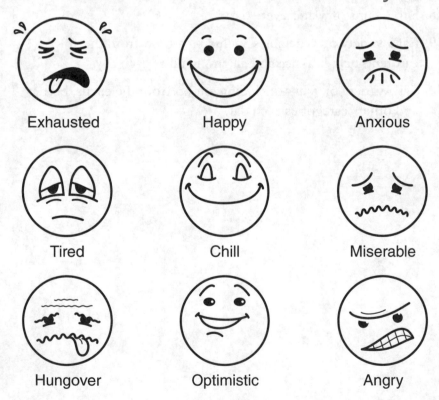

Exhausted   Happy   Anxious

Tired   Chill   Miserable

Hungover   Optimistic   Angry

(photo credits from left to right): © matthiasdrobeck/iStockphoto, ferrantraite/E+/Getty Images, Evgeniyaphotography/iStockphoto/Getty Images. From S.M. Kleiner and M. Greenwood-Robinson, *The New Power Eating* (Champaign, IL: Human Kinetics, 2019).

Power Eating Grocery Shopping List

Meal planning also includes grocery planning. I advise going to the grocery store with a list of Power Eating foods you'll need, week by week. Sticking to your list will help you stay on track. What follows is an example of a good shopping list, but feel free to customize it by adding your own favorites.

Lean Proteins

☐ Chicken

☐ Lean beef, lamb, pork

☐ Mixed beans

☐ Omega-3 eggs or regular eggs

☐ Other fish and shellfish

☐ Salmon

☐ Tofu, tempeh

☐ Tuna

☐ Turkey

☐ Veggie sausage links

Dairy

☐ Fat-free or low-fat milk

☐ Fat-free or low-fat plain Greek or regular yogurt

☐ Lower-fat hard cheeses like skim milk mozzarella, Swiss, and jack versus soft, ripened cheeses

☐ Low-fat sour cream (not fat-free, which is full of additives)

Fruits and Vegetables

☐ Broccoli, cauliflower, cabbage

☐ Carrots

☐ Cilantro

☐ Citrus fruit

☐ Cucumbers

☐ Fresh garlic

☐ Green beans

☐ Lemons

☐ Lettuce, kale

☐ Mint

☐ Mixed berries

☐ Onions

☐ Other fruits (apples, bananas, mangos)

☐ Other veggies (okra, plantains, sweet potatoes)

☐ Parsley

☐ Raw spinach

☐ Red and green peppers

☐ Tomatoes

☐ Whole mushrooms

Nuts and Seeds

☐ Mixed raw nuts (almonds, pecans)

☐ Other seeds

☐ Peanut or other nut butters

☐ Whole or ground flaxseed

Grains

- ☐ Brown rice
- ☐ High-protein pasta
- ☐ Oat bran
- ☐ Other grains
- ☐ Popcorn
- ☐ Quinoa grain
- ☐ Steel-cut oats
- ☐ Wheat bran
- ☐ Whole grain cereals
- ☐ Whole-grain bread
- ☐ Whole-wheat tortillas

Fats and Oils

- ☐ Avocados
- ☐ Butter, coconut oil, or spread
- ☐ Cooking spray (canola or olive)
- ☐ Extra-virgin olive oil
- ☐ Grapeseed, peanut
- ☐ Olives

Other

- ☐ Balsamic vinegar
- ☐ Black pepper
- ☐ Cayenne
- ☐ Chile
- ☐ Cinnamon
- ☐ Cumin
- ☐ Fajita seasoning
- ☐ Garlic powder
- ☐ Lemon juice
- ☐ Mustard
- ☐ Non-Dutched, nonalkali cocoa powder
- ☐ Paprika
- ☐ Raspberry vinegar
- ☐ Salsa
- ☐ Sea salt
- ☐ Stevia or Truvia
- ☐ Turmeric

14

Planning a Peak

Perhaps you've decided to fine-tune your physique to look more trim, fit, and muscular. Maybe you desire to take your strength training up a notch—to competitive bodybuilding, powerlifting, or weightlifting. Or perhaps you're already a competitive strength trainer who's searching for that extra edge. No matter what your ambition, proper nutrition is the key.

You may not realize it, but the same nutritional techniques that work for bodybuilders and other athletes can also be applied to recreational exercisers and strength trainers. That's because the goals are generally the same: increasing muscularity (degree of muscular bulk), etching in definition (absence of body fat), and training for symmetry (shape and size of muscles in proportion to each other).

Whether you're trying to get in shape for swimsuit season, preparing for a bodybuilding competition, cross-training to support another sport, or building strength for your sport, you strive to reduce body fat without sacrificing muscle mass so as to reveal as much muscular definition as possible. Or perhaps one of your chief goals is building strength and muscle mass, either for looks and health or because you're a competitive powerlifter and weightlifter. In these cases, your goal is to lift as much weight as possible when you train and compete.

If you're a competitor, you'll be required to make weight to qualify for a specific weight class. You must focus on gaining and preserving muscular weight and losing body fat to achieve your contest weight. Diet therefore plays a critical role in precontest preparation for all competitive strength trainers who want to achieve peak shape.

Until recently, most strength athletes partitioned their diets into two distinct phases: a bulking phase, in which the competitor eats huge amounts of food without much regard to sound nutrition practices or to the type of calories taken in from food, and a cutting phase, in which drastic measures such as starvation dieting and drugs are used to lose weight rapidly in the weeks before a contest. Even if you're not a competitor, you've probably done something similar: bulking up in the winter and then crash dieting to get in shape for summer.

Unless sound nutritional practices are followed, the cutting phase, much like a crash diet, can be unhealthy, rigid, monotonous, and damaging to performance. And bulking up tends to pile on fat weight, which is that much harder to lose when it comes time to get in shape or prepare for competition.

Today, though, more strength athletes choose to stay close to competition shape year-round. That way, it's easier to lose body fat because there's less to lose, and the process of cutting is much safer and more successful. And we all want to look our best all the time. You never know when you might have a photo shoot opportunity!

This chapter outlines a step-by-step diet strategy called tapering that lets you lose maximum body fat, retain hard-earned muscle, and perform at your best. This strategy works for exercisers, bodybuilders, and strength athletes—anyone who wants to become lean and muscular. The end of the chapter covers key issues for powerlifters and weightlifters.

Step 1: Plan Your Start Date

The length of time you spend dieting depends on how out of shape you are to begin with. If you've let yourself get too fat by bulking up, then you'll really have to stretch your dieting out by several months.

A caution for bodybuilding competitors: Don't start your dieting too close to your contest. You'll be too tempted to resort to crash dieting, which can result in loss of muscle, decreased strength and power, low energy, moodiness and irritability, and low immunity. Losing lots of fat in a short period of time is virtually impossible for most people, anyway. Physiologically, no one can lose more than 4 pounds (1.8 kg) of pure fat a week even by total fasting. Instead, take a gradual approach to dieting.

Start your diet or contest preparation about 10 to 12 weeks before your competition. During this period, make slight adjustments to your calorie and nutrient intake by increasing protein, as well as to your aerobic exercise level. In addition, supplement with creatine and drink one of my muscle-building formulas (see chapter 20).

Step 2: Determine a Safe Reduction in Calories

Getting cut is essential for achieving physique perfection, as well as for achieving competitive success in a sport such as bodybuilding. One way to begin this process is by slightly reducing your caloric intake. I use this strategy with any of my athlete clients who need to reduce body fat to enhance performance. By consuming fewer calories, you can gradually reduce body fat. However, you don't want to cut calories too much. A drastic reduction in calories will slow down your resting metabolic rate (RMR) for two reasons. The first has to do with the thermic effect of food (TEF), which is the increase in RMR after you eat a meal as food is digested and metabolized. Eating more calories increases the thermic effect of food and, along with it, your RMR. Likewise, cutting calories too much not only decreases the TEF but if you start to lose lean mass, your RMR will have an additional drop. Without enough calories to drive your metabolic processes, your body has a harder time burning calories to lose body fat.

Second, long periods of calorie deprivation—that is, diets under 1,200 calories a day—lower your RMR as a result of the low energy availability (LEA) or relative energy deficiency in sport (RED-S) response. This response simply means that your metabolism has slowed down to accommodate your lower caloric intake. Your body is stockpiling dietary fat and calories rather than burning them for energy. You can actually gain body fat on a diet of fewer than 1,200 calories a day.

The LEA response has been observed frequently in undernourished endurance athletes. In a study of triathletes, researchers found that these athletes weren't consuming enough calories to fuel themselves for training and competition. When calories were increased, the athletes' weight stayed the same. This occurred because their RMRs returned to normal with the introduction of ample calories. To keep your metabolism running in high gear, you have to eat enough calories to match your energy requirements.

When you drastically cut calories, you also slash your fat intake too much. That's a problem because you starve your brain of the fat it requires for nourishment. Consequently, your brain sends messages to your body to hang on to fat rather than burn it. In men, the low fat intake also diminishes the production of anabolic hormones, like testosterone. So there's no good reason to slash your fat intake.

While dieting, reduce your calories by up to 300 each day if you are a woman and 400 each day if you are a man. This is the ideal metabolic window for fat burning and will not adversely affect your RMR. (See chapter 5 for a discussion of this metabolic window.) At the same time, increase your aerobic exercise to burn up to 300 to 400 calories a day. This type of caloric manipulation will help you burn fat efficiently. You'll lose more fat in the initial weeks, and then you'll need to increase your exercise and probably lower your calories as you continue to shed body weight. I've designed the Power Eating fat-loss (chapter 18) and cutting (chapter 19) plans with exactly these scientific concepts in mind.

You might wonder, "Why can't I just crash diet for a few weeks to get in shape? After all, I'm training hard with weights. Shouldn't strength training protect me from losing muscle?" As logical as this argument sounds, scientific research proves otherwise. Case in point: In one study, overweight women were divided into two groups: a group that only dieted and a group that dieted and strength trained. The diet provided only 800 calories a day, and the study lasted four weeks. The results revealed that both groups lost the same amount of weight (11 lb, or 5 kg). Even the composition of the lost weight was the same. All the women lost 8 pounds (3.6 kg) of fat and 3 pounds (1.4 kg) of muscle. The bottom line is that strength training does not preserve muscle under these low-calorie dieting conditions, but it does when caloric restriction isn't so severe.

The implications are clear: In just four short weeks, you can lose precious muscle if you crash diet. Watch how low you go in decreasing your caloric intake. Research with bodybuilders confirms that you can lose muscle in just seven days on calories as low as 8.2 per pound (18 per kilogram) of body weight a day.

Step 3: Increase Aerobic Exercise

To sculpt a fit physique, increase the intensity and duration of your aerobic exercise. Aerobic exercise stimulates the activity of a fat-burning enzyme called *hormone-sensitive lipase*, which breaks down stored fat and moves it into circulation to be burned for energy. Aerobic exercise also increases $\dot{V}O_2$max—the capability to process oxygen and transport it to body tissues. Fat is burned most efficiently when sufficient oxygen is available.

If you put a lot of effort into your aerobic exercise, you may not have to reduce your calories. That's the conclusion of a recent study from West Virginia University. Women of normal weight were able to decrease their body fat within three months simply by exercising aerobically four days a week for about 45 minutes, each time at a heart rate between 80 and 90 percent of their maximum. They didn't cut calories, yet they still lost plenty of body fat. But they trained hard!

Here's some more good news: The better trained you are aerobically—and the leaner you are—the better your body can burn fat for energy. By increasing $\dot{V}O_2$max and thus the oxygen available to tissues, aerobic exercise enhances the ability of your muscles to combust fat as fuel. At the cellular level, the breakdown of fat speeds up, and it's released faster from storage sites in fat and muscle tissue.

In addition, focus on high-intensity interval training (HIIT), which alternates short bursts (one to two minutes) of high-intensity exercise with short bursts (one to two minutes) at a lower intensity. Research has shown this form of exercise to keep your metabolic rate elevated for several hours following your workout and is thus an effective fat-burning strategy. Plus, it maximizes your time in the gym and gives you a great whole-body workout.

Women's bodies can burn a lot of fat with regular aerobic exercise, which will result in their staying very lean. Most of the initial fat burned by women during endurance training is not from adipose tissue. Here's what I mean: There are droplets of fat stored in between muscle fibers (think of marbled meat). Women are better at storing fat in muscle, and accessing that fat during exercise, compared to men. But the longer you train aerobically, the more calories you burn, and the greater your deficit at the end of the day. So you get lean and stay lean. Of course, continue to resistance train to stay strong. Men, however, burn more carbohydrate through aerobic exercise proportionately compared to women. Men are also more prone to using protein as energy during endurance exercise than women are. So for men, maintaining muscle mass can be slightly more difficult if they are trying to get big and run long. I recommend that men hoping to build focus on HIIT three or four times a week for their aerobic capacity and calorie burning, and continue lifting to protect their muscle.

There's no doubt about it: Aerobic exercise, particularly when done in addition to HIIT, is a miracle worker when it comes to fat burning. Stay aerobically fit year-round and you'll have no trouble shedding those last few pounds of pudge. But here's the thing—aerobic training is not required! You've got a toolkit of options to choose from.

Step 4: Eat More Protein

To shed body fat, you should be eating at least 2.2 grams of protein per kilogram of body weight a day. This level will help you maintain muscle mass. Increasing your protein intake during a time of calorie reduction helps protect against muscle loss; the extra protein can be used as a backup energy source in case your body needs it.

Step 5: Plan Your Diet to Go From Heavy to Light

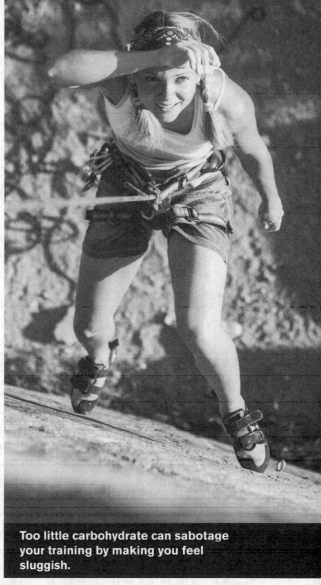

Too little carbohydrate can sabotage your training by making you feel sluggish.

pressmaster/fotolia.com

Eat your largest meal first thing in the morning. You guessed it: I'm talking about breakfast. Strength trainers and other health-conscious people need to take breakfast as seriously as they take their other meals and snacks.

Breakfast literally "breaks the fast" to get nutrients to your famished bodies. Plus, it can actually boost your metabolism. By contrast, there is also proof that skipping breakfast actually lowers your metabolic rate. The thermic effect of food—how many calories are used to digest your food—is higher in the morning and tapers off slightly throughout the day.

What makes a good breakfast? Complex, lightly processed or unprocessed carbohydrate such as that found in whole-grain cereal or bread and fresh fruit and some lean protein, with a little high-performance fat, make an excellent first meal of the day. Carbohydrate, in particular, helps with appetite control and boosts fat burning all day long. You don't have to be limited to breakfast foods, either. Enjoy some whole-grain bread and light cheese, or some chicken or fish, if you wish.

Here's one of my classic breakfast meal recommendations:

1 cup Puffed Kamut Cereal (puffed grains are super healthy and usually have nothing added)

1/2 banana

1/3 cup fresh blueberries or 1-2 tbsp raisins

1 1/2 tbsp flaxseed meal

1/2 tbsp chia seeds

1 cup nonfat milk

1 whole egg plus 2 egg whites fried with 1/2 tsp extra-virgin olive oil

428 calories; 53 g carbohydrate, 11 g fat, 30 g protein

You definitely won't be hungry after this!

Step 6: Time Your Meals and Exercise

When you are well fueled throughout the day, you can train harder and burn more calories. Before, during, and directly after exercise, put your fast carbohydrates to work for you. Depending on your goal, sometimes it is best to consume them during and after exercise. That's when your body can best burn them for the energy you need to build solid muscle. The rest of the day, focus on slow carbohydrate sources such as vegetables and beans.

After your workout, be sure to take in protein and carbohydrate to replenish your glycogen stores and create a hormonal environment in your body that is conducive to building muscle.

As you time your meals, be careful about overrestricting food. This can backfire and make you lose control by bingeing. It's better to allow yourself foods you consider treats than try to shun them altogether. Research supports the concept of "controlled cheating" to help you stay the course. I am not an advocate of cheat days, or cheat meals, because these are negative and self-defeating. Just plan to occasionally add the foods you love into your diet, or even just go ahead and splurge now and then. Either approach will get you to your goal with a much more positive attitude, and more sustainably. I encourage my clients to enjoy a few of their favorite foods every so often, but to try to eat them when they can best burn them off—say, at breakfast or after a workout. That way, these foods become recovery rewards. This optimistic attitude toward treats will keep you on track to meet your goals.

Step 7: Don't Neglect Carbohydrate

As far as the rest of your diet is concerned, don't cut too much carbohydrate, or you're going to be really sluggish and out of sorts. A lack of carbohydrate will adversely affect your energy levels and mood. It's critical to have some carbohydrate in your diet throughout the tapering phase. The best choices are slow carbohydrate sources such as veggies, whole grains, beans, and low-fat dairy.

I do, however, recommend cutting back on added sugars—sweets, nondiet sodas, and table sugar in your coffee or tea. As I've mentioned previously, added sugars are beneficial only around exercise when they're efficiently burned off for energy.

Solving the Problem of Added Sugars in Performance and Recovery

When fueling for exercise and recovery, fast carbohydrate sources are king. That means some combination of added sugar or engineered starch ingredients. These range from sucrose, glucose, and fructose to maltodextrin and amylopectin.

Ideally, if you are doing long-duration exercise, you should front-load your fuel with these types of products. But here is a red flag warning: Too much added sugar can cause stomach and GI discomfort—not a helpful feeling if you're competing in a marathon or triathlon and want to finish strong.

I don't give a shout-out to a specific brand unless it stands alone in terms of quality and research evidence. This is one of those times. A promising solution to the sugar issue is a patented amylopectin (starch) fraction used in the starch-based product Vitargo. Backed by a number of peer-reviewed research studies from the same laboratory that did work on carbohydrate loading, creatine, and beta-alanine, as well as from other labs, this unique starch fraction empties from the stomach and is delivered to the muscle cells nearly twice as fast as any other carbohydrate available. This is true even when compared to the fastest carbohydrate typically used in top sport drinks: maltodextrin plus multitransport sugars. A published performance study showed enhanced work output and endurance performance during a cycling time trial in subjects supplemented with Vitargo versus those taking a 98 percent maltodextrin and 2 percent sugar carbohydrate supplement or water.

Based on this research, I suggest Vitargo to my clients. It is not only very well tolerated as a sport supplement but also has enabled me to create even healthier diet plans. Because it is so rapidly emptied from the stomach, athletes can load carbohydrate before exercise better than they could before. They can therefore take in the majority of their dietary starch before, during, and after exercise to best support performance and recovery, without any gastrointestinal discomfort or bloat. Because they can minimize if not eliminate added sugar, they have lots of room for an abundance of vegetables all day long. They don't have to have so many added sugar and starch servings just to get in the levels of carbohydrate that they needed to previously, especially in building and cross-training diets.

If you want to try what I now do frequently in my practice, substitute grams of starch carbohydrate from Vitargo for grams of added sugar in sport drinks. In fact you'll know how many grams to use from the category "added carbohydrate or sugar" in the menu plans in chapters 15 through19. You'll be able to pack in much more, in fact, and perhaps minimize some of the starch servings in your diet the rest of the day as well. For fat and weight loss, this offers the edge you need.

With the recommended increase in your protein intake, for the peaking diet your total calories might look something like this: protein, 30 to 35 percent; carbohydrate, 40 percent; and fat, 25 to 30 percent. As long as you don't cut calories too drastically, you'll still have enough carbohydrate to support your training requirements. You can even have a minimal amount of added sugar (if you really can't live without it) and still meet the 40 percent carbohydrate requirement, although I prefer that you use your carbohydrate calories to eat nutritionally dense foods such as milk, grains, starchy and regular vegetables, and fruits.

Some very low-carbohydrate diets can hinder your training. Case in point: A study published in the *Journal of the International Society of Sports Nutrition* pointed out that the Atkins diet decreased exercise capacity in nine exercisers. Yes, they lost weight; however, they had a significant drop in their blood glucose levels, and this caused them to fatigue very early on during their workouts. This type of diet and others like it are neither appropriate nor necessary for active people.

Step 8: Focus on High-Performance Fat

When your goal is to build lean muscle mass (the building diet), there is plenty of room in your plan for the right types of dietary fat. However, when you are trying to peak in a fat-loss or cutting diet, there isn't any room for the wrong kinds of fat. Fat is critical to your success and should be eaten in the right proportions with protein and the right types of carbohydrate.

The key is to focus on healthy monounsaturated fat, including fat from vegetable oils, olives, nuts, and avocados. Continue to obtain your omega-3 polyunsaturated fat from fatty fish and a little flaxseed meal. And make sure to supplement with omega-3 (DHA and EPA) supplements. The key is variety with fats, just like with all food groups. It is with variety that you get the best array of nutritional opportunities.

Always avoid saturated and trans fat from processed snack foods, commercially baked goods, and fried foods, because they will sabotage your progress. If you enjoy the flavor and high smoke point of coconut oil, you can certainly include it as part of your fats and oils palette. You may find that the slightly higher concentration of medium-chain triglycerides in coconut oil help you consume more needed calories but stay a little leaner. However, it's not a panacea.

Step 9: Space Your Meals

Your body may better use its calories for energy, and especially protein for building, if you eat several small meals throughout the day. Most bodybuilders and other strength athletes eat five, six, or more meals a day. Spacing meals in this manner keeps you fueled throughout the day and may help you maintain better appetite control. Plus, the spacing of protein in 20- to 30-gram amounts throughout the day may give you better building results, as well as keep your metabolism revved all day. In other words, every time you eat, your metabolism accelerates. Eating multiple meals throughout the day is a good dietary practice for some, but it isn't a slam dunk for weight loss. Several studies have shown no difference in outcome with three large meals versus five to six smaller meals. It's the little packages of protein spaced throughout the day that may actually be more meaningful for building and recovery. In the end it's really more of what works best for you. It does take mindfulness to figure it out and then stick to your plan.

Step 10: Include Anti-Inflammatory Foods

Exercise can increase free radical production and inflammation in the body. However, you can mitigate these processes by choosing anti-inflammatory foods and immune-boosting foods, all of which are loaded with antioxidants. The key is to choose bright, colorful vegetables and fruits (I'm not talking about Fruit Loops or Trix cereals, either!), from green spinach to sweet oranges. You can also get many of these healing nutrients from dairy products, eggs, and fish. Fish is especially high in omega-3 fatty acids, which have very effective anti-inflammatory properties.

Here is a list of healing foods to consider:

Citrus fruits	Broccoli	Tomatoes
Carrots	Pineapples	Apples
Oranges	Bananas	Star fruits
Papayas	Mangos	Kiwi fruits
Blood oranges	Passion fruits	Prickly pears
Strawberries	Cherries	Cranberries
Raspberries	Blueberries	Red grapes
Black currants	Green tea	

At the same time, stay away from or limit "pro-inflammatory foods." These are foods that activate inflammation in your body. The biggest offender here is added sugar; by shunning processed foods and sweets, you automatically reduce harmful inflammation in your body. Pro-inflammatory foods include omega-6 fat sources, such as safflower oil, sunflower oil, soybean oil, cottonseed oil, and corn oil.

Step 11: Supplement Prudently

There are some real nutritional horror stories among people who crash diet or diet stringently for contests. They tend to suffer deficiencies in calcium, magnesium, zinc, vitamin D, and other nutrients. Generally, these deficiencies occur because dieters and bodybuilders eliminate dairy foods and red meat while dieting. I commonly hear about contest dieters eating only chicken breast and canned tuna, period. However, you don't need to shy away from any healthy foods. You can include red meat in your diet as long as it's lean and cooked appropriately. You can also include nonfat dairy foods, an important source of body-strengthening minerals, and fat-burning whey and casein proteins. Neither of these foods will make you gain fat, as long as you eat them in moderation.

Because calories are cut during diets, supplement with an antioxidant vitamin and mineral formula that contains at least 100 percent of the DRI for all essential nutrients. This type of supplement will help cover your nutritional bases. See chapters 9, 10, 11, and 12 for additional supplement recommendations.

Step 12: Watch Water Intake

Fitness-conscious people live in dread of water retention or bloating, medically known as edema. Water retention can keep you from looking lean even after you've pared down to physique perfection. Water causes certain areas to swell up, and you look like you have body fat even though it's only water weight.

How can you prevent water retention? Ironically, the best defense is to drink plenty of water throughout your tapering period. This means drinking at least 8 cups (2 L) of water or more daily. With ample fluid, your body automatically flushes itself of extra water. Not drinking enough water can make your body cling to as much fluid as it can, and you'll end up bloated. Dehydration can sap your energy, and you won't be able to work out as intensely.

Besides drinking plenty of water, follow these strategies to prevent water retention.

- *Be cautious with your sodium intake.* Sodium has gained a bad reputation, but it's an essential element in our diets. Our bodies have a minimum requirement of 500 milligrams a day. The body tightly regulates its electrolyte levels, including sodium. Decreasing sodium levels really doesn't have much of an effect; your body holds on to the amount of sodium it needs, even if you reduce your intake. It's essential to consume the minimum requirement to maintain fluid balance and electrolyte balance. Otherwise, nerve and muscle function will be impaired, and exercise performance will definitely diminish. Some bodybuilders have passed out just before their competitions because of dehydration and possible electrolyte imbalance.

  If you're sodium sensitive—that is, sodium causes you to retain water—you probably should reduce your intake slightly. Don't go to extremes, though. Simply avoid high-sodium foods such as snack foods, canned foods, salted foods, pickled foods, cured foods, and lunch meats. Certainly don't add any extra salt to your food. But eliminating natural, whole foods because of their sodium content is usually unnecessary. Concentrate your food choices on whole grains, fresh fruits and vegetables, nonfat dairy foods, and unprocessed meats.

- *Eat naturally diuretic vegetables.* Some foods naturally help the body eliminate water, including asparagus, cucumbers, parsley, and watercress. You might try eating these while dieting, especially if water retention is a concern. Add a serving or two of these foods to your diet every day. Avoid pharmacological forms of diuretics at all cost. Diuretic drugs flush sodium and other electrolytes from your body, causing life-threatening imbalances.

- *Continue aerobic exercise.* Aerobic exercise improves the resiliency and tone of blood vessels. Unless blood vessels are resilient, water can seep from them and collect in the tissues, and water retention is the result. A regular program of aerobics helps prevent this.

- *Add a hot yoga class or two to your weekly regimen.* Sweating is part of our natural fluid cycle rhythm and may help you stay in better fluid balance. So as long as you fully rehydrate, don't be afraid to sweat.

For Powerlifters and Weightlifters Only

As a powerlifter or weightlifter, you probably don't care much about getting ripped. Rather, you want to be as strong and as powerful as possible in your weight class. Here's what you should do to get strong for training and competition:

- *Load your muscles with energy sources.* Carbohydrate and creatine are your best bets. Stay on a carbohydrate-dense diet, supplemented with creatine. Take your creatine with carbohydrate, as recommended in chapter 10, to supercharge your muscles with energy. Numerous studies on creatine have shown that this supplement is a sure thing for boosting strength and power.

  You don't need to carbohydrate load. There's no scientific evidence that this method has any performance-enhancing benefit for strength athletes. Simply maintain a high-carbohydrate diet throughout your training and competition preparation. Going into competition well fueled is critical.

- *Manipulate your aerobics and carbohydrate intake.* Increase your aerobics and slightly lower your carbohydrate intake if you need to make weight. This will help you lose fat to qualify for your weight class. You may need to decrease your calories slightly, and you can do this by cutting carbohydrate. However, try to go no lower than 40 percent of your total calories. That way, you can reduce weight but maintain strength.

  Give yourself plenty of time to make weight—at least 10 to 12 weeks. If your contest is fast approaching, you can cut your calories down to 30 per kilogram of body weight a day. That will result in a loss of 3 to 4 pounds (1.4-1.8 kg) a week. But keep in mind that you may lose some muscle mass, too.

  If you do cut to 30 calories per kilogram of body weight a day, stay on this regimen for no longer than seven days. Prolonged restrictive dieting slows your RMR—and your ability to burn fat. You may also lose strength and power over time.

- *Avoid dangerous practices for making weight.* Before a meet, it's fairly common for some lifters to exercise in rubberized suits or sit in steam or sauna baths for extended periods—all without drinking much water. This practice can lead to dehydration so severe that it can harm the kidneys and heart. Dehydrated lifters also usually do poorly in competition.

  Fasting isn't a good idea, either, even for a day or two. You'll rapidly lose water, but then you'll gain the health problems caused by dehydration. Glycogen depletion sets in, too, making it virtually impossible to perform well on competition day.

Sport Nutrition Fact Versus Fiction: Night Eating—An Anabolic Secret

Eating at night used to be considered a no-no if you wanted to stay lean and muscular. This is a myth that I want to bust wide open. It probably exists because people mistakenly believe that when you're in bed and inactive, you don't burn off all the calories and fat from that meal you've eaten. The reality, however, is not that simple. On the contrary, it turns out that eating at night is another way to gain muscle mass, according to recent studies. Here's why: Your body actually stays in an anabolic condition throughout the night to support restoration and recovery in all areas. The reason is that, at night, testosterone (a muscle-building hormone) and growth hormone are naturally elevated. Thus, the right late-night snack can maximize the effects of these elevated hormones. Food also blunts cortisol (a fat-producing hormone) and boosts the availability of the building blocks for muscle such as branched-chain amino acids and glutamine.

The trick is to create the right anabolic late-night snack. It should feature a slowly digesting carbohydrate so it doesn't cause much insulin release, which could disturb your sleep and increase fat accumulation. Avoid fat, sugar, and processed sweets, too. Your snack should also focus on lean protein, such as milk, yogurt, or nuts. I recommend having a small casein protein shake made with low-fat milk, casein protein powder, and a couple of berries. If you prefer, you can just have 30 grams of casein protein mixed with milk. That simple mix gets the job done! *Warning:* If the food you eat at night is above and beyond your total calorie needs, it may not be muscle that you gain. These night-time calories still have to be part of your total energy needs for the day. Just remember: Eating the right food at night is a win-win for building muscle—while you sleep!

15

Maintaining Physique Menu Plans

The Power Eating maintaining physique diet outlined in this chapter is for exercisers; bodybuilders; and novice and recreational strength trainers, powerlifters, and weightlifters. Often during training you are not trying to gain or lose weight. Sometimes, it's a timing issue; you're just too busy to spend time in the gym. Sometimes, it is a planned part of your training schedule, such as after the competitive season. Whatever the reason, this menu plan will keep you right where you want to be.

   Please note: For all listings of added carbohydrate or sugar in each of these diet plans, you can choose to substitute starch. I will include grams of carbohydrate for pre-, during and post-workout sport drink and shake recommendations. Please review the sidebar Solving the Problem of Added Sugars in Performance and Recovery in chapter 14 before making the substitution.

Power Eating Maintaining Physique Diet

Workouts per week	Woman		Man	
	Three or four (novice)	Five or more (experienced)	Three or four (novice)	Five or more (experienced)
Calories/kg	29-33	38-40	33	42
Calories/lb	13-15	17-18	15	19
Protein				
g/kg	1.5	1.7	1.5	1.8
g/lb	0.7	0.8	0.7	0.8
Carbohydrate				
g/kg	3.5	5.5	4.5	5.5
g/lb	1.75	2.3	2.0	2.3
Fat*				
g/kg	~0.85-1.00	~1.00-1.30	~1.0	~1.4
g/lb	~0.39-0.45	~0.45-0.59	~0.45	~0.64

*Total fat varies based on total calories. To find your fat grams, determine your total calories, protein grams, and carbohydrate grams. Add your protein and carbohydrate calories (1 g protein = 4 calories, 1 g carbohydrate = 4 calories), subtract this total from the total calories, and divide by 9 (1 g fat = 9 calories). See chapter 13 for more information.

Power Eating Sample Maintaining Physique Menu Plans

130-POUND (59 KG) NOVICE WOMAN

(three or four workouts per week)

1,718 calories (33 calories/kg; based on top of kcal range); 89 grams protein; 228 grams carbohydrate; 50 grams fat

Food groups	Number of servings
Bread/starch	4
Fruit	5
Nonfat milk	3
Teaspoons of added carbohydrate or sugar	3
Vegetable	8
Protein:	
Very lean	5
Lean	3
Medium-fat	1
Fat	6

Food group servings	Menu
Breakfast	
1 bread/starch	1 cup (25 g) Kashi Whole Grain Puffs cereal
1 milk	1 cup (240 ml) fat-free milk
2 fruit	1/2 cup (120 ml) orange juice 3/4 cup (110 g) blueberries for cereal
2 vegetable	1 cup sautéed vegetables to scramble with egg
1 medium-fat protein	1 whole egg, scrambled in nonstick skillet
2 fat	1 tbsp ground flaxseed sprinkled on cereal 1 tsp oil for skillet
	Water
Snack	
1 fruit	8 dried apricot halves
1 vegetable	1 cup (128 g) mini carrots
1 fat	6 almonds
	Green tea (or other tea)
Lunch	
2 bread/starch	2 slices whole-grain (ideally sprouted grain) bread
2 vegetable	Fill sandwich with vegetable choices Veggie sticks
3 very lean protein	3 oz (90 g) turkey
1 fat	1/8 avocado
	Water
Preworkout snack	
1 milk	1 cup (230 g) plain yogurt
1 fruit	1 small banana
	Water
Workout	
	Water
Postworkout smoothie	
1 fruit	1 1/4 cups (180 g) whole strawberries
1 milk	1 cup (240 ml) nonfat milk
3 tsp added carbohydrate or sugar (12 g)	3 tsp honey
2 very lean protein	14 g whey protein isolate
Dinner	
1 bread/starch	1/2 baked sweet potato
3 vegetable	1 cup (180 g) steamed asparagus 2 cups (56 g) mixed green salad
3 lean protein	3 oz (90 g) wild salmon, grilled
2 fat	1 tsp olive oil for salmon 1 tsp butter or vegetable oil for potato 2 tbsp reduced-fat salad dressing
	Green tea (or other tea)

130-POUND (59 KG) EXPERIENCED WOMAN

(five or more workouts per week)

2,366 calories (40 calories/kg; based on top of kcal range); 100 grams protein; 325 grams carbohydrate; 74 grams fat

Food groups	Number of servings
Bread/starch	7
Fruit	7
Nonfat milk	3
Teaspoons of added carbohydrate or sugar	7
Vegetable	7
Protein:	
Very lean	5
Lean	3
Medium-fat	1
Fat	10

Food group servings	Menu
Breakfast	
2 bread/starch	2 slices whole-grain (ideally sprouted grain) bread
1 milk	1 cup (240 ml) fat-free milk
3 fruit	1 cup (240 ml) orange juice 3 tbsp no-sugar-added apple butter for bread
1 medium-fat protein	1 whole egg, scrambled
2 fat	1/8 avocado, sliced and cooked with eggs 1 tsp Heart Smart Omega margarine for cooking egg
	Water
Snack	
1 fruit	8 dried apricot halves
3 fat	18 almonds
	Green tea (or other tea)

Food group servings	Menu
Lunch	
3 bread/starch	6 in. (15 cm) Subway sandwich (choose from "Fresh Fit" list)
2 vegetable	Fill sandwich with vegetable choices
2 very lean protein	2 oz (60 g) meat included in sandwich
2 fat	2 tsp olive oil or 2 tbsp salad dressing
	Water
Preworkout snack	
1 milk	1 cup (230 g) plain yogurt
1 fruit	3/4 cup (110 g) blueberries
3 tsp added carbohydrate or sugar (12 g)	3 tsp honey
1 vegetable	Red pepper spears
	Water
Workout	
	Water
Postworkout smoothie	
1 fruit	1 1/4 cups (180 g) whole frozen strawberries
1 milk	1 cup (240 ml) nonfat milk
4 tsp added carbohydrate or sugar (16 g)	4 tsp sugar
3 very lean protein	21 g whey protein isolate
Dinner	
2 bread/starch	1 baked sweet potato
1 fruit	3 oz (about 15) red grapes
4 vegetable	1 cup (180 g) steamed asparagus 4 cups (112 g) mixed green salad
3 lean protein	3 oz (90 g) wild salmon, grilled
3 fat	1 tsp olive oil for salmon 1 tsp butter or vegetable for potato 2 tbsp reduced-fat salad dressing
	Green tea (or other tea)

180-POUND (82 KG) NOVICE MAN

(three or four workouts per week)

2,733 calories; 123 grams protein; 360 grams carbohydrate; 89 grams fat

Food groups	Number of servings
Bread/starch	8
Fruit	7
Nonfat milk	3
Teaspoons of added carbohydrate or sugar	16
Vegetable	9
Protein:	
Very lean	7
Lean	4
Medium-fat	1
Fat	11

Food group servings	Menu
Preworkout snack	
1 milk	1 cup (230 g) plain yogurt
1 fruit	3/4 cup (110 g) blueberries
3 tsp added carbohydrate or sugar (12 g)	3 tsp honey
	Water
Workout	
8 tsp added carbohydrate or sugar (32 g)	16 oz (480 ml) sport drink
	Water
Breakfast	
1 bread/starch	1 slice whole-grain bread
1 milk	1 cup (240 ml) fat-free milk
2 vegetable	1 cup sautéed vegetables in margarine, add eggs
2 fruit	1 cup (240 ml) orange juice
3 tsp added carbohydrate or sugar (12 g)	1 tbsp 100% fruit spread for bread
1 medium-fat protein	1 whole egg, scrambled in nonstick skillet

Food group servings	Menu
Breakfast *(continued)*	
2 very lean protein	4 egg whites, cooked with whole egg
2 fat	1/8 avocado, sliced and cooked with eggs 1 tsp Heart Smart Omega margarine for cooking eggs
	Water
Snack	
2 vegetable	2 cups (125 g) carrot and celery sticks (or others)
3 fat	1 1/2 tbsp natural peanut butter
Lunch	
5 bread/starch	12 in. (30 cm) Subway sandwich (choose from "Fresh Fit" list)
2 vegetable	Fill sandwich with vegetable choices
1 fruit	Banana
4 very lean protein	4 oz (115 g) meat included in sandwich
2 fat	2 tsp olive oil or 2 tbsp salad dressing
	Water
Snack	
2 fruit	16 dried apricot halves
1 milk	1 tall nonfat latté
1 very lean protein	1 reduced-fat string cheese stick
1 tsp added carbohydrate or sugar (4 g)	1 tsp sugar
2 fat	12 almonds
	Water
Dinner	
2 bread/starch	1 baked sweet potato
1 fruit	3 oz (~15) red grapes
1 tsp added carbohydrate or sugar (4 g)	1 tsp sugar or honey for tea
3 vegetable	1/2 cup (90 g) steamed asparagus 4 cups (112 g) mixed green salad
4 lean protein	4 oz (120 g) wild salmon, grilled
2 fat	1 tsp olive oil for salmon 2 tbsp reduced-fat salad dressing
	Green tea (or other tea)

180-POUND (82 KG) EXPERIENCED MAN

(five or more workouts per week)

3,413 calories; 148 grams protein; 451 grams carbohydrate; 113 grams fat

Food groups	Number of servings
Bread/starch	10
Fruit	9
Nonfat milk	3
Teaspoons of added carbohydrate or sugar	18
Vegetable	11
Protein:	
Very lean	11
Lean	4
Medium-fat	1
Fat	18

Food group servings	Menu
Preworkout snack	
1 milk	1 cup (230 g) plain yogurt
1 fruit	3/4 cup (110 g) blueberries
3 tsp added carbohydrate or sugar (12 g)	3 tsp honey
	Water
Workout	
8 tsp added carbohydrate or sugar (32 g)	16 oz (475 ml) sport drink
	Water
Breakfast	
2 bread/starch	2 slices whole-grain bread
1 milk	1 cup (240 ml) fat-free milk
3 vegetable	1 1/2 cups sautéed vegetables added to eggs
3 fruit	1 cup (240 ml) orange juice 1 cup (170 g) melon cubes
6 tsp added carbohydrate or sugar (24 g)	2 tbsp 100% fruit spread for bread
1 tsp added carbohydrate or sugar (4 g)	1 tsp sugar (for tea or coffee)
1 medium-fat protein	1 whole egg, scrambled in nonstick skillet

Food group servings	Menu
Breakfast (*continued*)	
2 very lean protein	4 egg whites, cooked with whole egg
5 fat	1/4 avocado, sliced and cooked with eggs 3 tsp butter or vegetable oil for cooking vegetables and eggs
	Tea or coffee
	Water
Snack	
2 bread/starch	8 whole-wheat crackers
2 vegetable	2 cups (125 g) carrot and celery sticks (or other vegetables)
1 very lean protein	1 reduced-fat string cheese
6 fat	3 tbsp natural peanut butter
	Water
Lunch	
5 bread/starch	12 in. (30 cm) Subway sandwich (choose from "Fresh Fit" list)
2 vegetable	Fill sandwich with vegetable choices
1 fruit	Banana
4 very lean protein	Included in sandwich
2 fat	2 tsp olive oil or 2 tbsp salad dressing
	Water
Snack	
2 fruit	16 dried apricot halves
1 milk	8 oz nonfat milk mixed with protein (can add water)
4 very lean protein	28 grams whey protein isolate (flavored)
2 fat	12 almonds
	Water
Dinner	
1 bread/starch	1/2 baked sweet potato
2 fruit	6 oz (~30) red grapes
4 vegetable	1 cup (180 g) steamed asparagus 4 cups (112 g) mixed green salad
4 lean protein	4 oz (120 g) wild salmon, grilled
3 fat	1 tsp olive oil for salmon 4 tbsp reduced-fat salad dressing
	Green tea (or other tea)

16

Building Muscle Menu Plans

My Power Eating diet for building muscle is for novice or experienced exercisers, bodybuilders, powerlifters, weightlifters, and other serious strength trainers who are interested in building quality muscle. The larger you are and the greater your muscle mass is, the more calories it will take for you to build muscle. If you are not seeing gains at these levels, increase your calories by 300 to 400 per day by primarily increasing carbohydrate (50 to 75 percent of the calorie increase) and secondarily increasing fat (25 to 50 percent of the caloric increase). If you are cross-training with intense aerobic exercise for long duration, increase your carbohydrate intake by another 1 to 2 grams per kilogram of body weight per day.

Your sport fuel is designated by teaspoons of added carbohydrate or sugar. You can use any number of available products that contain sugars or starches to meet these grams of added carbohydrate to fuel your training (1 tsp added sugar = 4 g carbohydrate).

Please note: For all listings of added carbohydrate or sugar in each of these diet plans, you can choose to substitute starch. I will include grams of carbohydrate for pre-, during and post-workout sport drink and shake recommendations. Please review the sidebar Solving the Problem of Added Sugars in Performance and Recovery in chapter 14 before making the substitution.

Power Eating Building Muscle Diet

Workouts per week	Woman		Man	
	Three or four (novice)	Five or more (experienced)	Three or four (novice)	Five or more (experienced)
Calories/kg	35-38	44-50	42	52+
Calories/lb	16-17	20-23	19	24+
Protein				
g/kg	2.0	2.2	2.2	2.5
g/lb	0.9	1.0	1.0	1.1
Carbohydrate				
g/kg	4.5	6.5	5.5	7.0
g/lb	2.1	3.0	2.5	3.2
Fat*				
g/kg	~1.0-1.3	~1.00-1.77	~1.33	1.77
g/lb	~0.45-0.59	~0.5-0.8	~0.6	0.8

*Total fat varies based on total calories. To find your fat grams, determine your total calories, protein grams, and carbohydrate grams. Add your protein and carbohydrate calories (1 g protein = 4 calories, 1 g carbohydrate = 4 calories), subtract this total from the total calories, and divide by 9 (1 g fat = 9 calories). See chapter 13 for more information.

Power Eating Sample Building Muscle Menu Plans

130-POUND (59 KG) NOVICE WOMAN

(three or four workouts per week)

2,076 calories (35 calories/kg; based on bottom of kcal range); 118 grams protein; 266 grams carbohydrate; 60 grams fat

Food groups	Number of servings
Bread/starch	6
Fruit	5
Nonfat milk	3
Teaspoons of added carbohydrate or sugar	3
Vegetable	8
Protein:	
Very lean	5
Lean	3
Medium-fat	1
Fat	9

Food group servings	Menu
Breakfast	
2 bread/starch	1 cup cooked oatmeal or other cooked cereal
1 milk	1 cup (240 ml) fat-free milk
2 fruit	1/2 cup (120 ml) orange juice
	3/4 cup (110 g) berries for cereal
1 medium-fat protein	1 whole egg, scrambled in nonstick skillet
1-2 seconds cooking spray	For cooking egg
1 fat	1 tbsp ground flaxseed sprinkled on cereal
	Water
Snack	
1 fruit	8 dried apricot halves
2 vegetable	1 cup (128 g) mini carrots
	1 cup (128 g) cherry tomatoes
2 fat	12 almonds
	Green tea (or other tea)
Lunch	
2 bread/starch	2 slices whole-grain (ideally sprouted grain) bread
3 vegetable	Fill sandwich with vegetable choices
	2 cups mixed green salad
3 very lean protein	2 oz (60 g) turkey
	1 oz (30 g) cheese
3 fat	1 fat included in cheese
	1/8 avocado
	1 tbsp salad dressing or 2 tbsp reduced-fat salad dressing
	Mustard for sandwich
	Water
Preworkout snack	
1 milk	1 cup (230 g) plain yogurt
1 fruit	1 small banana
	Water
Workout	
	Water
Postworkout smoothie	
1 fruit	1 1/4 cups (180 g) whole strawberries
1 milk	1 cup (240 ml) nonfat milk
3 tsp added carbohydrate or sugar (12 g)	3 tsp honey
2 very lean protein	14 g whey protein isolate
Dinner	
2 bread/starch	1 baked sweet potato
3 vegetable	1 cup (180 g) steamed asparagus
	4 cups (112 g) mixed green salad
3 lean protein	3 oz (90 g) wild salmon, grilled
3 fat	1 tsp olive oil for salmon
	1 tsp butter or vegetable oil for potato
	4 tbsp reduced-fat salad dressing
	Green tea (or other tea)

130-POUND (59 KG) EXPERIENCED WOMAN

(five or more workouts per week)

2,947 calories (50 calories/kg, based on top of kcal range); 130 grams protein; 384 grams carbohydrate; 99 grams fat

Food groups	Number of servings
Bread/starch	8
Fruit	8
Nonfat milk	3
Teaspoons of added carbohydrate or sugar	18
Vegetable	7
Protein:	
Very lean	5
Lean	4
Medium-fat	1
Fat	16

Food group servings	Menu
Breakfast	
2 bread/starch	2 slices whole-grain bread
1 milk	1 cup (240 ml) fat-free milk
2 fruit	1 cup (240 ml) orange juice
4 tsp added carbohydrate or sugar (16 g)	4 tsp 100% fruit spread for bread
1 vegetable	1/2 cup (28 g) sautéed mushrooms added to egg
1 medium-fat protein	1 whole egg, scrambled
4 fat	1/4 avocado, sliced and cooked with egg 2 tsp butter or vegetable oil for cooking mushrooms and egg
	Water
Snack	
2 fruit	16 dried apricot halves
3 fat	18 almonds
	Green tea (or other tea)

Food group servings	Menu
Lunch	
3 bread/starch	6 in. (18 cm) Subway sandwich (choose from "Fresh Fit" list)
2 vegetable	Fill sandwich with vegetable choices
2 very lean protein	2 oz (60 g) meat included in sandwich 1 oz (30 g) cheese
3 fat	1 fat serving included in cheese 2 tsp olive oil or 2 tbsp salad dressing
	Water
Preworkout snack	
1 milk	1 cup (230 g) plain yogurt
1 fruit	3/4 cup (110 g) blueberries
3 tsp added carbohydrate or sugar (12 g)	3 tsp honey
	Water
Workout	
8 tsp added carbohydrate or sugar (32 g)	16 oz (480 ml) sport drink
	Water
Postworkout smoothie	
1 fruit	1 1/4 cups (180 g) whole strawberries
1 milk	1 cup (240 ml) nonfat milk
3 tsp added sugar	3 tsp honey
3 very lean protein	21 g whey protein isolate
1 fat	1/8 avocado
Dinner	
3 bread/starch	1 baked sweet potato 1/2 cup (98 g) brown rice
2 fruit	6 oz (~30) red grapes
4 vegetable	1 cup (180 g) steamed asparagus 4 cups (112 g) mixed green salad
4 lean protein	4 oz (120 g) wild salmon, grilled
5 fat	1 tsp olive oil to rub on salmon 4 tbsp salad dressing
	Green tea (or other tea)

180-POUND (82 KG) NOVICE MAN

(three or four workouts per week)

3,420 calories; 180 grams protein; 450 grams carbohydrate; 100 grams fat

Food groups	Number of servings
Bread/starch	10
Fruit	8
Nonfat milk	3
Teaspoons of added carbohydrate or sugar	24
Vegetable	9
Protein:	
Very lean	10
Lean	6
Medium-fat	1
Fat	14

Food group servings	Menu
Preworkout snack	
1 milk	1 cup (230 g) plain yogurt
1 fruit	3/4 cup (110 g) blueberries
3 tsp added carbohydrate or sugar (12 g)	3 tsp honey
2 very lean protein	14 g whey protein isolate whisked into yogurt
	Water
Workout	
16 tsp added sugar	32 oz (950 ml) sport drink
	Water
Breakfast	
2 bread/starch	2 slices whole-grain bread
1 milk	1 cup (240 ml) fat-free milk
2 fruit	1 cup (240 ml) orange juice
4 tsp added sugar	4 tsp 100% fruit spread for bread
2 vegetable	1 cup sautéed vegetables to add to eggs
1 medium-fat protein	1 whole egg, scrambled

Food group servings	Menu
Breakfast *(continued)*	
2 very lean protein	4 egg whites, cooked with whole egg
4 fat	1/4 avocado, sliced and cooked with eggs 2 tsp olive oil for cooking vegetables and eggs
	Water
Snack	
2 bread/starch	8 whole-wheat crackers
1 lean protein	1 oz (30 g) cheese
1 vegetable	1 cup (124 g) celery sticks
3 fat	1 1/2 tbsp natural peanut butter
	Water
Lunch	
5 bread/starch	12 in. (30 cm) Subway sandwich (choose from "Fresh Fit" list)
2 vegetable	Fill sandwich with vegetable choices
1 fruit	Banana
6 very lean protein	4 oz (120 g) meat included in sandwich 2 oz (60 g) cheese
3 fat	2 fat servings included in cheese 1 tsp olive oil or 1 tbsp salad dressing
	Water
Snack	
2 fruit	16 dried apricot halves
1 milk	1 tall nonfat latté
1 tsp added carbohydrate or sugar (4 g)	1 tsp sugar
2 fat	12 almonds
	Water
Dinner	
1 bread/starch	1/2 baked sweet potato
2 fruit	6 oz (about 30) red grapes
4 vegetable	1 cup (180 g) steamed asparagus 4 cups (112 g) mixed green salad
5 lean protein	5 oz (150 g) wild salmon, grilled
2 fat	1 tsp olive oil for salmon 4 tbsp reduced-fat salad dressing
	Green tea (or other tea)

180-POUND (82 KG) EXPERIENCED MAN

(five or more workouts per week)

4,249 calories; 205 grams protein; 576 grams carbohydrate; 125 grams fat

Food groups	Number of servings
Bread/starch	13
Fruit	10
Nonfat milk	3
Teaspoons of added carbohydrate or sugar	30
Vegetable	9
Protein:	
Very lean	13
Lean	5
Medium-fat	1
Fat	24

Food group servings	Menu
Preworkout snack	
1 milk	1 cup (230 g) plain yogurt
1 fruit	3/4 cup (110 g) blueberries
3 tsp added carbohydrate or sugar (12 g)	3 tsp honey
3 very lean protein	21 g whey protein isolate whisked into yogurt
	Water
Workout	
16 tsp added carbohydrate or sugar (64 g)	32 oz (950 ml) sport drink
	Water
Breakfast	
2 bread/starch	2 slices whole-grain bread
1 milk	1 cup (240 ml) fat-free milk (make a smoothie with milk, juice, fruit, whey protein)
3 fruit	1/2 cup (120 ml) orange juice 1 1/2 cups frozen fruit
6 tsp added carbohydrate or sugar (24 g)	2 tbsp 100% fruit spread for bread
2 vegetable	1 cup sautéed mushrooms and red peppers
1 medium-fat protein	1 whole egg, scrambled
4 very lean protein	4 egg whites, cooked with whole egg 14 g whey protein isolate (for smoothie)
6 fat	1/2 avocado, sliced and cooked with eggs 2 tsp vegetable oil for cooking eggs and vegetables
	Water

Food group servings	Menu
Snack	
2 bread/starch	8 whole-wheat crackers
2 fruit	2/3 cup (158 ml) Concord grape juice (make a spritzer by mixing with sparkling water)
1 vegetable	1 cup (124 g) celery sticks
6 fat	3 tbsp natural peanut butter
	Water
Lunch	
5 bread/starch	12-in. (36 cm) Subway sandwich (choose from "Fresh Fit" list)
2 vegetable	Fill sandwich with vegetable choices
1 fruit	Banana
6 very lean protein	4 oz (120 g) meat included in sandwich 2 oz (60 g) cheese
4 fat	2 fat servings included in cheese 2 tsp olive oil or 2 tbsp salad dressing
	Water
Snack	
2 fruit	16 dried apricot halves
1 milk	1 tall nonfat latté
2 tsp added carbohydrate or sugar (8 g)	2 tsp sugar
2 fat	12 almonds
	Water
Dinner	
4 bread/starch	1 baked sweet potato 1 cup cooked quinoa
3 fruit	1 cup (124 g) raspberries and 1 cup (165 g) cubed mango; put on top of ice cream
3 tsp added carbohydrate or sugar (12 g)	1/2 cup light ice cream
4 vegetable	1 cup (180 g) steamed asparagus 4 cups (112 g) mixed green salad
5 lean protein	5 oz (150 g) wild salmon, grilled
6 fat	1 fat serving included in ice cream 1 tsp olive oil for salmon 4 tbsp salad dressing
Free (no calories)	1 tbsp whipped cream to top fruit and ice cream
	Water

VERY IMPORTANT: These calorie levels reflect the needs of people who consistently train very hard. If that's not you, then these calorie levels will be too high. If that's the case, use the menu for those doing fewer workouts per week, use female calorie levels if you're a man, or use a maintenance plan from chapter 15. If you need to drop only a few calories, then cut out the added carbohydrate or sugar everywhere except around training.

POWER PROFILE: Weight Gain

Are you a hard gainer—unable to put on any appreciable muscle weight no matter how hard you try?

That was the case of Scott E., a 44-year-old business executive who, at 6 feet 3 inches (191 cm) and 177 pounds (80 kg), had not been able to gain weight in 20 years. To make matters worse, he had no appetite; plus he had stomach problems caused by stress, infections, and overtreatment with antibiotics. I placed him on my Power Eating muscle-building diet.

Before beginning this diet, Scott was consuming only about 2,800 calories a day and not enough vitamins, minerals, or fluids. I increased his calories to 3,560 calories daily, plus added more protein (113 g daily) and carbohydrate (570 g daily). He started supplementing with a good antioxidant, eating multiple meals throughout the day, and consuming healthier fat from fish and plant sources. He also decreased his alcohol intake.

In addition, I recommended that Scott supplement with Kleiner's Updated Easy Muscle-Building Formula (see chapter 20), take 400 milligrams of vitamin E, and continue taking acidophilus, a supplement that restores intestinal flora after antibiotic treatment. I also suggested that Scott try a natural supplement, Prelief, to help reduce stomach irritation.

In only six weeks, Scott's energy levels soared, and he felt energetic enough to begin a regular exercise program. He gained 15 pounds (7 kg) of pure muscle—with no increase in his waist measurement. Scott felt that the Prelief helped him eat the extra calories without stomach irritation.

As Scott put it, "In the first three weeks, I gained 14 pounds (6 kg), from 180 (82 kg) to 194 (88 kg). To put this in perspective, I have not weighed over 184 (83 kg) in 20 years and have been trying to gain weight for the past two to three years." What's more, most of his stomach problems were resolved.

This highlights the problems that athletes can face when food intake needs to be high. Natural products like Prelief are very important in your training diet toolkit. Two other similarly natural products are Beano and Lactaid. The natural enzymes found in Beano work to prevent gas by breaking down the complex carbohydrate found in many foods such as beans, vegetables, and whole grains, making eating the foods you need to eat in abundance more enjoyable. Lactaid is a lactase-enzyme replacement supplement. Today you can buy the brand name, or any number of house-brand products, that help digest the milk sugar lactose, which many people cannot digest well. You can also try milk and other dairy products that have been pretreated with Lactaid and are much lower in lactose than the original versions.

There are no side effects to any of these three products, and if you find that the recommended dose of Beano or Lactaid doesn't work for you, try more. There is no harm in consuming more of these enzymes. I am a big advocate of using them to support a healthy diet abundant in the foods that help to build a strong body.

17

Cross-Training Menu Plans

If you're really interested in performance, or even high-level fitness, you probably cross-train with a variety of fitness activities. This chapter is for everyone who strength trains to enhance power for an endurance sport. Unlike the other menu plans, which are focused squarely on building strength and power and cutting fat, these menu plans will help you fine-tune your diet to build power yet still enhance endurance.

Because you're focusing on building strength and endurance, you'll use more carbohydrate to fuel your cardiorespiratory exercise. And because athletes who race don't want to add size and weight to their frames, you won't need the amount of protein that it takes to build muscle size. You want just enough to increase power and recover fully. And of course, you'll need the right amount of fat to fuel your endurance and allow for important joint cushioning and lubrication, hormonal balance, cellular recovery, anti-inflammatory functions, and brain support, for which fat is key.

Fat Adaptation

When you exercise in an endurance event, your body starts out by burning carbohydrate, moves into fat burning for the majority of the middle of the event, and then as you tire, you return to burning carbohydrate for the final sprint to the finish. The better trained you are, the better your body is at switching from carbohydrate to fat at the beginning of the race, and the longer you will use fat for fuel before you begin to tire and return to carbohydrate. This final switch actually determines how much endurance you really have, and how much power you'll have for the last lap or final sprint to the finish line. If you could get your body to switch to fat metabolism more quickly, stay there longer, and preserve more carbohydrate for the very end of the race, you'd definitely have a competitive edge. That's the whole theory behind fat adaptation.

The question is whether well-trained athletes could use fat adaptation to their benefit and extend endurance time before exhaustion hits. Although sport nutrition scientists are always studying how we can better match the diets of endurance athletes to their performance potential, the world of self-appointed experts continues to doubt the veracity of these investigations, and they claim that there is a conspiracy to push carbohydrate over fat as fuel for endurance exercise performance. In the words (or rant) of one of the leading sports scientists today, Dr. Trent Stellingwerff wrote: "I am paid to work with elite athletes to try and make them go faster in Olympic events within the rules of sport . . . if there was evidence that all I needed to do was change and shift an athlete's macronutrient intake to LCHF [low carbohydrate high fat] to turn them into world beaters do you not think I would *immediately* do this?" (@TStellingwerff, 1/4/2018).

At this point we know that fat adaptation actually happens. Some people adapt more sustainably to the diet than others, but in those who respond well, a high-fat, low-carbohydrate diet followed for five days to two weeks can stretch the body's ability to burn fat instead of carbohydrate. The nature of the diet, only 15 percent of calories from carbohydrate (below 50 g/day) and 70 percent from fat, leaves you with very low carbohydrate stores, regardless of the fact that there is no scientific data that this diet has ever led to enhanced athletic performance. To remedy that losing situation, scientists have created and tested a "dietary periodization" model in which you follow the high-fat protocol with one to three days of carbohydrate restoration. During this restoration period, you flip the carbohydrate–fat ratios to 70:15 and taper your exercise. Your ability to oxidize fat for fuel drops slightly but is still elevated well above where it would be without the fat adaptation diet strategy, and you partially regain your ability to burn carbohydrate when you need it. The bottom line is that we can't be great at both carbohydrate and fat metabolism at the same time. As we diminish carbohydrate consumption we up-regulate fat metabolism, meaning as we getter better at burning fats we down-regulate our carbohydrate metabolism and thus our ability to quickly utilize carbohydrate at high-intensity training levels when we need it to ride hills or sprint to the finish.

Despite the fact that this all really does happen in responsive subjects, the measures of performance have been disappointing. It is not clear at all whether altering metabolic profiles actually improves performance. Some studies showed a small but insignificant amount of improvement in the real world, others showed no change, and some recorded a decrement in cycling performance.

The concept of fat adaptation is still very much in the testing phase. To paraphrase Dr. Stellingwerff, it would be awesome if we could get it to work! But all indications so far are that it doesn't. You can try it out and see whether you are a responder, and whether you can tolerate the diet as well as the metabolic changes. I'll be honest: It's not an easy diet to follow, especially if your calorie needs are high. And because we still have no data to support the fat adaptation theory for enhanced performance, the menus in this chapter focus on the well-established and scientifically supported higher-carbohydrate diet for endurance athletes.

Protein During Training and Events

Just about anyone who is active has heard that you refuel, recover, rebuild, and grow much better if you have carbohydrate and protein soon after exercise. More recent data have begun to support the idea that the carbohydrate–protein combo prior to exercise also enhances muscle recovery and growth. And in fact having it either before or after is probably what's important, not necessarily one or the other. But the question of whether protein is helpful during exercise when it is taken along with carbohydrate has been hanging around for at least a decade. The first studies on the use of protein, or amino acids, during exercise focused on endurance activity and the question of whether, when given during exercise, protein positively affects the brain and the lengthening of time to exhaustion during exercise. That question has still not been answered. But as we have developed better laboratory tests for muscle protein synthesis and breakdown, the research into protein consumption with carbohydrate during endurance exercise has moved in that direction. As athletes have begun to cross-train to support their endurance activities, interest in the area of carbohydrate–protein consumption during exercise has grown as well, offering opportunity for more research to support product development.

The most recent evidence appears to lean toward positive effects from the use of some protein with carbohydrate during exercise; however, it is not definitely clear. A peer-reviewed sophisticated study investigated the impact of carbohydrate–protein coingestion during endurance exercise on muscle protein balance and synthesis. During exercise on a cycle ergometer, the subjects were given either a carbohydrate-only beverage (1 g/kg/h carbohydrate) or a calorically identical beverage of both carbohydrate (0.8 g/kg/h) and casein protein hydrolysate (0.2 g/kg/h). The study demonstrated that muscle protein synthesis rates improved with either beverage beyond a fasting state, but that the addition of protein did not further augment rates of muscle protein synthesis.

A separate study examined the influence of carbohydrate–protein coingestion on running capacity toward the end of a soccer-specific intermittent exercise protocol. The subjects ran three trials while randomly consuming either a placebo, a 6.9 percent carbohydrate solution, or a solution that was 4.8 percent carbohydrate and 2.1 percent protein. All beverages were matched for color and taste. The carbohydrate–protein beverage resulted in longer run times to fatigue compared to those in the other two test trials. The subjects recovered faster between sets of intermittent exercise to better endurance capacity and perceived a lower rate of exertion during exercise when they ingested the carbohydrate–protein beverage.

A third study tested the effect of a carbohydrate–protein beverage during competitive endurance exercise in the heat. Twenty-eight cyclists competing in the eight-day Transalp mountain bike race were the subjects of the study and were randomly assigned either a carbohydrate-only placebo (76 g/L) or a carbohydrate–protein beverage (72 g/L carbohydrate; 18 g/L protein). Carbohydrate–protein supplementation significantly prevented body mass loss, enhanced body temperature regulation, and improved competitive exercise performance compared to the placebo. The combination did not have an effect on muscle damage or soreness. The flaw in this study is that the placebo and the test beverage were not of the same caloric value. The carbohydrate–protein beverage contained more calories, or more energy. So it is difficult to assess whether the total energy or the presence of protein actually made the difference in the results.

There is a practical consideration with protein supplementation during exercise: Many people cannot tolerate protein or amino acids in their fluid-replacement or sport drinks, commonly experiencing stomach upset and nausea. If that happens to you, clearly it will not improve your performance. If you tolerate the protein in your beverage during exercise, then I think it's worth trying, especially if you are an ultradistance athlete. More protein is burned as fuel during these long duration events than in any other form of exercise. If you don't observe any benefits after a few weeks, then you might do well to drop it. There's no use in wasting money on something that doesn't work.

Caffeine Works

Caffeine has been used before exercise for decades, but a new twist was presented by a study that investigated the effect of adding caffeine to a postexercise carbohydrate drink on subsequent high-intensity interval running capacity. In this study the six subjects first exercised to exhaustion to deplete their muscles of glycogen (stored carbohydrate). Immediately following the workout and at one, two, and three hours after exercise, they consumed either water, a carbohydrate-only solution (1.2 g/kg of body weight), or a similar carbohydrate solution with 8 milligrams per kilogram of body weight of caffeine added. All beverages looked and tasted the same. After four hours of recovery, the subjects performed a shuttle test (test of high-intensity running capacity) to exhaustion. All six subjects improved performance in the carbohydrate–caffeine trial compared with the other two trials. Although for years word on the street has been that this is a winning strategy for those who can tolerate caffeine, it's very good to have data to back up the common knowledge. And because the half-life of caffeine is five to seven hours, it's not really all that surprising that an efficacious dose of caffeine, an acknowledged performance-enhancing aid, helps in the second round of performance.

Please note: For all listings of added carbohydrate or sugar in each of these diet plans, you can choose to substitute starch. I will include grams of carbohydrate for pre-, during and post-workout sport drink and shake recommendations. Please review the sidebar Solving the Problem of Added Sugars in Performance and Recovery in chapter 14 before making the substitution.

Power Eating Cross-Training Diet*

Workouts per week	Woman		Man	
	Three or four (novice)	Five or more (experienced)	Three or four (novice)	Five or more (experienced)
Calories/kg	35-37+	44-51+	37-41+	50-58+
Calories/lb	16-16.8+	20-23.2+	16.8-18.6+	22.7-26.4+
Protein				
g/kg	1.5	1.8	1.5	1.8
g/lb	0.6	0.72-0.82	0.6	0.72-0.82
Carbohydrate				
g/kg	5-7	6-10+	5-7	6-10+
g/lb	2.3-3.2	2.7-4.6+	2.3-3.2	2.7-4.6+
Fat**				
g/kg	~1.2	~1.8	0.7	~1.0
g/lb	~0.55	~0.82	~0.32	~0.45

*The distribution of calories and nutrients for the cross-training plan will vary based on the volume and intensity of training in total and from day to day. Adjust your total calories and carbohydrate intake to meet your day's needs, from rest days to long-distance, high-intensity, multiple-workout days, and as you near race day. This is a diet recommendation for daily training. Specific competition preparation and race day nutrition are highly individualized and variable. Seek expert advice from a sport nutritionist for customized planning.

**Total fat varies based on total calories. To find your fat grams, determine your total calories, protein grams, and carbohydrate grams. Add your protein and carbohydrate calories (1 g protein = 4 calories, 1 g carbohydrate = 4 calories), subtract this total from the total calories, and divide by 9 (1 g fat = 9 calories). See chapter 13 for more information.

Power Eating Sample Cross-Training Menu Plans

130-POUND (59 KG) NOVICE WOMAN

(three or four workouts per week)

2,136 calories (36 calories/kg; based on middle of kcal range); 89 grams protein; 355 grams carbohydrate; 40 grams fat

Power Eating Cross-Training Diet

Food groups	Number of servings
Bread/starch	7
Fruit	6
Nonfat milk	3
Teaspoons of added carbohydrate or sugar	20
Vegetable	8
Protein:	
Very lean	4
Lean	3
Medium-fat	1
Fat	5

Food group servings	Menu
Breakfast	
2 bread/starch	1 cup cooked oatmeal or other cooked cereal
1 milk	1 cup (240 ml) fat-free milk
2 fruit	1/2 (120 ml) cup orange juice 3/4 cup (110 g) berries for cereal
1 medium-fat protein	1 whole egg, scrambled in nonstick skillet
1-2 seconds cooking spray	For cooking egg
1 fat	1 tbsp ground flaxseed sprinkled on cereal
	Water
Snack	
1 bread/starch	3/4 oz (23 g) pretzels
1 fruit	4 dried apricots
2 vegetable	1 cup (128 g) mini carrots 1 cup (128 g) cherry tomatoes
1 fat	6 almonds
	Green tea (or other tea)

Food group servings	Menu
Lunch	
2 bread/starch	2 slices whole-grain (ideally sprouted grain) bread
1 fruit	Apple
3 vegetable	Fill sandwich with vegetable choices 2 cups (112 g) mixed green salad
2 very lean protein	2 oz (60 g) turkey
1 fat	1/8 avocado Mustard for sandwich
	Water
Preworkout snack	
1 milk	1 cup (230 g) plain yogurt
1 fruit	1 small banana
	Water
Workout	
12 tsp added carbohydrate or sugar (48 g)	32 oz (950 ml) typical sport drink
Postworkout smoothie	
1 fruit	1 1/4 cups (180 g) frozen whole strawberries
1 milk	1 cup (240 ml) nonfat milk
8 tsp added carbohydrate or sugar (32 g)	6 tsp sugar and 2 tsp honey
2 very lean protein	14 g whey protein isolate
Dinner	
2 bread/starch	1 baked sweet potato
3 vegetable	1 cup (180 g) steamed asparagus 4 cups (122 g) mixed green salad
3 lean protein	3 oz (90 g) wild salmon, grilled
2 fat	1 tsp olive oil for salmon 2 tbsp reduced-fat salad dressing
	Green tea (or other tea)

130-POUND (59 KG) EXPERIENCED WOMAN

(five or more workouts per week)

2,856 calories (48 calories/kg; based on middle of kcal range); 106 grams protein; 473 grams carbohydrate; 60 grams fat

PLUS: 0.2 g/kg/h protein combined with added carbohydrate or sugar in beverage *during* exercise; in this case, add about 12 g protein/h. If you prefer to try essential amino acids (EAAs) instead of whey protein isolate, the formula is 0.2 g of EAA per 1 g total protein.

Food groups	Number of servings
Bread/starch	9
Fruit	9
Nonfat milk	3
Teaspoons of added carbohydrate or sugar	32
Vegetable	8
Protein:	
Very lean	5
Lean	4
Medium-fat	1
Fat	9

Food group servings	Menu
Breakfast	
2 bread/starch	2 slices whole-grain bread
1 milk	1 cup (240 ml) fat-free milk
2 fruit	1 cup (240 ml) orange juice
4 tsp added carbohydrate or sugar (16 g)	4 tsp 100% fruit spread for bread
2 vegetable	1 cup sautéed mushrooms and onions added to egg
1 medium-fat protein	1 whole egg, scrambled
2 fat	1/8 avocado, spread on bread 1 tsp canola oil for cooking vegetables and egg
	Water

Food group servings	Menu
Snack	
2 fruit	16 dried apricot halves
3 fat	18 almonds
	Green tea (or other tea)
Lunch	
3 bread/starch	6 in. (15 cm) Subway sandwich (choose from "Fresh Fit" list)
2 vegetable	Fill sandwich with vegetable choices
2 very lean protein	2 oz (60 g) meat included in sandwich
1 fat	1 tsp olive oil or 1 tbsp salad dressing
	Water
Preworkout snack	
1 bread/starch	3/4 oz (21 g) pretzels
1 milk	1 cup (230 g) plain low-fat yogurt
1 fruit	3/4 cup (110 g) blueberries
3 tsp added carbohydrate or sugar (12 g)	3 tsp honey
	Water
Workout	
16 tsp added carbohydrate or sugar (64 g)	32 oz (950 ml) sport drink
11 g protein isolate/h	Casein or whey protein isolate (typically 1/2 serving)
	Water
Postworkout smoothie	
2 fruit	1 1/4 cups (180 g) frozen whole strawberries 1 frozen medium banana
1 milk	1 cup (240 ml) nonfat milk
9 tsp added carbohydrate or sugar (36 g)	6 tsp sugar and 3 tsp honey
3 very lean protein	21 g whey protein isolate
Dinner	
3 bread/starch	1 baked sweet potato 1/2 cup brown rice
2 fruit	6 oz (~30) red grapes
4 vegetable	1 cup (180 g) steamed asparagus 4 cups (112 g) mixed green salad
4 lean protein	4 oz (120 g) wild salmon, grilled
3 fat	1 tsp olive oil to rub on salmon 4 tbsp reduced-fat salad dressing
	Green tea (or other tea)

180-POUND (82 KG) NOVICE MAN

(three or four workouts per week)

3,275 calories (40 calories/kg; based on middle of kcal range); 123 grams protein; 491 grams carbohydrate; 91 grams fat

Food groups	Number of servings
Bread/starch	12
Fruit	9
Nonfat milk	3
Teaspoons of added carbohydrate or sugar	23
Vegetable	9
Protein:	
Very lean	7
Lean	5
Medium-fat	1
Fat	8

Food group servings	Menu
Preworkout snack	
1 milk	1 cup (230 g) plain yogurt
1 fruit	3/4 cup (110 g) blueberries
2 tsp added carbohydrate or sugar (8 g)	2 tsp honey
2 very lean protein	14 g whey protein isolate whisked into yogurt
	Water
Workout	
16 tsp added carbohydrate or sugar (64 g)	32 oz (950 ml) sport drink
	Water
Breakfast	
2 bread/starch	2 slices whole-grain bread
1 milk	1 cup (240 ml) fat-free milk
2 fruit	1 cup (240 ml) orange juice
4 tsp added carbohydrate or sugar (16 g)	4 tsp 100% fruit spread for bread
2 vegetable	1 cup sautéed vegetables added to eggs

Food group servings	Menu
Breakfast *(continued)*	
1 medium-fat protein	1 whole egg, scrambled
1 very lean protein	2 egg whites, cooked with whole egg
2 fat	1/4 avocado, spread on bread
	1 tsp olive oil for cooking vegetables and eggs
	Water
Snack	
2 bread/starch	8 whole-wheat crackers
1 fruit	3 tbsp no-sugar-added apple butter
1 vegetable	1 cup (124 g) celery sticks
3 fat	1 1/2 tbsp natural peanut butter
	Water
Lunch	
5 bread/starch	12 in. (30 cm) Subway sandwich (choose from "Fresh Fit" list)
2 vegetable	Fill sandwich with vegetable choices
1 fruit	Banana
4 very lean protein	4 oz (120 g) meat included in sandwich
1 fat	1 tsp olive oil or 1 tbsp salad dressing
	Water
Snack	
2 fruit	16 dried apricot halves
1 milk	1 tall nonfat latté
1 tsp added carbohydrate or sugar	1 tsp sugar
	Water
Dinner	
3 bread/starch	1 baked sweet potato
	1/2 cup brown rice
2 fruit	6 oz (~30) red grapes
4 vegetable	1 cup (180 g) steamed asparagus
	4 cups (112 g) mixed green salad
5 lean protein	5 oz (150 g) wild salmon, grilled
2 fat	1 tsp olive oil for salmon
	4 tbsp reduced-fat salad dressing
	Green tea (or other tea)

180-POUND (82 KG) EXPERIENCED MAN

(five or more workouts per week)

4,500 calories (55 calories/kg; based on middle of kcal range)); 147 grams protein; 654 grams carbohydrate; 144 grams fat

PLUS: 0.2 g/kg/h protein combined with added carbohydrate or sugar in beverage *during* exercise; in this case, add about 16 g protein/h. If you prefer to try essential amino acids (EAAs) instead of whole protein isolate, the formula is 0.2 g of EAA per 1 g total protein.

Food groups	Number of servings
Bread/starch	15
Fruit	13
Nonfat milk	3
Teaspoons of added carbohydrate or sugar	39
Vegetable	9
Protein:	
Very lean	9
Lean	6
Medium-fat	1
Fat	14

Food group servings	Menu
Preworkout snack	
1 milk	1 cup (230 g) plain yogurt
1 fruit	3/4 cup (110 g) blueberries
6 tsp added carbohydrate or sugar (24 g)	6 tsp honey
3 very lean protein	21 g whey protein isolate whisked into yogurt
	Water
Workout	
16 tsp added carbohydrate or sugar (64 g)	32 oz (950 ml) sport drink
16 g protein isolate/h	Casein or whey protein isolate
	Water
Breakfast	
4 bread/starch	2 slices whole-grain bread 1 cup cooked oatmeal
1 milk	1 cup (240 ml) fat-free milk (make a smoothie with milk, juice, fruit, sugar, whey protein)
4 fruit	1/2 cup (120 ml) orange juice 1 1/2 cups frozen fruit 2 tbsp raisins or 1/2 cup fresh fruit for oatmeal
12 tsp added carbohydrate or sugar (48 g)	2 tbsp 100% fruit spread for bread 2 tbsp sugar for smoothie

Food group servings	Menu
Breakfast *(continued)*	
2 vegetable	1 cup sautéed mushrooms and red peppers added to eggs
1 medium-fat protein	1 whole egg, scrambled
2 very lean protein	4 egg whites, cooked with whole egg 14 g whey protein isolate (for smoothie)
4 fat	1/4 avocado, sliced and cooked with eggs 1 tsp butter or vegetable oil for cooking eggs and vegetables
	Water
Snack	
2 bread/starch	8 whole-wheat crackers
2 fruit	2/3 cup (158 ml) Concord grape juice (make a spritzer by mixing with sparkling water)
1 vegetable	1 cup (124 g) celery sticks
4 fat	2 tbsp natural peanut butter
	Water
Lunch	
5 bread/starch	12 in. (30 cm) Subway sandwich (choose from "Fresh Fit" list)
2 vegetable	Fill sandwich with vegetable choices
1 fruit	Banana
4 very lean protein	4 oz (120 g) meat included in sandwich
1 fat	1 tsp olive oil or 1 tbsp salad dressing
	Water
Snack	
2 fruit	16 dried apricot halves
1 milk	1 tall nonfat latté
2 tsp added carbohydrate or sugar (8 g)	2 tsp sugar
	Water
Dinner	
4 bread/starch	1 baked sweet potato 1 cup cooked quinoa
3 fruit	1 cup (124 g) raspberries and 1 cup (165 g) cubed mango; put on top of ice cream
3 tsp added carbohydrate or sugar (12 g)	1/2 cup light ice cream
4 vegetable	1 cup (180 g) steamed asparagus 4 cups (112 g) mixed green salad
6 lean protein	6 oz (180 g) wild salmon, grilled
5 fat	1 fat serving included in ice cream 1 tsp olive oil for salmon 3 tbsp salad dressing
Free (no calories)	1 tbsp whipped cream to top fruit and ice cream
	Water

18

Fat-Loss Menu Plans

The diets in this chapter for losing fat are for novice and experienced exercisers, bodybuilders, athletes, and virtually anyone who wants to lose body fat in a safe, controlled manner—without losing precious muscle. Caloric levels differ for men and women because it is more difficult for women to lose fat than it is for men.

Please note: For all listings of added carbohydrate or sugar in each of these diet plans, you can choose to substitute starch. I will include grams of carbohydrate for pre-, during and post-workout sport drink and shake recommendations. Please review the sidebar Solving the Problem of Added Sugars in Performance and Recovery in chapter 14 before making the substitution.

Power Eating Fat-Loss Diet

Workouts per week	Woman		Man	
	Three or four (novice)	Five or more (experienced)	Three or four (novice)	Five or more (experienced)
Calories/kg	25	35	28	38
Calories/lb	11.4	16.0	12.7	17.3
Protein				
g/kg	2.2	2.2	2.2	2.2
g/lb	1.0	1.0	1.0	1.0
Carbohydrate				
g/kg	2.5	3.5	3.0	4.0
g/lb	1.1	1.6	1.4	1.8
Fat*				
g/kg	~0.7	~1.4	~0.8	~1.5
g/lb	~0.32	~0.64	~0.36	~0.68

*Total fat varies based on total calories. To find your fat grams, determine your total calories, protein grams, and carbohydrate grams. Add your protein and carbohydrate calories (1 g protein = 4 calories, 1 g carbohydrate = 4 calories), subtract this total from the total calories, and divide by 9 (1 g fat = 9 calories). See chapter 13 for more information.

Power Eating Sample Fat-Loss Menu Plans

130-POUND (59 KG) NOVICE WOMAN

(three or four workouts per week)

1,472 calories; 130 grams protein; 148 grams carbohydrate; 40 grams fat

Food groups	Number of servings
Bread/starch	3
Fruit	3
Nonfat milk	3
Teaspoons of added carbohydrate or sugar	0
Vegetable	4
Protein:	
Very lean	7
Lean	5
Medium-fat	1
Fat	4

Food group servings	Menu
Breakfast	
1 bread/starch	1 cup (25 g) Kashi Whole Grain Puffs cereal
1 milk	1 cup (240 ml) fat-free milk
1 fruit	3/4 cup (110 g) blueberries for cereal
1 medium-fat protein	1 whole egg, scrambled in nonstick skillet
1 very lean protein	2 egg whites, scrambled with whole egg
1 fat	1 tbsp ground flaxseed sprinkled on cereal
	Water
Snack	
1 vegetable	1 cup (128 g) mini carrots
1 fat	6 almonds
	Green tea (or other tea)
Lunch	
1 bread/starch	Subway Turkey Breast Wrap
2 vegetable	Fill sandwich with vegetable choices
4 very lean protein	3 oz (90 g) turkey included 1 oz (30 g) cheese
1 fat	1 fat serving included in cheese
Free (no calories)	Dijon mustard
	Water
Preworkout snack	
1 milk	1 cup (230 g) plain yogurt
1 fruit	1 small banana
	Water
Workout	
	Water
Postworkout smoothie	
1 fruit	3/4 cup (112 g) frozen whole strawberries 1/4 cup (60 ml) orange juice
1 milk	1 cup (240 ml) nonfat milk
2 very lean protein	14 g whey protein isolate
Dinner	
1 bread/starch	1/2 baked sweet potato
1 vegetable	1/2 cup (90 g) steamed asparagus
5 lean protein	5 oz (150 g) wild salmon, grilled
1 fat	1 tsp olive oil for salmon
	Green tea (or other tea)

130-POUND (59 KG) EXPERIENCED WOMAN

(five or more workouts per week)

2,068 calories; 130 grams protein; 207 grams carbohydrate; 80 grams fat

Food groups	Number of servings
Bread/starch	5
Fruit	4
Nonfat milk	3
Teaspoons of added carbohydrate or sugar	0
Vegetable	8
Protein:	
Very lean	6
Lean	4
Medium-fat	1
Fat	11

Food group servings	Menu
Breakfast	
2 bread/starch	2 slices whole-grain bread
1 milk	1 cup (240 ml) fat-free milk
1 fruit	1/2 cup (120 ml) orange juice
2 vegetable	1 cup sautéed vegetables for eggs
1 medium-fat protein	1 whole egg, scrambled
3 fat	1/8 avocado, spread on bread 2 tsp olive oil for cooking eggs and vegetables
	Water
Snack	
1 fruit	8 dried apricot halves
3 fat	18 almonds
	Green tea (or other tea)

Food group servings	Menu
Lunch	
1 bread/starch	Subway Turkey Breast Wrap
2 vegetable	Fill sandwich with vegetable choices
4 very lean protein	3 oz (90 g) turkey included in sandwich 1 oz (30 g) cheese
2 fat	1 fat serving included in cheese 1 tsp olive oil or 1 tbsp salad dressing
	Water
Preworkout snack	
1 bread/starch	3/4 oz (23 g) whole-wheat pretzels
1 milk	1 cup (230 g) plain yogurt
1 fruit	3/4 cup (110 g) blueberries
	Water
Workout	
	Water
Postworkout smoothie	
1 fruit	1 1/4 cups (180 g) frozen whole strawberries
1 milk	1 cup (240 ml) nonfat milk
2 very lean protein	14 g whey protein isolate
Dinner	
1 bread/starch	1/2 baked sweet potato
4 vegetable	1 cup (180 g) steamed asparagus 4 cups (112 g) mixed green salad
4 lean protein	4 oz (120 g) wild salmon, grilled
3 fat	1 tsp olive oil for salmon 4 tbsp reduced-fat salad dressing
	Green tea (or other tea)

180-POUND (82 KG) NOVICE MAN

(three or four workouts per week)

2,294 calories; 180 grams protein; 245 grams carbohydrate; 66 grams fat

Food groups	Number of servings
Bread/starch	6
Fruit	6
Nonfat milk	3
Teaspoons of added carbohydrate or sugar	0
Vegetable	9
Protein:	
Very lean	11
Lean	6
Medium-fat	1
Fat	8

Food group servings	Menu
Preworkout snack	
1 milk	1 cup (230 g) plain yogurt
1 fruit	3/4 cup (110 g) blueberries
	Water
Workout	
	Water
Breakfast	
1 bread/starch	1 slice whole-grain bread
1 milk	1 cup (240 ml) fat-free milk
2 fruit	1/2 cup (120 ml) orange juice 1/2 cup frozen mango or other fruit
2 vegetable	1 cup sautéed vegetables for eggs
1 medium-fat protein	1 whole egg, scrambled in nonstick skillet
5 very lean protein	4 egg whites, cooked with whole egg 21 g whey protein isolate added to milk and orange juice and blended
1 fat	1/8 avocado, spread on bread

Food group servings	Menu
Breakfast *(continued)*	
1-2 seconds cooking spray	For eggs
	Water
Snack	
1 vegetable	1 cup (124 g) celery sticks
1 very lean protein	1/2 cup (90 g) edamame or 1 serving (~1/3 of bag) of soy crisps
1 bread/starch	Included in the edamame or soy crisps
2 fat	1 tbsp natural peanut butter
	Water
Lunch	
3 bread/starch	6 in. (15 cm) Subway sandwich (choose from "Fresh Fit" list)
2 vegetable	Fill sandwich with vegetable choices
1 fruit	Banana
5 very lean protein	2 oz (60 g) included in sandwich; request double meat 1 oz (30 g) cheese
1 fat	1 fat serving included in cheese
Free (no calories)	Dijon mustard
	Water
Snack	
1 fruit	8 dried apricot halves
1 milk	1 tall nonfat latté
2 fat	12 almonds
	Water
Dinner	
1 bread/starch	1/2 baked sweet potato
1 fruit	3 oz (about 15) red grapes
4 vegetable	1 cup (180 g) steamed asparagus 4 cups(112 g) mixed green salad
6 lean protein	6 oz (180 g) wild salmon, grilled
2 fat	1 tsp olive oil for salmon 2 tbsp reduced-fat salad dressing
	Green tea (or other tea)

180-POUND (82 KG) EXPERIENCED MAN

(five or more workouts per week)

3,108 calories; 180 grams protein; 327 grams carbohydrate; 120 grams fat

Food groups	Number of servings
Bread/starch	8
Fruit	8
Nonfat milk	3
Teaspoons of added carbohydrate or sugar	0
Vegetable	9
Protein:	
Very lean	10
Lean	6
Medium-fat	1
Fat	21

Food group servings	Menu
Preworkout snack	
1 milk	1 cup (230 g) plain yogurt
1 fruit	3/4 cup (110 g) blueberries
	Water
Workout	
	Water
Breakfast	
2 bread/starch	2 slices whole-grain bread
1 milk	1 cup (240 ml) fat-free milk
3 fruit	1 cup (240 ml) orange juice 3/4 cup frozen berries 1/2 frozen medium banana
2 vegetable	1 cup sautéed vegetables for eggs
1 medium-fat protein	1 whole egg, scrambled
4 very lean protein	4 egg whites, cooked with whole egg 14 g whey protein isolate, blended with milk, orange juice, and fruit

Food group servings	Menu
Breakfast *(continued)*	
4 fat	1/4 avocado, spread on bread 2 tsp olive oil for cooking vegetables and eggs
	Water
Snack	
1 vegetable	1 cup (124 g) celery sticks
2 very lean protein	1 cup (180 g) edamame or 2 servings (~2/3 of the bag) of soy crisps
2 bread/starch	Included in edamame or soy crisps
6 fat	3 tbsp natural peanut butter
	Water
Lunch	
3 bread/starch	6 in. (15 cm) Subway sandwich (choose from "Fresh Fit" list)
2 vegetable	Fill sandwich with vegetable choices
1 fruit	Banana
4 very lean protein	2 oz (60 g) meat included in sandwich; request double meat
2 fat	2 tsp olive oil or 2 tbsp salad dressing
	Water
Snack	
2 fruit	16 dried apricot halves
1 milk	1 tall nonfat latté
3 fat	18 almonds
	Water
Dinner	
1 bread/starch	1/2 baked sweet potato
1 fruit	3 oz (about 15) red grapes
4 vegetables	1 cup (180 g) steamed asparagus 4 cups (112 g) mixed green salad
6 lean protein	6 oz (180 g) wild salmon, grilled
6 fat	8 large black olives 1 tsp olive oil for rubbing on salmon and drizzling on asparagus 4 tbsp salad dressing
	Green tea (or other tea)

POWER PROFILE: Fat Loss

Several years ago, I was asked to work with a 28-year-old basketball player after his physical conditioning and performance had markedly diminished over a period of a year.

At our initial meeting, the 6-foot 11-inch (211 cm) player weighed 276 pounds (125 kg) and had 23 percent body fat. Seriously concerned about his condition and his performance, he reported that he had been desperately trying to lose weight, particularly because his contract required him to maintain a certain weight and body fat; his ultimate goal was 257 pounds (116.5 kg) and 13 percent body fat.

His diet consisted of 1,700 calories, with 30 percent coming from protein, 27 percent from carbohydrate, 32 percent from fat, and 11 percent from alcohol. These are clearly not optimal percentages for an athlete, particularly one who is trying to lose weight and retain muscle.

Because of his poor diet, he was fatigued, even unable to eat when he got home from practice. What's more, he was afraid to eat, fearing that food would show up the next day on the scale. He truly was in the beginning stages of an eating disorder. And the less he ate, the higher his body fat percentage climbed.

With only five weeks to go until his first goal-weight deadline, I placed him on the Power Eating diet for losing fat. This initially included 4,019 calories (33 calories per kilogram), 222 grams of protein, 603 grams of carbohydrate, and 80 grams of fat. In addition, he drank a gallon (4 L) of fluid a day and supplemented with 500 milligrams of vitamin E. During his workout, he sipped 48 ounces (1.4 L) of a glucose–electrolyte solution; after his workout, he consumed a serving of Kleiner's Essential Muscle-Building Formula for Men or Kleiner's Muscle-Building Formula.

After several weeks and some success, I discontinued the glucose–electrolyte solution during his aerobic workouts to enhance fat-burning during exercise because he was required to make weight by a contract deadline. This was the only major change I made. I also decreased his daily calories by 100 to activate further weight loss.

In five weeks, he made amazing progress, reaching 263.5 pounds (119.5 kg) and 12.75 percent body fat. A few weeks later, he weighed in at 261 pounds (118 kg) and 12.9 percent body fat. Both the team and the athlete were excited about the outcome, and he returned to successful full-court play.

Power profile update: The most noteworthy change in this diet was the massive increase in calories that allowed the athlete to actually have the energy to get out of bed and get to practice. His performance in workouts and games returned to very close to his all-star performances. And his body dropped the extra fat that it was preserving, allowing energy and protein to be used for performance and building. Alcohol was also a huge deficit to his performance. That remained a struggle to the end of his career, but during this time when we worked together, he got his head in the game and followed my guidance perfectly. His story is a testament to the power of evidence-based sport nutrition.

19

Getting Cut Menu Plans

To lean out—either for additional body-fat reduction or for a bodybuilding competition—tweak your diet using my Power Eating seven-day cutting diet. (It's particularly useful for bodybuilders who must lean out the week before a competition.) The distribution of nutrients for the cutting plan is based on getting enough protein and fat within the restricted number of calories. This forces a limited amount of carbohydrate, which allows for rapid weight loss. Some of that weight loss is fluid, because as you deplete stored muscle glycogen you lose fluid from muscle cells. Use this approach only when absolutely necessary. Because women have more difficulty losing fat than men do, calorie levels are different for them. Stay on this diet no longer than 14 days.

Please note: For all listings of added carbohydrate or sugar in each of these diet plans, you can choose to substitute starch. I will include grams of carbohydrate for pre-, during and post-workout sport drink and shake recommendations. Please review the sidebar Solving the Problem of Added Sugars in Performance and Recovery in chapter 14 before making the substitution.

Power Eating Getting Cut Diet

Workouts per week	Woman		Man	
	Three or four (novice)	Five or more (experienced)	Three or four (novice)	Five or more (experienced)
Calories/kg	22	30	25	32
Calories/lb	10	13.6	11.4	14.5
Protein				
g/kg	2.3	2.5	2.3	2.5
g/lb	1.05	1.1	1.05	1.1
Carbohydrate				
g/kg	1.8	2.9	2.3	3.0
g/lb	0.82	1.32	1.05	1.36
Fat*				
g/kg	~0.6	~0.9	~0.7	~1.1
g/lb	~0.27	~0.41	~0.32	~0.5

*Total fat varies based on total calories. To find your fat grams, determine your total calories, protein grams, and carbohydrate grams. Add your protein and carbohydrate calories (1 g protein = 4 calories, 1 g carbohydrate = 4 calories), subtract this total from the total calories, and divide by 9 (1 g fat = 9 calories). See chapter 13 for more information.

Power Eating Sample Getting Cut Menu Plans

130-POUND (59 KG) NOVICE WOMAN

(three or four workouts per week)

1,301 calories; 136 grams protein; 106 grams carbohydrate; 37 grams fat

Food groups	Number of servings
Bread/starch	1
Fruit	2
Nonfat milk	3
Teaspoons of added carbohydrate or sugar	0
Vegetable	5
Protein:	
Very lean	10
Lean	4
Medium-fat	1
Fat	4

Food group servings	Menu
Breakfast	
1 bread/starch	1 cup (25 g) Kashi puffed cereal
1 milk	1 cup (240 ml) fat-free milk
1 fruit	3/4 cup (110 g) blueberries for cereal
1 medium-fat protein	1 whole egg, scrambled in nonstick skillet
2 very lean protein	4 egg whites, scrambled with whole egg
1 fat	1 tbsp (12 g) ground flaxseed sprinkled on cereal
	Water
Snack	
1 vegetable	1 cup (128 g) mini carrots
1 fat	6 almonds
	Green tea (or other tea)
Lunch	
2 vegetable	Subway Grilled Chicken Breast and Spinach Salad
6 very lean protein	3 oz (90 g) chicken included in salad; request double meat
1 fat	2 tbsp (30 ml) reduced-fat dressing
	Water
Preworkout snack	
1 milk	1 cup (230 g) plain yogurt
1 fruit	1 small banana
	Water
Workout	
	Water
Postworkout smoothie	
1 milk	1 cup (240 ml) nonfat milk
2 very lean protein	14 g whey protein isolate, blended with milk and 3 or 4 ice cubes
Dinner	
2 vegetable	1/2 cup (90 g) steamed asparagus 2 cups (56 g) mixed green salad
4 lean protein	4 oz (120 g) wild salmon, grilled
1 fat	1 tsp (5 ml) olive oil for salmon
Free (no or insignificant number of calories)	2 tbsp (30 ml) fat-free Italian dressing
	Green tea (or other tea)

130-POUND (59 KG) EXPERIENCED WOMAN
(five or more workouts per week)

1,762 calories; 148 grams protein; 171 grams carbohydrate; 54 grams fat

Food groups	Number of servings
Bread/starch	3
Fruit	4
Nonfat milk	3
Teaspoons of added carbohydrate or sugar	0
Vegetable	6
Protein:	
Very lean	10
Lean	5
Medium-fat	1
Fat	7

Food group servings	Menu
Breakfast	
1 bread/starch	1 slice whole-grain bread
1 milk	1 cup (240 ml) fat-free milk
1 fruit	1/2 cup (120 ml) orange juice
1 medium-fat protein	1 whole egg, scrambled in nonstick skillet
2 very lean protein	4 egg whites, cooked with whole egg
1 fat	1/8 avocado, spread on bread
	Water
Snack	
1 fruit	4 dried apricots
1 vegetable	1 cup (128 g) mini carrots
2 very lean protein	1 1/2 oz turkey jerky
2 fat	12 almonds
	Green tea (or other tea)

Food group servings	Menu
Lunch	
1 bread/starch	Subway Turkey Breast Wrap
2 vegetable	Fill wrap with vegetable choices
4 very lean protein	3 oz (90 g) turkey included in wrap 1 oz (30 g) cheese included in wrap
2 fat	1 fat included in cheese 1 tsp (5 ml) olive oil or 1 tbsp (15 ml) salad dressing
	Water
Preworkout snack	
1 milk	1 cup (230 g) plain yogurt
1 fruit	3/4 cup (110 g) blueberries
	Water
Workout	
	Water
Postworkout smoothie	
1 fruit	3/4 cup (112 g) whole frozen strawberries
1 milk	1 cup (240 ml) fat-free milk
2 very lean protein	14 g whey protein isolate
Dinner	
1 bread/starch	1/2 baked sweet potato
3 vegetable	1/2 cup (90 g) steamed asparagus 4 cups (112 g) mixed green salad
5 lean protein	5 oz (150 g) wild salmon, grilled
2 fat	1 tsp (5 ml) olive oil for salmon 2 tbsp (30 ml) reduced-fat salad dressing
	Green tea (or other tea)

180-POUND (82 KG) NOVICE MAN

(three or four workouts per week)

2,044 calories; 188 grams protein; 188 grams carbohydrate; 60 grams fat

Food groups	Number of servings
Bread/starch	5
Fruit	3
Nonfat milk	3
Teaspoons of added carbohydrate or sugar	0
Vegetable	6
Protein:	
Very lean	11
Lean	8
Medium-fat	1
Fat	8

Food group servings	Menu
Preworkout snack	
1 milk	1 cup (230 g) plain yogurt
1 fruit	3/4 cup (110 g) blueberries
	Water
Workout	
	Water
Breakfast	
1 bread/starch	1 slice whole-grain bread
1 milk	1 cup (240 ml) fat-free milk
1 fruit	1/2 cup (120 ml) orange juice
1 medium-fat protein	1 whole egg, scrambled in nonstick skillet
5 very lean protein	4 egg whites, cooked with whole egg 21 g whey protein isolate, blended with milk, orange juice, and 3 or 4 ice cubes
1 fat	1/8 avocado, sliced and cooked with eggs
	Water

Food group servings	Menu
Snack	
1 vegetable	1 cup (124 g) celery sticks
2 very lean protein	1 cup (180 g) edamame or 2 servings (about 2/3 bag) of soy crisps
2 bread/starch	Included in the edamame or soy crisps
2 fat	1 tbsp (16 g) natural peanut butter
	Water
Lunch	
1 bread/starch	Subway Turkey Breast Wrap
2 vegetable	Fill wrap with vegetable choices
4 very lean protein	3 oz (90 g) turkey included in wrap 1 oz (30 g) cheese included in wrap
1 fat	1 fat included in cheese
Free (no calories)	Dijon mustard
	Water
Snack	
1 fruit	4 dried apricots
1 milk	1 tall nonfat latté
2 fat	12 almonds
	Water
Dinner	
1 bread/starch	1/2 baked sweet potato
3 vegetable	1/2 cup (90 g) steamed asparagus 4 cups (112 g) mixed green salad
8 lean protein	8 oz (240 g) wild salmon, grilled
2 fat	1 tsp (5 ml) olive oil for salmon 2 tbsp (30 ml) reduced-fat salad dressing
	Green tea (or other tea)

180-POUND (82 KG) EXPERIENCED MAN

(five or more workouts per week)

2,625 calories; 202 grams protein; 245 grams carbohydrate; 93 grams fat

Food groups	Number of servings
Bread/starch	5
Fruit	6
Nonfat milk	3
Teaspoons of added carbohydrate or sugar	0
Vegetable	9
Protein:	
Very lean	12
Lean	8
Medium-fat	1
Fat	13

Food group servings	Menu
Preworkout snack	
1 milk	1 cup (230 g) plain yogurt
1 fruit	3/4 cup (110 g) blueberries
	Water
Workout	
	Water
Breakfast	
1 bread/starch	1 slice whole-grain bread
1 milk	1 cup (240 ml) fat-free milk for smoothie
2 fruit	1/2 cup (120 ml) orange juice for smoothie 1/2 cup frozen mango or other fruit for smoothie
2 vegetable	1 cup sautéed vegetables for eggs
1 medium-fat protein	1 whole egg, scrambled
4 very lean protein	4 egg whites, cooked with whole egg 14 g whey protein isolate, blended with milk, orange juice, fruit, and 3 or 4 ice cubes

Food group servings	Menu
Breakfast (*continued*)	
3 fat	1/4 avocado, spread on bread 1 tsp (5 ml) olive oil for cooking vegetables and eggs
	Water
Snack	
1 vegetable	1 cup (124 g) celery sticks
2 very lean protein	1 cup (180 g) edamame or 2 servings (~2/3 bag) of soy crisps
2 bread/starch	Included in edamame or soy crisps
4 fat	2 tbsp (32 g) natural peanut butter
	Water
Lunch	
1 bread/starch	Subway Turkey Breast Wrap
2 vegetable	Fill wrap with vegetable choices
4 very lean protein	3 oz (90 g) turkey included in wrap 1 oz (30 g) cheese included in wrap
1 fat	1 fat serving included in cheese
Free (no calories)	Dijon mustard
	Water
Snack	
2 fruit	1/2 cup orange juice 1 frozen small banana
1 milk	1 cup nonfat milk
2 very lean protein	14 g whey protein isolate
2 fat	1 tbsp nut butter, blended with juice, banana, milk, whey, and 3 or 4 ice cubes
	Water
Dinner	
1 bread/starch	1/2 baked sweet potato
1 fruit	3 oz (90 g, or ~15) red grapes
4 vegetable	1 cup (180 g) steamed asparagus 4 cups (112 g) mixed green salad
8 lean protein	8 oz (240 g) wild salmon, grilled
3 fat	8 large black olives 1 tsp (5 ml) olive oil for salmon
Free (no or insignificant number of calories)	1 tbsp (15 ml) reduced-fat Italian salad dressing
	Green tea (or other tea)

Special Advice to Competitors

Many strength athletes worry about being too full just as they go into competition. However, it's critical to have enough fluid, calories, and nutrients to feel strong and look great. Probably the best way to do this is to supplement your diet with liquid meal replacements. These will charge you up but pass through your digestive system more quickly than solid foods.

Whatever meal-replacement brand and product you choose, make sure it is third-party tested and certified for purity. The company should guarantee that it is absolutely free of banned substances and contaminants! This is not the time to get caught with a positive reading on a doping test. Protein and meal-replacement supplements are notorious for being intentionally or unintentionally spiked with performance-enhancing drugs.

Because each serving of a meal replacement is about the same number of calories as a small meal or snack, you should drink it 90 minutes to 2 hours before your competition to feel your best during the contest. If you feel comfortable, you can also add some low-fiber foods throughout the day to increase your nutritional intake and avoid the boredom of just drinking. Then, eat a variety of foods after the competition to round out your nutrition for the day.

20

Power Eating Recipes

Although there are many supplements on the market, I always like to use fresh ingredients whenever possible. These recipes were designed for the strength-training clients and teams I have worked with over many years. Try them all to find out which ones are your favorites. They've been created for busy people, so each recipe should only take a few minutes to prepare and a few more minutes to cook. If you've been a reader of earlier editions of *Power Eating*, you'll notice that some of the recipes have been updated, using new formulations and new ingredients. And there are some awesome brand new ones that I know you're going to love!

Power Drinks

While smoothie recipes get fancier and more complicated by the minute, my goal with these essential drinks is to give you what you need as fast as possible, from easy-to-access ingredients. These are the basics. You can gussy them up when you've got more time.

Kleiner's Essential Muscle-Building Formula for Women

1 cup (240 ml) nonfat milk or soy milk fortified with calcium
   and vitamins A and D

1/4 cup (60 ml) calcium-fortified orange juice

1/4 cup (37 g) frozen strawberries

14 g whey protein isolate

Blend until smooth.

One serving contains:

Nutrients	Food Group Servings
224 calories (265 if use regular soy milk)	1 fruit serving
29 g carbohydrate	3 very lean protein servings
27 g protein	1 nonfat milk serving
0 fat (1 fat if use regular soy milk)	
<1 g fiber	

Kleiner's Essential Muscle-Building Formula for Men

1 cup (240 ml) nonfat milk or soy milk fortified with calcium
   and vitamins A and D

1/2 cup (120 ml) calcium-fortified orange juice

1 tbsp (21 g) honey

1/4 cup (37 g) frozen strawberries

21 g whey protein isolate

Blend until smooth.

One serving contains:

Nutrients	Food Group Servings
360 calories (400 if use regular soy milk)	1 1/2 fruit servings
54 g carbohydrate	4 very lean protein servings
36 g protein	1 nonfat milk serving
0 fat	4 tsp (20 g) added sugar
1 g fiber	

Kleiner's Updated Easy Muscle-Building Formula

While the original recipe started my shake-making days for high school foot-
ballers in North Carolina in 1988, the ease of instant breakfast (the mainstay
ingredient) had to give way to a more healthful option. I apologize if you're
going to miss the old stand-by, but try this one, you'll like it! You'll get a great
start to your day, or a great postworkout boost.

1 cup (240 ml) nonfat milk or soy milk fortified with calcium
  and vitamins A and D

1/2 cup (120 ml) natural coconut water

1/2 cup (120 ml) plain kefir

1 frozen medium banana

1/2 cup (133 g) frozen mango

1 tbsp (16 g) almond butter

1/2 tbsp (1 g) chia seeds

(Optional: Add 20 g whey protein isolate and 80 calories.)

Blend until smooth.

One serving contains:

Nutrients	Food Group Servings
469 calories (509 if use regular soy milk)	1 1/2 nonfat milk servings
72 g carbohydrate	3 1/2 fruit servings
20 g protein	3 very lean protein servings
12 g fat	2 fat servings
6 g fiber	

Kleiner's Muscle-Building Formula

1 cup (150 g) frozen strawberries

1 cup (230 g) nonfat strawberry yogurt

15 g whey protein isolate

1 tbsp (21 g) honey

1 cup (240 ml) nonfat milk

1 cup (240 ml) calcium-fortified orange juice

Blend until smooth.

One serving contains:

Nutrients	Food Group Servings
529 calories	3 fruit servings
100 g carbohydrate	2 very lean protein servings
31 g protein	2 nonfat milk servings
1 g fat	6 tsp (30 g) added sugar
4 g fiber	

Kleiner's Muscle Formula Plus

20 g whey protein isolate or 25 g plant protein

1 cup (150 g) frozen unsweetened strawberries

1 medium banana

1 cup (240 ml) light vanilla soy milk fortified with calcium
and vitamins A and D

3/4 cup (180 ml) calcium-fortified orange juice

1/4 cup (60 ml) tart cherry juice

1/2 tbsp (1 g) chia seeds

1/2 tbsp (1 g) flaxseed meal

Blend until smooth.

One serving contains:

Nutrients	Food Group Servings
524 calories	5 fruit servings
91 g carbohydrate	4 very lean protein servings
34 g protein	1 nonfat milk serving
5 g fat	1 fat serving
8 g fiber	1 tsp (5 g) added sugar

Kleiner's Muscle Formula Plus Light

20 g whey protein isolate or plant protein

1/2 cup (75 g) frozen unsweetened strawberries

1/2 medium banana

1 cup (240 ml) light vanilla soy milk fortified with calcium
and vitamins A and D

1/2 cup (120 ml) calcium-fortified orange juice

1/4 cup (60 ml) tart cherry juice

1/2 tbsp (1 g) chia seeds

Blend until smooth.

One serving contains:

Nutrients	Food Group Servings
392 calories	3 fruit servings
62 g carbohydrate	3 very lean protein servings
30 g protein	1 nonfat milk serving
3 g fat	1/2 fat serving
6 g fiber	1/2 tsp (2 g) added sugar

Bone-Builder Smoothie

1 cup (240 ml) nonfat milk

1/2 cup (120 ml) calcium-fortified orange juice

1/2 cup (115 g) nonfat vanilla yogurt

1 cup (150 g) mixture of frozen mango, blueberries, strawberries

1/2 cup (15 g) chopped fresh or frozen kale

1 tbsp (15 g) nonfat dry milk powder

14 g whey protein isolate

Blend until smooth.

One serving contains:

Nutrients	Food Group Servings
440 calories	3 fruit servings
80 g carbohydrate	1/2 vegetable serving
30 g protein	2 very lean protein servings
0 g fat	2 nonfat milk servings
6 g fiber	3 tsp (15 g) added sugar

Mocha Breakfast Smoothie

1 cup (240 ml) nonfat milk or light unsweetened soy milk

1/2 cup (120 ml) strongly brewed coffee, chilled

2 tbsp (32 g) natural peanut butter

1/2 large banana

2 scoops USANA Whey or Plant Protein MySmartShake*

10 ice cubes

Blend until smooth.

One serving contains:

Nutrients	Food Group Servings
497 calories	1 fruit serving
43 g carbohydrate	2 1/2 very lean protein servings
34 g protein	2 nonfat milk servings
22 g fat	4 fat servings
5 g fiber	

*I specifically like USANA brand MySmartShake as the base for these recipes because it contains very high quality ingredients and is very lightly flavored, allowing the use of fruits and vegetables to give the full flavor to the recipe.

Soyful Smoothie (Lactose Free)

1/3 block (5 oz, or 150 g) soft tofu

3/4 cup (112 g) frozen strawberries

1/2 medium banana

1/2 cup (120 ml) vanilla nonfat soy milk fortified with vitamins A and D and calcium

1/2 cup (120 ml) calcium-fortified orange juice

2 tsp (14 g) honey

Cream tofu in blender until smooth. Add the next five ingredients and blend until smooth.

One serving contains:

Nutrients	Food Group Servings
321 calories	3 fruit servings
61 g carbohydrate	1 medium-fat protein serving
11 g protein	1/2 nonfat milk serving
5 g fat	2 tsp (10 g) added sugar
4 g fiber	

Phytochemical Phenomenon II

1 cup (150 g) frozen mixture of mango and papaya

1/2 medium kiwifruit, peeled and quartered

1/2 cup (115 g) plain nonfat yogurt

1/3 cup (79 ml) pomegranate juice

2/3 cup (158 ml) pineapple juice

1 cup (240 ml) nonfat milk or unflavored soy milk

Blend until smooth.

One serving contains:

Nutrients	Food Group Servings
383 calories	5 fruit servings
83 g carbohydrate	3 very lean protein servings
16 g protein	1 1/2 nonfat milk servings
1 g fat	
4 g fiber	

Zesty Citrus Smoothie

This smoothie will help replenish fluids and electrolytes, particularly on hot days.

  2 in. (6 cm) piece of fresh ginger
  1 cup (148 g) lemon sorbet
  2 cups (480 ml) cold, unflavored sparkling water
  2 tbsp (30 ml) lemon juice
  1 tbsp (15 ml) lime juice
  1/8 tsp (0.75 g) salt
  2 tbsp (30 g) sugar*
  15 ice cubes
  Zest of 1 large lemon (~2 tbsp, or 30 g)

*If you prefer a sweeter drink, add more sugar, agave syrup, or stevia.

Grate the ginger and squeeze the juice from the grated ginger. Blend the ginger juice with the remaining ingredients until the mixture reaches the consistency of a frozen margarita drink. For a lower-calorie beverage, make one recipe for two servings.

One serving contains:

Nutrients
150 calories
38 g carbohydrate
1 g protein
0 g fat
1 g fiber

Food Group Servings
9 1/2 tsp (48 g) added sugar

Piña Colada Smoothie

1 cup (240 ml) nonfat milk

1/2 cup (120 ml) natural coconut water

2 scoops USANA Whey or Plant Protein MySmartShake

6 oz (170 g) low-fat piña colada yogurt (or other coconut and pineapple yogurt)

1/2 cup (120 ml) crushed pineapple in natural juice

2 tbsp (30 ml) light coconut milk

1/2 tsp (3 ml) rum extract

4 ice cubes

Blend until smooth.

One serving contains:

Nutrients	Food Group Servings
512 calories	1 fruit serving
75 g carbohydrate	3 nonfat milk servings
33 g protein	2 fat servings
10 g fat	6 tsp (30 g) added sugar
1 g fiber	

Antioxidant Advantage

1 cup (240 ml) nonfat milk

1/3 cup (79 ml) Concord grape juice

1 tbsp (15 ml) lime juice

1/2 cup (115 g) plain nonfat yogurt

1/2 cup (75 g) frozen strawberries

1/4 cup (37 g) frozen blueberries

5 g creatine monohydrate

Blend until smooth.

One serving contains:

Nutrients	Food Group Servings
255 calories	2 fruit servings
50 g carbohydrate	1 very lean protein
18 g protein	1 1/2 nonfat milk servings
0 g fat	3 g fiber

Morning Pick-Me-Up

2 tsp (10 g) chai tea leaves
2 cups (480 ml) nonfat milk
1/3 cup (40 g) nonfat dry milk powder
1 1/2 tbsp (32 g) honey
1/8 tsp (0.5 g) nutmeg
4 ice cubes

Simmer the tea in milk for 5 to 8 minutes. Cool in the refrigerator. Pour the milk into a blender, straining out the tea leaves. Add the remaining ingredients. Blend until smooth.

One serving contains:

Nutrients	Food Group Servings
350 calories	3 nonfat milk servings
62 g carbohydrate	6 tsp (30 g) added sugar
25 g protein	
1 g fat	
0 g fiber	

Caribbean Crush

11 1/2 oz (340 ml, or 1 can) papaya juice
1/3 cup (80 ml) crushed pineapple in natural juice
1/2 medium banana
21 g whey protein isolate
6 ice cubes

Blend until smooth.

One serving contains:

Nutrients	Food Group Servings
364 calories	4 1/2 fruit servings
69 g carbohydrate	3 very lean protein servings
23 g protein	
1 g fat	
4 g fiber	

Apple Pie à la Mode

1 cup (240 ml) unfiltered apple juice

1/2 cup (115 g) unsweetened applesauce

1/3 cup (48 g) vanilla nonfat frozen yogurt

2 tbsp (30 g) toasted wheat germ

1/3 cup (40 g) nonfat dry milk powder

10 g whey protein isolate

Blend until smooth.

One serving contains:

Nutrients	Food Group Servings
399 calories	3 fruit servings
74 g carbohydrate	2 very lean protein servings
25 g protein	1 nonfat milk serving
2 g fat	3 tsp (15 g) added sugar
4 g fiber	

Lemon-Lime Zinger Sport Drink

To fuel and hydrate your body, drink this power booster within two hours before exercise. It's also a great fluid replenisher during or after exercise or anytime during an active day.

1 in. (3 cm) piece of fresh ginger

2 cups (480 ml) cold unflavored sparkling water

1 tbsp (15 ml) lemon juice

2 tsp (10 ml) lime juice

2 tbsp (30 g) sugar

Scant 1/8 tsp (0.75 g) salt

Grate the ginger and squeeze out the juice. Blend the ginger juice with the remaining ingredients for 20 seconds. Serve immediately.

One serving contains:

Nutrients	Food Group Servings
109 calories	7 tsp (35 g) added sugar
28 g carbohydrate	
0 g protein	
0 g fat	
0 g fiber	

Anti-Inflammatory Recovery Shake Recipes

I use the USANA Nutrimeal here because it is a nicely designed meal replacement that boosts your total nutrition, is guaranteed pure, and allows for the nutritional profile that I desire. Whatever brand you use, look for a guarantee of purity.

Combine the following ingredients in a blender, blend on high speed, and enjoy.

Apple Ginger Spinach Berry

1 cup (240 ml) all-natural 100% apple juice

1 tbsp (~1 in., or 3 cm, piece) fresh chopped ginger

2 cups (56 g) baby spinach

1/2 cup (72 g) fresh or frozen blueberries

3 scoops chocolate USANA Nutrimeal

1 scoop whey protein isolate

Makes 2 servings.

One serving contains (includes apple juice):

Nutrients	Food Group Servings
323 calories	2 fruit servings
48 g carbohydrate	1 vegetable serving
21 g protein	2 1/2 very lean protein servings
3 g fat	1/2 nonfat milk serving
7 g fiber	1/2 fat serving
	3 tsp (15 g) added sugar

Raspberry Plum Basil

1 cup (240 ml) water or 100% natural juice (apple, berry, etc.)

1/2 cup (75 g) fresh or frozen raspberries

2 medium plums, sliced

1 tbsp fresh basil (1 tsp, or 0.3 g, dried)

3 scoops vanilla USANA Nutrimeal

1 scoop whey protein isolate

Makes 2 servings.

One serving contains (includes apple juice):

Nutrients	Food Group Servings
370 calories	2 1/2 fruit servings
61 g carbohydrate	2 1/2 very lean protein servings
21 g protein	1/2 nonfat milk serving
4 g fat	1/2 fat serving
7 g fiber	3 tsp (15 g) added sugar

Banana Beet Orange

1 cup (240 m) water or 100% all-natural orange juice

1 tsp (2.4 g) cinnamon

1/4 tsp (0.6 g) ground nutmeg

1/4 tsp (0.6 g) turmeric

1 small banana

1/2 cup (68 g) beets, chopped (~2 or 3 beets)

3 scoops vanilla USANA Nutrimeal

1 scoop whey protein isolate

Makes 2 servings.

One serving contains (includes orange juice):

Nutrients	Food Group Servings
318 calories	2 fruit servings
52 g carbohydrate	2 1/2 very lean protein servings
22 g protein	1/2 nonfat milk serving
3 g fat	1/2 fat serving
5 g fiber	3 tsp (15 g) added sugar

Almond Peach

1 cup (240 ml) water or almond milk

1 cup (250 g) frozen peaches

1 tbsp (16 g) nut butter

1 tsp (2.4 g) cinnamon

3 scoops vanilla USANA Nutrimeal

1 scoop whey protein isolate

Makes 2 servings.

One serving contains (includes almond milk):

Nutrients	Food Group Servings
275 calories	1/2 fruit serving
30 g carbohydrate	2 1/2 very lean protein servings
22 g protein	1/2 nonfat milk serving
10 g fat	2 fat servings
7 g fiber	3 tsp (15 g) added sugar

Pump Up Your Power Drink

You can create your own designer drink by adding certain natural ingredients and nutritional supplements. Here's a rundown:

Fiber. With a goal of 25 to 35 grams per day, getting enough fiber is often difficult. Commercial juices and smoothies are usually devoid of fiber, but they don't have to be. Increase the fiber content of your power drinks by using fruit, fruit with skins or seeds, ground flaxseed meal (golden flaxseed melts right into the drink), chia seeds, or wheat germ. You can also eat whole-wheat crackers or breads with your drink to easily increase fiber.

Protein. Protein powders boost the protein content of your drink when you don't want to increase any other nutrients. If you just want to add protein, use whey, or, if you prefer plant-based sources, soy isolates or other plant protein products that you like.

Probiotic. If you use a powdered probiotic and don't like to just take it plain like I do (it's tangy like natural yogurt), your daily shake or smoothie is a great place to hide it.

Energy. To pack in energy and macronutrients, shake and meal-replacement powders work well. If you are lactose intolerant, choose lactose-free, energy-boosting supplement powders and meal replacements.

Creatine monohydrate. My opinion is that the motherload of evidence suggests that almost anyone can benefit from creatine supplementation, from performance enhancements to brain protection. Add creatine to your diet to enhance your performance. Especially after exercise, a power drink is a great way to get in one of your four daily 5-milligram doses, or your single 5-milligram dose for the day.

Power Breakfasts

Indian Breakfast Salad

This delicious salad is served as a side dish in India but makes a fast and fabulous breakfast. It is spiced with cardamom, but because cardamom is expensive, you may prefer to use cinnamon.

1/2 tsp (2 g) butter

2 tbsp (14 g) slivered almonds

2 medium bananas, thinly sliced

4 tbsp (61 g) low-fat plain yogurt

3 tbsp (45 g) light sour cream

1 tbsp (21 g) honey

1/8 tsp (0.25 g) ground cardamom or 1/4 tsp (0.6 g) ground cinnamon

1. Melt the butter in a small nonstick skillet over medium heat. Toast almonds, stirring frequently, until golden, about 3 minutes.

2. Meanwhile, in a medium bowl, mix bananas with yogurt, sour cream, honey, and cardamom. Add almonds and enjoy.

Makes 2 servings.

One serving contains:

Nutrients	Food Group Servings
250 calories	2 fruit servings
42 g carbohydrate	1 lean protein serving
6 g protein	1 fat serving
8 g fat	3 tsp (15 g) added sugar
4 g fiber	

Breakfast Parfait

2 cups (480 g) fat-free Greek yogurt
1 cup (110 g) muesli, unsweetened
1 1/4 cups (180 g) fresh berries
2 tbsp flaxseed meal (13 g ground flaxseeds)
2 tbsp toasted chopped nuts (your choice)

1. In two 16 oz (480 ml) glass or plastic cups, layer the ingredients by adding 1/4 of the yogurt, 1/4 of the muesli, 1/4 of the flaxseed meal, and 1/4 of the berries.

2. Repeat step 1, reserving a dollop of the yogurt for the top, and top with 1/2 the chopped nuts.

Makes 2 servings.

One serving contains:

Nutrients	Food Group Servings
340 calories	2 bread servings
50 g carbohydrate	1/2 fruit serving
24 g protein	1 milk serving
7 g fat	3 very lean protein servings
8 g fiber	1 fat serving

Peach Melba Yogurt Pops

These delicious pops can be prepared the night before to make a great light breakfast that you can easily hit the road with on a warm summer morning. If you don't want to bother with adding the sticks, just poke a fork into the pop when you're ready to eat.

1 cup (247 g) sliced canned peaches in light syrup*
1 cup (230 g) low-fat raspberry yogurt
1 cup (240 ml) orange juice

1. Blend ingredients until smooth. Pour into four 10 oz (300 ml) plastic cups. Place in the freezer.

2. When mixture is partly frozen, insert sticks or plastic spoons.

*If you prefer and have access to fresh peaches, quickly scald them, remove skin, slice and add 5 tsp simple syrup or maple syrup.

Makes 2 servings.

One serving contains:

Nutrients	Food Group Servings
280 calories	2 fruit servings
64 g carbohydrate	1 nonfat milk serving
6 g protein	5 tsp (25 g) added sugar
1 g fat	
3 g fiber	

Orange Cinnamon French Toast

This toast takes only slightly longer to prepare than the standard version that pops out of the toaster.

2 large eggs, lightly beaten
2 tbsp (30 ml) orange juice
1/4 tsp (0.6 g) ground cinnamon
4 slices whole-grain bread
Vegetable cooking spray

1. In a shallow bowl, combine eggs, orange juice, and cinnamon.

2. Spray a nonstick skillet and heat over medium heat for 1 to 2 minutes, until hot.

3. Dip bread into the mixture to coat both sides. Place bread slices in the skillet, pouring any extra egg mixture over them. Cook for about 2 minutes on each side or until browned.

Makes 2 servings.

One serving contains:

Nutrients
220 calories
28 g carbohydrate
12 g protein
7 g fat
4 g fiber

Food Group Servings
2 bread servings
1 medium-fat protein serving

Pineapple Cheese Danish

4 slices raisin bread

4 tbsp (62 g) canned, unsweetened, crushed pineapple, drained

1/2 cup (4 oz, or 120 g) part-skim ricotta cheese

1 tsp (5 g) brown sugar

Dash ground cinnamon

1. Spread each slice of bread with 1 oz (30 g) of cheese and top with pineapple. Combine brown sugar and cinnamon and sprinkle on top of the pineapple.

2. Broil in toaster oven or under the broiler until sugar starts to bubble, about 2 minutes.

Makes 2 servings.

One serving contains:

Nutrients	Food Group Servings
246 calories	2 bread servings
35 g carbohydrate	1/3 fruit serving
11 g protein	1/2 medium-fat protein serving
7 g fat	1/2 fat serving
3 g fiber	

Fruit 'n' Cheese Wraps

1 small red apple, cored and sliced

1 small d'Anjou or Bartlett pear, cored and sliced

2 oz (60 g) thinly sliced cheddar cheese

4 small soft tortillas

1. Place apple and pear slices on tortillas. Cover with cheese.

2. Place under broiler or in toaster oven for 1 to 2 minutes or until cheese melts and bubbles. Wrap and enjoy!

Makes 2 servings.

One serving contains:

Nutrients	Food Group Servings
322 calories	2 bread servings
47 g carbohydrate	1 fruit serving
13 g protein	1 medium-fat protein serving
12 g fat	1 fat serving
7 g fiber	

Asparagus, Spinach, and Feta Omelet

1 cup (240 ml) pure egg whites
1 whole egg
4 asparagus spears, trimmed
1/2 cup (14 g) fresh baby spinach leaves, chopped
1 oz (30 g) low-fat feta cheese
Canola oil spray
Ground black pepper (to taste)
Sea salt (to taste)

1. Wash and chop baby spinach. Whisk egg and egg whites together. Lightly spray frying pan with canola oil and heat. When pan is hot, pour in egg mixture; when egg mix bubbles, flip with spatula.

2. Lower the heat by 50 percent, and place asparagus spears and spinach leaves evenly on one half of the omelet. Crumble feta over the top and season with a little salt and pepper. Continue cooking until egg mixture is almost cooked.

3. Using a flat, wide-lipped spatula, fold the uncovered half omelet over spinach, asparagus, and feta. Place the spatula on top of omelet for 15 seconds (this allows the feta to melt). Serve immediately.

Makes 2 servings.

One serving contains:

Nutrients
294 calories
5 g carbohydrate
41 g protein
10 g fat
2 g fiber

Food Group Servings
1 vegetable serving
2 very lean protein servings
2 medium-fat protein servings

Recipe created by Shar Sault. Used with permission of Metabolic Precision, www.mp-body.com.

Dr. K's Favorite Frittata

I love frittatas because you can use whatever vegetables you've got in the fridge, and get creative with other ingredients that happen to be around. They also work for a meal at any time of day.

1 tsp (5 g) olive oil
1/2 small onion, chopped
1/2 red pepper, chopped
2 button or crimini mushrooms, sliced
1 whole egg
1/3 cup (80 ml) egg whites
2 tsp (5 g) sun-dried tomato pesto
2 tsp (5 g)chevre goat cheese
A few sprigs of curly parsley
Freshly ground black pepper

1. Sauté onion and pepper in olive oil in a small oven-safe skillet for a few minutes over medium heat.
2. Add mushrooms and sauté until soft.
3. Meanwhile turn on oven broiler with rack on top setting.
4. Beat egg with egg whites and pour over cooking vegetables and cover.
5. When eggs are cooked around the edges and partially cooked on top, remove from heat, uncover and dot with sun-dried tomato pesto.
6. Place pan under broiler for a few minutes, until eggs cook and turn lightly golden brown and slightly puffy. Do not let them burn.
7. Remove from oven, slide frittata out of pan onto plate, and dot eggs with chevre. Add a sprig or two of parsley and freshly ground black pepper, then enjoy.

Makes 1 serving.

One serving contains:

Nutrients	Food Group Servings
247 calories	2 vegetable servings
12 g carbohydrate	3 medium-fat protein servings
19 g protein	
14 g fat	

Easy Main Courses

Chicken in Orange Sauce With Pistachios

8 skinless, boneless chicken breast halves
4 tbsp (34 g) cake flour
1 1/2 cups (360 ml) fresh orange juice
1/4 cup (60 ml) white wine
1/4 cup (60 ml) white wine vinegar
1/2 cup (120 ml) minced shallots
2 tbsp (30 g) brown sugar
2 tbsp (30 ml) olive oil
2 tbsp (24 g) unsalted butter, cut into small pieces
3 tbsp (63 g) honey
8 orange slices
8 tbsp (62 g) unsalted pistachio nuts to garnish
Salt and pepper to taste
Wax paper

1. Trim chicken breasts and pound thick ends under wax paper to cook evenly. Combine salt, pepper, and cake flour. Dust on chicken breasts.

2. In a saucepan, bring orange juice, wine, vinegar, shallots, and brown sugar to a boil. Simmer and reduce to about 1 cup. Keep warm.

3. Heat olive oil in a large skillet over medium heat. Sauté chicken breasts in batches until springy to the touch, 4 minutes per side. Transfer to an ovenproof casserole dish and set aside.

4. Remove sauce from heat and whisk in cold butter pieces. Pour over chicken and keep chicken warm in oven set at 250 degrees F (121 degrees C). Chicken may be chilled or frozen at this point.

5. To serve, thoroughly reheat chicken in oven at 325 degrees F (163 degrees C), basting well with the sauce.

6. Heat honey with 2 tbsp (30 ml) of the orange sauce. Sprinkle each breast with 1 tbsp (8 g) of pistachios. Coat orange slice with heated honey and sauce to garnish chicken.

Makes 8 servings.

One serving contains:

Nutrients
334 calories
22 g carbohydrate
30 g protein
13 g fat
2 g fiber

Food Group Servings
4 very lean protein servings
2 fat servings
1/2 fruit serving
1 tsp (5 g) added sugar

Here are two recipes that give you the mood-boosting effects of omega-3 fat and the metabolism-boosting benefits of cayenne pepper. If you can stand the heat, add cayenne to your diet on a daily basis to help you stay lean but not mean.

Pan-Fried Cajun Catfish

1/2 cup (69 g) cornmeal
1 tsp (0.3 g) dried parsley flakes
1/2 tsp (1 g) paprika
1/8 tsp (0.2 g) cayenne pepper (or to taste)
1/8 tsp (0.2 g) white pepper
1/8 tsp (0.2 g) black pepper
1/2 tsp (3 g) salt
1/4 tsp (0.4 g) thyme
1/2 tsp (1.4 g) garlic powder
1/4 tsp (0.6 g) onion powder
1 whole egg
2 1/2 tbsp (37 ml) water
12 oz (360 g) catfish fillets
Nonstick cooking spray
Lemon wedges

1. Mix together the cornmeal, herbs, and spices in a flat dish. In a separate dish, beat the egg with the water.

2. Heat a nonstick frying pan over medium-high heat for 30 seconds. Generously spray the pan with cooking spray. Dip each fillet in the egg–water mixture and then coat generously in the cornmeal mixture. Place skin side down in the frying pan for 5 to 6 minutes, or until the bottom is golden brown. Turn the fish and cook another 6 to 7 minutes. Turn again if needed and remove promptly. Watch the fish closely as it cooks. Do not let the oil smoke or the coating burn. Fish should be tender inside, crisp and brown on the outside. Serve hot with lemon wedges.

Makes 3 servings.

One serving contains:

Nutrients	Food Group Servings
281 calories	4 lean protein servings
18 g carbohydrate	1 bread serving
25 g protein	
11 g fat	
2 g fiber	

Lemon Sole With Mustard Sauce

This is a great fish recipe for those who don't love fish, as well as for those who do.

1 lb (480 g) lemon sole fillets
1/4 cup (60 ml) lemon juice
1/4 cup (60 ml) white wine
1 tsp (5 ml) cornstarch dissolved in 1/8 cup (30 ml) cold water
1 cup (240 ml) water
1/4 cup (60 ml) apple juice
2 tsp (10 ml) dry white wine
1 tsp (3 g) minced garlic
1 tbsp (15 ml) lime juice sweetened with 1 tsp (5 g) sugar
2 tsp (10 g) prepared yellow mustard
1 tsp (5 ml) Worcestershire sauce
1/8 tsp (0.2 g) cayenne pepper (or to taste)

1. Place the fish, lemon juice, and 1/4 cup (60 ml) white wine in a pan and bake at 400 degrees F (200 degrees C) for 20 minutes, or until the fish is flaky and white.

2. Combine the dissolved cornstarch, water, apple juice, dry white wine, and garlic in a saucepan. Heat over medium heat to thicken, stirring often.

3. In a small bowl, whisk together the sweetened lime juice, mustard, Worcestershire sauce, and cayenne pepper. Add the mustard mixture to the cornstarch mixture and whisk until well blended. Allow the mixture to continue cooking until thickened.

4. Place the fish on a platter, pour the mustard sauce over it, and serve.

Makes 4 servings.

One serving contains:

Nutrients
170 calories
6 g carbohydrate
26 g protein
2 g fat
0 g fiber

Food Group Servings
1/2 fruit serving
4 very lean protein servings

Tuna Supreme

This is great in a salad or in a wrap. In less than 5 minutes you can make tuna interesting enough to look forward to every day. I always double the ingredients when I make this meal so that I know I always have plenty on hand every day. Preparation and forward planning makes life so much easier when maintaining a great nutrition plan.

2 celery sticks, finely diced (add leaves)
1/2 red pepper, diced
1/2 red onion, finely diced
1/2 cup (120 ml) finely chopped parsley
2 cans (7 oz each; 400 g total) tuna in spring water (drained)
1/2 cup (73 g) corn kernels
2 tbsp (20g) low-fat mayonnaise
1/2 tsp (2.5 g) Dijon mustard
Fresh ground pepper to season

1. First prepare and finely dice celery, pepper, red onion, and parsley.
2. Drain tuna and place into a bowl.
3. Add all chopped ingredients; then add corn, pepper, mayonnaise, and mustard.
4. Mix together well, making sure the mayonnaise and mustard are dispersed evenly throughout.
5. Serve on rice cakes, with a salad, or in a tortilla wrap.

This meal is quick 'n' easy, tastes great, and is full of protein.

Makes 2 servings.

One serving contains:

Nutrients	Food Group Servings
292 calories	3 vegetable servings
18 g carbohydrate	7 very lean protein servings
55 g protein	1/2 fat serving
4 g fat	
3 g fiber	

Recipe created by Shar Sault. Used with permission of Metabolic Precision, www.mp-body.com.

Mediterranean Brussels Sprouts With Tuna

Brussels sprouts are one of the most nutritious vegetables you can add to your plan. They belong to the cruciferous family and are rich in vitamins C and E, folate, beta-carotene, and iron, and contain a unique spectrum of phytonutrients and fiber.

When sprayed with a little olive oil and seasoned with fresh herbs, garlic, and spices, these Brussels sprouts are simply delicious.

1 tbsp (15 ml) virgin olive oil or canola oil spray

1 red pepper, sliced into 2 in. (6 cm) long, thin strips

2 cloves garlic, finely chopped

3 cans (7 oz each; 600 g total) albacore tuna chunks in spring water (drained)

1 cup (225 g) Roma tomatoes, peeled and chopped

1 tsp (5 g) brown or raw sugar

1 2/3 cups (375 g) Brussels sprouts, washed well and sliced in halves or quarters

1/2 cup (~24) pitted kalamata olives, sliced

2 tbsp (30 ml each) fresh basil and cilantro, both finely chopped

Cracked black pepper (to taste)

Pine nuts to garnish (optional)

1. Heat oil in frying pan or wok, and stir-fry pepper and garlic for 2 to 3 minutes.

2. Add tuna, Roma tomatoes, sugar, Brussels sprouts, olives, and fresh herbs.

3. Cover and cook for 5 to 7 minutes. Stir frequently.

4. Season with pepper and serve immediately. Sprinkle pine nuts as garnish (optional).

Makes 4 servings.

One serving contains:

Nutrients	Food Group Servings
291 calories	4 vegetable servings
20 g carbohydrates	5 very lean protein servings
37 g protein	1/2 fat serving
7 g fat	
5 g fiber	

Recipe created by Shar Sault. Used with permission of Metabolic Precision, www.mp-body.com.

Five-Minute Tuna Cakes

Our household should have shares in a tuna cannery with the amount of tuna we consume. These tuna cakes are fast, delicious, and nutritious! They can be eaten hot or cold and served with salad or vegetables. Make up a large batch of these tuna cakes and store them in the freezer. They come in really handy when you want a fast meal!

2 (7 oz each; 400 g total) cans of albacore tuna in spring water, drained

1 onion, finely chopped

1 tbsp (1 in., or 3 cm, root) fresh ginger, finely chopped

1 clove garlic, finely chopped

2 tbsp (30 ml) cilantro, chopped

2 tbsp (30 ml) parsley, chopped

1 whole egg

Canola oil spray

Freshly ground black pepper

1. Heat frying pan and spray lightly with oil.
2. Add onion, ginger, and garlic, and cook for 1 minute, stirring frequently.
3. Remove from heat. Cool.
4. Place tuna into a bowl.
5. Add cilantro, parsley, black pepper, and the cooked onion mixture. Add egg and mix well to combine.
6. Shape into small cakes.
7. Heat fry pan used earlier. Spray lightly with oil.
8. Place patties in pan and cook on high for 2 to 3 minutes on each side until brown. Tuna cakes should be moist and a little pink in the center when cooked.

Makes 8 cakes.

One serving contains:

Nutrients
79 calories
2 g carbohydrate
14 g protein
2 g fat
<1 g fiber

Food Group Servings
2 very lean protein servings

Recipe created by Shar Sault. Used with permission of Metabolic Precision, www.mp-body.com.

Just Like Summertime Grilled Chicken

1 cup (240 ml) plain, whole-milk yogurt
1 tsp (6 g) each: salt, ground pepper, cumin, freshly grated ginger
2-3 cloves garlic, minced
2 tbsp (30 ml) lime juice
2 lb (900 g) bone-in chicken pieces (your choice: legs, thighs, breasts)

1. Mix ingredients except chicken into yogurt to make marinade. Poke chicken pieces in several places with a fork, then cover chicken with yogurt. Marinate, covered in refrigerator, for 8 to 12 hours.
2. Remove from refrigerator 30 minutes prior to cooking.
3. Microwave until partially cooked. Timing depends on the power of your microwave.
4. Finish on grill until chicken is completely cooked.

Makes 6 servings.

One serving contains:

Nutrients	Food Group Servings
174 calories	4 very lean protein servings
2 g carbohydrate	
28 g protein	
6 g fat with skin removed (9 g with skin)	

Ready-to-Serve Vegetables

Irene's Marinated Broccoli

This is the easiest recipe to prepare for yourself or for entertaining. It makes the best-tasting raw broccoli you could imagine! It's great alone, or you could add the optional dip for a special occasion. If you drain well, the fat content will be lower.

1 bunch (~3 cups, or 213 g) broccoli, cut into small florets

Marinade:
1/4 cup (60 ml) cider or wine vinegar
3/4 cup (180 ml) virgin olive oil
2 cloves garlic, split (or more if desired)
1 tsp (5 g) sugar
2 tsp (2 g) fresh dill

Put broccoli in resealable bag and cover with marinade. Marinate in bag, refrigerated, overnight. Drain.

Optional Dip*
2 cups (448 g) light canola mayonnaise (also works with half mayo and half plain yogurt, the way I actually make it at home)
1 1/2 tsp (3 g) curry powder
1 tsp (5 g) ketchup
1/4 tsp (1 ml) Worcestershire sauce

Mix together. Serve with drained broccoli. Makes 6 servings.

One serving without dip contains:

Nutrients
90 calories
2 g carbohydrate
1 g protein
9 g fat
1 g fiber

Food Group Servings
1/2 vegetable serving
2 fat servings

*Add 1 fat serving for every 1 tbsp (15 ml) dip (45 calories).

Alotta Onions Soup

Whenever I've shared this recipe with anyone, the description has always started out with "a lot of onions." The water and electrolyte content makes it a great fluid replacer after exercise. This recipe, which serves only two or three, is pared down from the army-sized version we make at home.

2 cloves fresh garlic, minced
1 tbsp (15 ml) canola oil
1/2 tbsp (7 ml) sesame oil
1 1/2 large yellow onions, thinly sliced
6 cups (1.4 L) water
1 1/2 tbsp (22 ml) soy sauce
1/4 tsp (1 ml) freshly ground black pepper
4-6 tsp (8-12 g) freshly grated Parmesan cheese

1. Sauté the garlic in the oils in a shallow nonstick pan over medium heat until slightly soft, about 3 to 5 minutes. Add onions and cook, stirring occasionally, until slightly caramelized, about 20 minutes.

2. Transfer the onions and garlic to a soup pot. Add the water, soy sauce, and pepper. Bring to a low boil over high heat; then reduce the heat to low and simmer uncovered for 15 minutes.

3. Serve in full bowls sprinkled with 2 tsp (4 g) of Parmesan cheese.

Makes 3 servings.

One serving contains:

Nutrients	Food Group Servings
109 calories	1 1/2 vegetable servings
8 g carbohydrate	1 1/2 fat servings
2 g protein	
8 g fat	
1 g fiber	

Great Grains

Easy Energy Couscous

4 tbsp (27 g) slivered almonds
4 tbsp (40 g) golden raisins
12 dried apricots, quartered
8 dried figs, quartered
1/2 tsp (1.2 g) cinnamon
1/2 cup (120 ml) fresh orange juice
1 1/2 cups (360 ml) water
1/4 tsp (1 ml) salt
1 tbsp (12 g) butter
1 cup (173 g) whole-wheat couscous

1. Place the almonds, raisins, apricots, and figs in a bowl with the cinnamon. Cover with the orange juice and refrigerate for a minimum of 30 minutes and up to overnight.
2. In a saucepan, bring the water, salt, and butter to a boil. Stir in the couscous. Cover and simmer over low heat for 5 minutes. Remove from heat and let stand 5 minutes. Fluff the couscous lightly with a fork.
3. Transfer the fruit and nut mixture to a saucepan and warm thoroughly over medium-low heat. Turn into a mixing bowl and add the cooked couscous. Mix well. Couscous can be served warm or cold.

Makes 6 servings.

One serving contains:

Nutrients	Food Group Servings
258 calories	2 fruit servings
49 g carbohydrate	1 bread serving
5 g protein	1 fat serving
5 g fat	
7 g fiber	

Seashore Buckwheat

2/3 cup (70 g) whole-wheat pasta shells
1 tbsp (15 ml) canola oil
1 cup (70 g) sliced mushrooms
1 small onion, diced
2 cups (480 ml) chicken stock
1 whole egg, slightly beaten
1 cup (164 g) preroasted buckwheat kernels or groats
Pinch of white pepper and salt to taste

1. Cook the pasta shells until al dente according to package directions; drain and set aside.

2. Heat the oil in a nonstick pan over medium heat. Add the mushrooms and onion and sauté until the onion is translucent, about 7 minutes. Set aside.

3. Heat the stock to boiling. In a small mixing bowl, combine the egg with the buckwheat until the kernels are coated. Turn the buckwheat into a medium-sized skillet. Stir the egg and buckwheat mixture over medium-high heat for 3 to 4 minutes until it is hot and slightly toasted and the egg-coated kernels are well separated. Reduce the heat to low and carefully stir in the boiling stock, sautéed mushrooms and onions, and pepper and salt. Cover tightly and simmer 10 to 12 minutes, or until the buckwheat kernels are tender and all the liquid has been absorbed.

4. Turn into an oven-safe casserole dish and mix in the pasta shells. Place uncovered under an oven broiler for 3 to 5 minutes, just to brown the top. Watch closely and remove promptly.

Makes 4 servings.

One serving contains:

Nutrients	Food Group Servings
232 calories	2 bread servings
39 g carbohydrate	2 vegetable servings
9 g protein	1/2 very lean protein serving
6 g fat	1/2 fat serving
5 g fiber	

Appendix A

Three- to Seven-Day Food Record

When working with clients, I always want to know what they are eating *before* they learn what I have to say. If you are my client, I'll have you record your usual diet for each of your different typical days, with typical days broken out as training days, rest days, work days, nonwork days, school days, weekend days, even travel days if they are part of your usual diet on some regular basis. With this tool, you'll record your usual diet for as many different typical days as possible. My goal is to always keep as much of your usual diet in place as possible, then adjust timing, combining, and altering food selections and supplements where needed. The more you can keep in place, the more likely you are to stick with the new plan.

To get down to work, choose at least three days and up to seven days in the following 24-hour diet log. If you record for longer than seven days, you most likely will not record complete data, and once it's not complete, it's not helpful. You can make copies of the diet log that follows. Try to record the food as you eat it or just afterward; it is often difficult to remember in the evening exactly what you ate eight hours before. Record everything you eat and drink, including water, and be as detailed as possible.

When you are finished recording, translate all the foods from a single day into food groups, and then into calories and grams of protein, carbohydrate, and fat by plugging them into the diet analysis table that follows. Use the food group tables from chapter 13 to get the nutrient details about each food group.

You can do this yourself by hand, the old-fashioned way, and really learn the details of your diet. Online and mobile apps vary in content, data quality, and ease of use, but they keep improving. Those with fees may have better database content than those that are free to use. Whichever works for you is the better choice. Even with the digital programs, make sure to record right after you eat to get the most reliable data.

Finally, go back and review the columns that contain information about where and why you ate. Sometimes you will see clues to solving problem areas in your diet or barriers to your ability to stick with your plan. Note those clues, and add them into your overall plan to create more successful habits. Recording your diet and training is one of the best ways to change old habits into new habits. You can build your new plan into your Success Tracker from chapter 13.

24-Hour Diet Log

Time of day	Food eaten	Description	Quantity	Location	Why you ate

From S.M. Kleiner and M. Greenwood-Robinson, *The New Power Eating* (Champaign, IL: Human Kinetics, 2019).

Diet Analysis Table

Diet record date: _____

Food groups	Number of servings	Carbohydrate (g)	Protein (g)	Fat (g)	Calories
Bread/starch					
Fruit					
Nonfat milk					
Low-fat milk					
Teaspoons of added carbohydrate or sugar					
Vegetable					
Very lean protein					
Lean protein					
Medium-fat protein					
Fat protein					
Totals					

From S.M. Kleiner and M. Greenwood-Robinson, *The New Power Eating* (Champaign, IL: Human Kinetics, 2019).

Appendix B

Restaurant Guide and Healthy Fast Food

Dining out does not have to mean diet disaster. You can take control of your menu and your meals at restaurants. The trick is to have a game plan before you go.

To start with, choose a restaurant that serves nutritious choices: chicken, fish, salads, baked potatoes, and steamed vegetables, to name just a few. Avoid all-you-can-eat buffets and restaurants that offer only high-calorie, high-fat foods. Before arriving at the restaurant, decide what you'll order, and how you'd like it prepared—grilled chicken, baked or grilled fish, or lean red meat, for example.

Beware of "feel bad" fat hiding in certain restaurant foods. Sauces, condiments, butter, oil, mayonnaise, creams, and rich cheeses all add a lot of pro-inflammatory fat to appetizers, entrees, and side dishes. Ask the serving staff to leave out high-fat ingredients. Another option is to make a substitution, such as a baked potato for French fries.

Request that sauces, salad dressings, and sour cream be served on the side so you can control the amount you use. Request that a menu item be prepared using an alternative method, such as broiling instead of frying.

Be inquisitive! Ask questions about foods on the menu. Be specific! How is the food prepared? What are the ingredients? To help you, consult the following menu guide, which shows what to choose and what to avoid. Of course, it is fine to use some of these higher-fat techniques and ingredients when you are cooking at home and can control the amounts you use. It's the dousing of foods with butters, sauces, and creams at restaurants that makes them undesirable as regulars in your diet.

Menu Guide

Choose	Avoid
Entrees	
In their own juices	Fried
Boiled	Sautéed
Grilled	Au gratin
Baked	Buttery, buttered
Roasted	Creamed, cream sauce

Choose	Avoid
Entrees *(continued)*	
Poached	Hollandaise
Lean meats (e.g., round, sirloin, tenderloin, flank steak, filet mignon)	Parmesan
Garden fresh	Marinated (in oil)
Tomato juice	Casserole
	Gravy
	Hash
	Potpie
	Crispy
Appetizers	
Steamed seafood (e.g., mussels, clams, crabs, lobsters, shrimp)	Swimming in butter
Raw or steamed vegetables	Cheese
Vegetable antipasto	
Soups	
Gazpacho, consommé, broth-type	Creamed
Vegetables	
Fresh, raw, steamed	Fried
Baked potato or yams	Heavily buttered, creamed, in cheese sauce
Salads	
With clear or reduced-fat dressings	With creamy dressings
	With meat, bacon, cheese, croutons
Breads	
Dry (no butter)	Baked with butter, shortening, or cheese
Whole grain or sprouted grain with seeds	Sweet rolls
Sandwiches	
Tuna, chicken, turkey, seafood, lean cooked beef	Processed lunch meats, hard cheese, fried foods
	Sandwiches with sauces, gravies, mayonnaise, or bacon
Desserts	
Fruit, sorbet, sherbet, low-fat ice creams and frozen yogurt, angel food cake, other specially made low-fat and low-sugar items	Commercial pies, cakes, pastries, ice cream, candies

Top 10 Fast-Food Restaurants and Best Choices

The establishments listed in this section have made an effort to stand above the crowd. And then, of course, sometimes you just can't do any better than one of the big fast-food chains. So here are my top choices and the best menu options when you're on the road.

Menus and recipes change so quickly that nutrition information in a book is outdated in a heartbeat. All of these restaurants have nutrition information available both on the premises and online.

The following are in alphabetical order (not best to worst).

Au Bon Pain

Best choices: Whole grains, salads, small plates, fresh fruit, vegetarian options

Chipotle

Best choices: protein selections, burritos, burrito bowls, rice or beans depending on your need, salsa, lettuce, cheese or guacamole (you can check out their nutrition calculator at www.chipotle.com)

Einstein Bros. Bagels

Best choices: Good Grains Bagel, high-fiber Veg Out, reduced-fat shmears, hummus, peanut butter, half or whole-sized salad

McDonald's (sometimes it's the only place you've got)

Best choices: Grilled Chicken Classic and wraps (skip the mayo or sauce), salad, Egg McMuffin

Panera Bread

Best choices: broth bowls, whole grains, fresh fruit, full or half-size portions, salads, vegetarian options

Qdoba

Best choices: Craft 2–Naked Burrito (customize your size and ingredients), fresh produce, vegetarian choices

Starbucks

Best choices: Protein Boxes with a good ratio of carbohydrate to protein; some selections to include are fresh fruit, veggies, hard boiled eggs, pb&j with a cheese stick, turkey club; Sous vide egg bites

Subway

Best choices: all items with 6 grams of fat or less (their Fresh Fit selections) on a wheat roll with extra veggies and double protein on a 6-inch roll (skip the mayo and use mustard, vinegar, and oil); chicken salad; for higher energy needs, a foot-long can be a good bet (sometimes requesting double protein is necessary)

Taco Del Mar

Best choices: fresh produce, fish, whole grains, chicken burritos, vegetarian options

Wendy's

Best choices: baked potato topped with chili, broccoli, and chives (skip the sour cream, cheese, and Buttery Best Spread)

Works Consulted

Abramowicz, W.N., et al. 2005. Effects of acute versus chronic L-carnitine L-tartrate supplementation on metabolic responses to steady state exercise in males and females. *International Journal of Sport Nutrition and Exercise Metabolism* 15: 386-400.

Achten, J., et al. 2004. Higher dietary carbohydrate content during intensified running training results in better maintenance of performance and mood state. *Journal of Applied Physiology* 96: 1331-1340.

Ajmol, A., et al. 2016. The influence of caffeine ingestion on strength and power performance in female team-sport players. *Journal of the International Society of Sports Nutrition* 13: 46.

Akermark, C., I. Jacobs, M. Rasmusson, and J. Karlsson. 1996. Diet and muscle glycogen concentration in relation to physical performance in Swedish elite ice hockey players. *International Journal of Sport Nutrition* 6: 272-284.

Alkhenizan, A.H., et al. 2004. The role of vitamin E in the prevention of coronary events and stroke. Meta-analysis of randomized controlled trials. *Saudi Medical Journal* 25: 1808-1814.

Allen, J.D., et al. 1998. Ginseng supplementation does not enhance healthy young adults' peak aerobic exercise performance. *Journal of the American College of Nutrition* 17: 462-466.

American Dietetic Association. 1995. Position of the American Dietetic Association: Phytochemicals and functional foods. *Journal of the American Dietetic Association* 95: 493-496.

American Dietetic Association. 1998. Position of the American Dietetic Association: Use of nutritive and non-nutritive sweeteners. *Journal of the American Dietetic Association* 98: 580-588.

American Dietetic Association. 2009. Position of the American Dietetic Association: Functional foods. *Journal of the American Dietetic Association* 98: 735-746.

American Heart Association and American College of Cardiology Foundation. 2013. Lifestyle management to reduce cardiovascular risk. *Circulation* 129: S76-S99

American Institute for Cancer Research. (n.d.). Coconut water: Health or hype? http://preventcancer.aicr.org/site/News2?page=NewsArticle&id=19168&news_iv_ctrl=2303.

Anderson, G.H., et al. 2002. Inverse association between the effect of carbohydrates on blood glucose and subsequent short-term food intake in young men. *American Journal of Clinical Nutrition* 76: 1023-1030.

Anderson, J.W., et al. 2009. Health benefits of dietary fiber. *Nutrition Reviews* 67: 188-205.

Andersson, B., X. Xuefan, M. Rebuffe-Scrive, K. Terning, et al. 1991. The effects of exercise training on body composition and metabolism in men and women. *International Journal of Obesity* 15: 75-81.

Anomasiri, W., et al. 2004. Low dose creatine supplementation enhances sprint phase of 400 meters swimming performance. *Journal of the Medical Association of Thailand* 87: S228-S232.

Antonio, J., et al. 1999. Glutamine: A potentially useful supplement for athletes. *Canadian Journal of Applied Physiology* 24: 1-14.

Antonio, J., et al. 2015. A high protein diet (3.4 g/kg/d) combined with a heavy resistance training program improves body composition in healthy trained men and women: A follow-up investigation. *Journal of the International Society of Sports Nutrition* 12: 39.

Antonio, J., et al. 2018. High protein consumption in trained women: Bad to the bone? *Journal of the International Society of Sports Nutrition* 15: 6.

Applegate, L. 1992. Protein power. *Runner's World*, June 22-24.

Aragon, et al. 2017. *Journal of the International Society of Sports Nutrition* 14: 16.

Araújo, J.R., et al. 2017. Impact of high-fat diet on the intestinal microbiota and small intestinal physiology before and after the onset of obesity. *Biochimie* 141: 97-106.

Arkadianos , I., et al. 2007. Improved weight management using genetic information to personalize a calorie controlled diet. *Nutrition Journal*, October 18.

Arkadianos, J., et al. 2017. Improved weight management using genetic information to personalize a calorie controlled diet. *Nutrition Journal* 6: 29.

Armstrong, L.E. 2002. Caffeine, body fluid-electrolyte balance, and exercise performance.

International Journal of Sport Nutrition and Exercise Metabolism 12: 189-206.

Asrih, M., et al. 2015. Ketogenic diet impairs FGF21 signaling and promotes differential inflammatory responses in the liver and white adipose tissue. *PLoS One* 14: e0126364.

Aulin, K.P., et al. 2000. Muscle glycogen resynthesis rate in humans after supplementation of drinks containing carbohydrates with low and high molecular masses. *European Journal of Applied Physiology* 81: 346-351.

Avery, N.G., et al. 2003. Effects of vitamin E supplementation on recovery from repeated bouts of resistance exercise. *Journal of Strength and Conditioning Research* 17: 801-809.

Azadbakht, L., et al. 2007. Soy inclusion in the diet improves features of the metabolic syndrome: A randomized crossover study in postmenopausal women. *American Journal of Clinical Nutrition* 85: 735-741.

Bachman, J.G., L.D. Johnston, and P.M. O'Malley. 2011. *Monitoring the future: Questionnaire responses from the nation's high school seniors, 2010.* Ann Arbor, MI: Institute for Social Research.

Backhouse, S.H., et al. 2005. Effect of carbohydrate and prolonged exercise on affect and perceived exertion. *Medicine & Science in Sports & Exercise* 37: 1768-1773.

Bahrke, M.S., et al. 1994. Evaluation of the ergogenic properties of ginseng. *Sports Medicine* 18: 229-248.

Bahrke, M.S., et al. 2004. Abuse of anabolic androgenic steroids and related substances in sport and exercise. *Current Opinion in Pharmacology* 4: 614-620.

Balon, T.W., J.F. Horowitz, and K.M. Fitzsimmons. 1992. Effects of carbohydrate loading and weight-lifting on muscle girth. *International Journal of Sport Nutrition* 2: 328-334.

Balsom, P.D., et al. 1998. Carbohydrate intake and multiple sprint sports: With special reference to football (soccer). *International Journal of Sports Medicine* 20: 48-52.

Baranov, A.I. 1982. Medicinal uses of ginseng and related plants in the Soviet Union: Recent trends in the Soviet literature. *Journal of Ethnopharmacology* 6: 339-353.

Barth, C.A., and U. Behnke. 1997. Nutritional physiology of whey components. *Nahrung* 41: 2-12.

Bazzarre, T.L., et al. 1992. Plasma amino acid responses of trained athletes to two successive exhaustive trials with and without interim carbohydrate feeding. *Journal of the American College of Nutrition* 11 (5): 501-511.

Bean, A. 1996. Here's to your immunity. *Runner's World, February 23.*

Bellisle, F., and C. Perez. 1994. Low-energy substitutes for sugars and fats in the human diet: Impact on nutritional regulation. *Neuroscience Behavioral Review* 18: 197-205.

Belza, A., et al. 2007. Body fat loss achieved by stimulation of thermogenesis by a combination of bioactive food ingredients: A placebo-controlled, double-blind 8-week intervention in obese subjects. *International Journal of Obesity* 31: 121-130.

Bemben, M.G., et al. 2005. Creatine supplementation and exercise performance: Recent findings. *Sports Medicine* 35: 107-125.

Benardot, D. 2007. Timing of energy and fluid intake: New concepts for weight control and hydration. *ACSM's Health & Fitness Journal* 11: 13-19.

Benardot, D. 2009. Fear of calories: Part I. *Peak Running Performance.* 18 (2): 11-15.

Benardot, D. 2009. Fear of calories: Part II. *Peak Running Performance.* 18 (3): 2-5.

Benardot, D. 2013. Energy thermodynamics revisited: Energy intake strategies for optimizing body composition and performance. *Energy Thermodynamics and Sports* 11: 1-13.

Benton, D., et al. 2001. The influence of phosphatidylserine supplementation on mood and heart rate when faced with an acute stressor. *Nutritional Neuroscience* 4: 169-178.

Biolo, G., et al. 1997. An abundant supply of amino acids enhances the metabolic effect of exercise on muscle protein. *American Journal of Physiology* 273: E122-E129.

Bird, S.P., et al. 2006. Effects of liquid carbohydrate/essential amino acid ingestion on acute hormonal response during a single bout of resistance exercise in untrained men. *Nutrition* 22: 367-375.

Birketvedt, G.S., et al. 2005. Experiences with three different fiber supplements in weight reduction. *Medical Science Monitor* 11: P15-P18.

Bjorntorp, P. 1991. Importance of fat as a support nutrient for energy: Metabolism of athletes. *Journal of Sports Sciences* 9: 71-76.

Blankson, H., et al. 2000. Conjugated linoleic acid reduces body fat mass in overweight and obese humans. *Journal of Nutrition* 130: 2943-2948.

Blesso, C.N., et al. 2013. Effects of carbohydrate restriction and dietary cholesterol provided by eggs on clinical risk factors in metabolic syndrome. *Journal Clinical Lipidology* 7 (5): 463-471.

Blesso, C.N. 2015. Egg phospholipids and cardiovascular health. *Nutrients* 7: 2731-2747.

Blomstrand, E. 2006. A role for branched-chain amino acids in reducing central fatigue. *Journal of Nutrition* 136: 544S-547S.

Blomstrand, E., et al. 2006. Branched-chain amino acids activate key enzymes in protein synthesis after physical exercise. *Journal of Nutrition* 136: 269S-273S.

Bloomer, R.J., et al. 2000. Effects of meal form and composition on plasma testosterone, cortisol, and insulin following resistance exercise. *International Journal of Sport Nutrition and Exercise Metabolism* 10: 415-424.

Blumenthal, M., ed. 1998. *The complete German Commission E monographs.* Austin, TX: American Botanical Council.

Blumenthal, M., ed. 2000. *Herbal medicine: Expanded Commission E monographs.* Austin, TX: *American Botanical Council, Integrative Medicine Communications.*

Bogardus, C., et al. 1981. Comparison of carbohydrate-containing and carbohydrate-restricted hypocaloric diets in the treatment of obesity. Endurance and metabolic fuel homeostasis during strenuous exercise. *The Journal of Clinical Investigation* 68: 399-404.

Borsheim, E., et al. 2002. Essential amino acids and muscle protein recovery from resistance exercise. *American Journal of Physiology, Endocrinology, and Metabolism* 4 (283): E648-E657.

Borsheim, E., et al. 2004. Effect of an amino acid, protein, and carbohydrate mixture on net muscle protein balance after resistance exercise. *International Journal of Sport Nutrition and Exercise Metabolism* 14: 255-271.

Brantsaeter, A.L., et al. 2017. Organic food in the diet: Exposure and health implications. *Annual Review Public Health* 38: 295-313.

Brass, E.P. 2004. Carnitine and sports medicine: Use or abuse? *Annals of the New York Academy of Sciences* 1033: 67-78.

Bremner, K., et al. 2002. The effect of phosphate loading on erythrocyte 2,3-bisphosphoglycerate levels. *Clinica Chimica Acta* 323: 111-114.

Brilla, L.R., and V. Conte. 1999. Effects of zinc-magnesium (ZMA) supplementation on muscle attributes of football players. *Medicine & Science in Sports & Exercise* 31 (Suppl 5): Abstract No. 483.

Brilla, L.R., and T.F. Haley. 1992. Effect of magnesium supplementation on strength training in humans. *Journal of the American College of Nutrition* 11: 326-329.

Brooks, G.A., et al. 2005. Exercise physiology: Human bioenergetics and its applications, 4th ed. Boston: McGraw-Hill Companies.

Brown, G.A., et al. 2000. Effects of anabolic precursors on serum testosterone concentrations and adaptations to resistance training in young men. *International Journal of Sport Nutrition and Exercise Metabolism* 10: 340-359.

Brown, J., M.C. Crim, V.R. Young, and W.J. Evans. 1994. Increased energy requirements and changes in body composition with resistance training in older adults. *The American Journal of Clinical Nutrition* 60: 167-175.

Bruyère, O., et al. 2018. Inappropriate claims from non-equivalent medications in osteoarthritis: a position paper endorsed by the European Society for Clinical and Economic Aspects of Osteoporosis, Osteoarthritis and Musculoskeletal Diseases (ESCEO). *Aging Clinical and Experimental Research* 30: 111–117.

Bryner, R.W., R.C. Toffle, I.H. Ullrich, and R.A. Yeager. 1997. The effects of exercise intensity on body composition, weight loss, and dietary composition in women. *Journal of the American College of Nutrition* 16: 68-73.

Bucci, L.R. 2000. Selected herbals and human exercise performance. *The American Journal of Clinical Nutrition* 72 (Suppl. 2): 624S-636S.

Buckley, J.D., et al. 1998. Effect of an oral bovine colostrum supplement (Intact) on running performance. Abstract, 1998 Australian Conference of Science and Medicine in Sport, Adelaide, South Australia.

Buckley, J.D., et al. 1999. Oral supplementation with bovine colostrum (Intact) increases vertical jump performance. Abstract, 4th Annual Congress of the European College of Sport Science, Rome.

Bujko, J., et al. 1997. Benefit of more but smaller meals at a fixed daily protein intake. *Zeitschrift Fur Ernahrungswissenschaft* 36: 347-349.

Burke, E.R. 1999. *D-ribose: What you need to know.* Garden City Park, NY: Avery.

Burke, L.E., et al. 2008. A randomized clinical trial of a standard versus vegetarian diet for weight loss: The impact of treatment preference. *International Journal of Obesity* 32: 166-176.

Burke, L.M. 1997. Nutrition for post-exercise recovery. *International Journal of Sport Nutrition* 1: 214-224.

Burke, L.M., et al. 1998. Carbohydrate intake during prolonged cycling minimizes effect of glycemic index of preexercise meal. *Journal of Applied Physiology* 85: 2220-2226.

Burke, L.M., et al. 2017. Low carbohydrate, high fat diet impairs exercise economy and negates the performance benefit from intensified training in elite race walkers. *Journal of Physiology* 595: 2785-2807.

Butterfield, G., et al. 1991. Amino acids and high protein diets. In *Perspectives in exercise science and sports medicine, vol. 4*, ed. D. Lamb and M. Williams, 87-122. Madison, WI: Brown & Benchmark.

Calder, A., et al. 2011. A review on the dietary flavonoid kaempferol. *Mini Reviews in Medicinal Chemistry* 11: 298-344.

Campbell, B.I., et al. 2004. The ergogenic potential of arginine. *Journal of the International Society of Sports Nutrition* 1: 35-38.

Campbell, W.W., M.C. Crim, V.R. Young, et al. 1995. Effects of resistance training and dietary protein intake on protein metabolism in older adults. *American Journal of Physiology* 268: E1143-E1153.

Campbell, W.W., et al. 1999. Effects of an omnivorous diet compared with a lactoovovegetarian diet on resistance-training-induced changes in body composition and skeletal muscle in older men. *American Journal of Clinical Nutrition* 70: 1032-1039.

Carli, G., et al. 1992. Changes in exercise-induced hormone response to branched chain amino acid administration. *European Journal of Applied Physiology* 64: 272-277.

Carlson, J.J., et al. 2011. Dietary fiber and nutrient density are inversely associated with the metabolic syndrome in US adolescents. *Journal of the American Dietetic Association* 111: 1688-1695.

Castell, L.M. 1996. Does glutamine have a role in reducing infections in athletes? *European Journal of Applied Physiology* 73: 488-490.

Center for Science in the Public Interest. 2006. Choosing safer beef to eat. www.cspinet.org/foodsafety/saferbeef.html.

Chandler, R.M., H.K. Byrne, J.G. Patterson, and J.L. Ivy. 1994. Dietary supplements affect the anabolic hormones after weight-training exercise. *Journal of Applied Physiology* 76: 839-845.

Charley, H. 1982. *Food science*. New York: John Wiley & Sons.

Chilibeck, P.D., et al. 2004. Effect of creatine ingestion after exercise on muscle thickness in males and females. *Medicine & Science in Sports & Exercise* 36: 1781-1788.

Chilibeck, P.D., et al. 2005. Creatine monohydrate and resistance training increase bone mineral content and density in older men. *The Journal of Nutrition, Health & Aging* 9: 352-353.

Clancy, S.P., P.M. Clarkson, M.E. DeCheke, et al. 1994. Effects of chromium picolinate supplementation on body composition, strength, and urinary chromium loss in football players. *International Journal of Sport Nutrition* 4: 142-153.

Clark, N. 1993. Athletes with amenorrhea. *The Physician and Sportsmedicine* 21: 45-48.

Clarkson, P.M. 1991. Nutritional ergogenic aids: Chromium, exercise, and muscle mass. *International Journal of Sport Nutrition* 1: 289-293.

Clarkson, P.M. 1996. Nutrition for improved sports performance: Current issues on ergogenic aids. *Sports Medicine* 21: 393-401.

Cleo, G., et al. 2017. Could habits hold the key to weight loss maintenance? A narrative review. *Journal Nutrition Human Diet* 30 (5), 655-664.

Coleman, E. 1997. Carbohydrate unloading: A reality check. *The Physician and Sportsmedicine* 25: 97-98.

Collomp, K. 1991. Effects of caffeine ingestion on performance and anaerobic metabolism during the Wingate Test. *International Journal of Sports Medicine* 12: 439-443.

Collomp, K., A. Ahmaidi, M. Audran, and C. Prefaut. 1992. Benefits of caffeine ingestion on sprint performance in trained and untrained swimmers. *European Journal of Applied Physiology* 64: 377-380.

Colson, S.N., et al. 2005. Cordyceps sinensis- and Rhodiola rosea-based supplementation in male cyclists and its effect on muscle tissue oxygen saturation. *Journal of Strength and Conditioning Research* 19: 358-363.

Conjugated linoleic acid overview. 2001, March 1. Professional monographs: Herbal, mineral, vitamin, nutraceuticals. Westlake Village, CA: Intramedicine.

Convertino, V.A., et al. 1996. ACSM position stand. Exercise and fluid replacement. *Medicine & Science in Sports & Exercise* 28: i-vii.

Coyle, E.F. 1991. Timing and method of increased carbohydrate intake to cope with heavy training, competition and recovery. *Journal of Sports Sciences* 9 Spec No: 29-51.

Coyle, E.F. 1995. Fat metabolism during exercise. *Sports Science Exchange* 8: 1-7.

Coyle, E.F. 1997. Fuels for sport performance. In *Perspectives in exercise science and sports medicine,* ed. D. Lamb and R. Murray. Carmel, IN: Cooper.

Craciun, A.M., et al. 1998. Improved bone metabolism in female elite athletes after vitamin K supplementation. *International Journal of Sports Medicine* 19: 479-484.

Crouter, S.E. et al. 2012. Relationship between physical activity, physical performance, and iron status in adult women. *Applied Physiology, Nutrition, and Metabolism* 37: 697-705.

Daley, C.A., et al. 2010. A review of fatty acid profiles and antioxidant content in grass-fed and grain-fed beef. *Nutrition Journal* 9: 10.

Dalton, R.A., et al. 1999. Acute carbohydrate consumption does not influence resistance exercise performance during energy restriction. *International Journal of Sport Nutrition* 9: 319-332.

Davis, J.M., et al. 1999. Effects of branched-chain amino acids and carbohydrate on fatigue during intermittent, high-intensity running. *International Journal of Sports Medicine* 20: 309-314.

Delzenne, N.M., et al. 2011. Modulation of the gut microbiota by nutrients with prebiotic properties: Consequences for host health in the context of obesity and metabolic syndrome. *Microbial Cell Factories* 10 (Suppl 1): S10.

DeMarco, H.M., et al. 1999. Pre-exercise carbohydrate meals: Application of glycemic index. *Medicine & Science in Sports & Exercise* 31: 164-170.

Deschenes, M.R., and W.J. Kraemer. 1989. The biochemical basis of muscular fatigue. *National Strength and Conditioning Association Journal* 11: 41-44.

Deutz, R.C., et al. 2000. Relationship between energy deficits and body composition in elite female gymnasts and runners. *Medicine & Science in Sports & Exercise* 32: 659-668.

Diepvens, K., et al. 2006. Metabolic effects of green tea and of phases of weight loss. *Physiology & Behavior* 87: 185-191.

Diepvens, K., et al. 2007. Obesity and thermogenesis related to the consumption of caffeine, ephedrine, capsaicin, and green tea. *American Journal of Physiology* 292: R77-R85.

Dimeff, R.J. 1993. Steroids and other performance enhancers. In *Clinical preventive medicine,* ed. R.N. Matzen and R.S. Lang. St. Louis: Mosby-Year Book, Inc.

Dimeff, R.J., 1996. Drugs and sports: Prescription and non-prescription. Presented at Sports Medicine for the Rheumatologist, American College of Rheumatology, Phoenix, Arizona, May 19.

Doherty, M., et al. 2005. Effects of caffeine ingestion on rating of perceived exertion during and after exercise: A meta-analysis. *Scandinavian Journal of Medicine & Science in Sports* 15: 69-78.

Dowling, E.A., et al. 1996. Effect of Eleutherococcus senticosus on submaximal and maximal performance. *Medicine & Science in Sports & Exercise* 28: 482-489.

Drew, M., et al. 2018. Prevalence of illness, poor mental health and sleep quality and low energy availability prior to the 2016 Summer Olympic Games. *British Journal of Sports Medicine* 52: 1-8.

Duhita, M.R., et al. 2017. Oral contraceptive pill alters acute dietary protein-induced yhermogenesis in young women. *Obesity* 25: 1482-1485.

Dulloo, A.G. 1999. Efficacy of a green tea extract rich in catechin polyphenols and caffeine in increasing 24-h energy expenditure and fat oxidation in humans. *The American Journal of Clinical Nutrition* 70: 1040-1045.

Duncan, S.H., and Belenguer, A. 2007. Reduced dietary intake of carbohydrates by obese subjects results in decreased concentrations of butyrate and butyrate-producing bacteria in feces. *Applied and Environmental Microbiology* 73: 1073-1078.

Earnest, C.P., et al. 2004. Effects of a commercial herbal-based formula on exercise performance in cyclists. *Medicine & Science in Sports & Exercise* 36: 504-509.

Ebbeling, C.B., et al. 2012. Effects of dietary composition on energy expenditure during weight-loss maintenance. *Journal of the American Medical Association* 307: 2627-2634.

Eelderink, C., et al. 2012. The glycemic response does not reflect the in vivo starch digestibility of fiber-rich wheat products in healthy men. *Journal of Nutrition* 142: 258-263.

Eelderink, C., et al. 2012. Slowly and rapidly digestible starch foods can elicit a similar glycemic response because of differential tissue glucose uptake in healthy men. *American Journal of Clinical Nutrition* 96: 1017-1024.

Engels, H.J., et al. 1997. No ergogenic effects of ginseng during graded maximal aerobic exercise. *Journal of the American Dietetic Association* 97: 1110-1115.

Ergogenic aids: Reported facts and claims. 1997. *Scan's Pulse Supplement, Winter,* 15-19.

Essen-Gustavsson, B., and P.A. Tesch. 1990. Glycogen and triglyceride utilization in relation to muscle metabolic characteristics in men performing heavy-resistance exercise. *European Journal of Applied Physiology* 61: 5-10.

Evans, W. 1996. The protective role of antioxidants in exercise induced oxidative stress. Keynote address, 13th Annual SCAN Symposium, Scottsdale, Arizona, April 28.

Fairfield, K.M., and R.H. Fletcher. 2002. Vitamins for chronic disease prevention in adults. *Journal of the American Medical Association* 287: 3116-3126.

Farinatti, P., et al. 2016. Oxygen consumption and substrate utilization during and after resistance exercises performed with different muscle mass. *International Journal of Exercise Science* 9: 77-88.

Fawcett, J.P., S.J. Farquhar, R.J. Walker, et al. 1996. The effect of oral vanadyl sulfate on body composition and performance in weight-training athletes. *International Journal of Sport Nutrition* 6: 382-390.

Fedor, D., and D.S. Kelley. 2009. Prevention of insulin resistance by n-3 polyunsaturated fatty acids. *Current Opinion in Clinical Nutrition and Metabolic Care* 12: 138-146.

Ferreira, M., et al. 1997. Effects of conjugated linoleic acid supplementation during resistance training on body composition and strength. *Journal of Strength and Conditioning Research* 11: 280.

Firth, G., and Manzo, L.G. 2004. Alcohol and athletic performance. Reprinted with permission: *For the Athlete: Alcohol and Athletic Performance.* University of Notre Dame.

Fogarty, M.C., et al. 2013. Acute and chronic watercress supplementation attenuates exercise-induced peripheral mononuclear cell DNA damage and lipid peroxidation. *British Journal of Nutrition* 109: 293-301.

Fogelholm, M. 1992. Micronutrient status in females during a 24-week fitness-type exercise program. *Annals of Nutrition and Metabolism* 36: 209-218.

Fogt, D.L., et al. 2000. Effects of post exercise carbohydrate-protein supplement on skeletal muscle glycogen storage. *Medicine & Science in Sports & Exercise* 2 (Suppl): Abstract No. 131.

Foley, D. 1984, April. Best health bets from the B team. *Prevention,* 62-67.

Frentsos, J.A., and J.R. Baer. 1997. Increased energy and nutrient intake during training and competition improves elite triathletes' endurance performance. *International Journal of Sport Nutrition* 7: 61-71.

Frey-Hewitt, K.M., K.M. Vranizan, D.M. Dreon, and P.D. Wood. 1990. The effect of weight loss by dieting or exercise on resting metabolic rate in overweight men. *International Journal of Obesity* 14: 327-334.

Friedl, K.E., R.J. Moore, L.E. Martinez-Lopez, et al. 1994. Lower limit of body fat in healthy active men. *Journal of Applied Physiology* 77: 933-940.

Galgani, J.E., et al. 2010. Effect of dihydrocapsiate on resting metabolic rate in humans. *American Journal of Clinical Nutrition* 92: 1089-1093.

Gaullier, J.M., et al. 2007. Six months supplementation with conjugated linoleic acid induces regional-specific fat mass decreases in overweight and obese. *British Journal of Nutrition* 97: 550-560.

Gerster, H. 1989. The role of vitamin C in athletic performance. *Journal of the American College of Nutrition* 8: 636-643.

Gerster, H. 1991. Function of vitamin E in physical exercise: A review. *Zeitschrift fur Ernahrungswissenschaft* 30: 89-97.

Gibala, M. 2009. Molecular responses to high-intensity interval exercise. *Applied Physiology, Nutrition, and Metabolism* 34: 428-432.

Gillette, C.A., R.C. Bullough, and C.L. Melby. 1994. Postexercise energy expenditure in response to acute aerobic or resistive exercise. *International Journal of Sport Nutrition* 4: 347-360.

Gillman, M.W., L.A. Cupples, D. Gagnon, et al. 1995. Protective effect of fruits and vegetables on development of stroke in men. *Journal of the American Medical Association* 273: 1113-1117.

Giovannucci, E., A. Ascherio, E.B. Rimm, et al. 1995. Intake of carotenoids and retinol in relation to risk of prostate cancer. *Journal of the National Cancer Institute* 87: 1767-1776.

Gisolfi, C.V., et al. 1992. Guidelines for optimal replacement beverages for different athletic events. *Medicine & Science in Sports & Exercise* 24: 679-687.

Goldfarb, A.H. 1999. Nutritional antioxidants as therapeutic and preventive modalities in exercise-induced muscle damage. *Canadian Journal of Applied Physiology* 24: 249-266.

Goldstein, E.R., et al. 2010. International Society of Sports Nutrition position stand: Caffeine and performance. *Journal of the International Society of Sports Nutrition* 7: 5.

Gornall, J., and R.G. Villani. 1996. Short-term changes in body composition and metabolism with severe dieting and resistance exercise. *International Journal of Sport Nutrition* 6: 285-294.

Goulet, E.D., et al. 2005. Assessment of the effects of eleutherococcus senticosus on endurance performance. *International Journal of Sport Nutrition and Exercise Metabolism* 15: 75-83.

Graef, J.L., et al. 2009. The effects of four weeks of creatine supplementation and high-intensity interval training on cardiorespiratory fitness: A randomized controlled trial. *Journal of the International Society of Sports Nutrition* 6: 18.

Green, A.L., E. Hultman, I.A. MacDonald, D.A. Sewell, and P.L. Greenhaff. 1996. Carbohydrate ingestion augments skeletal muscle creatine accumulation during creatine supplementation in humans. *American Journal of Physiology* 271: E821-E826.

Green, N.R., and A.A. Ferrando. 1994. Plasma boron and the effects of boron supplementation in males. *Environmental Health Perspective Supplement* 7: 73-77.

Groeneveld, G.J., et al. 2005. Few adverse effects of long-term creatine supplementation in a placebo-controlled trial. *International Journal of Sports Medicine* 26: 307-313.

Gross, M., et al. 1991. Ribose administration during exercise: Effects on substrates and products of energy metabolism in healthy subjects and a patient with myoadenylate deaminase deficiency. *Klinische Wochenschrift* 69: 151-155.

Guest N, et al. 2018. Caffeine, CYP1A2 Genotype, and Endurance Performance in Athletes. *Medicine & Science in Sports & Exercise.* doi: 10.1249/MSS.0000000000001596. [Epub ahead of print]

Haaz, S., et al. 2006. Citrus aurantium and synephrine alkaloids in the treatment of overweight and obesity: An update. *Obesity Reviews* 7: 79-88.

Habeck, M. 2002. A succulent cure to end obesity. *Drug Discovery Today* 7: 280-281.

Haff, G.G., et al. 1999. The effect of carbohydrate supplementation on multiple sessions and bouts of resistance exercise. *Journal of Strength and Conditioning Research* 13: 111-117.

Haff, G.G., et al. 2000. Carbohydrate supplementation attenuates muscle glycogen loss during acute bouts of resistance exercise. *International Journal of Sport Nutrition and Exercise Metabolism* 10: 326-339.

Hanausek, M., et al. 2003. Detoxifying cancer causing agents to prevent cancer. *Integrative Cancer Therapies* 2: 139-144.

Harberson, D.A. 1988. Weight gain and body composition of weightlifters: Effect of high-calorie supplementation vs. anabolic steroids. In *Report of the Ross Laboratories Symposium on muscle development: Nutritional alternatives to anabolic steroids,* ed. W.E. Garrett Jr. and T.E. Malone, 72-78. Columbus, OH: Ross Laboratories.

Hargreaves, M. 2000. Skeletal muscle metabolism during exercise in humans. *Clinical and Experimental Pharmacology and Physiology* 27: 225-228.

Hartung, G.H., J.P. Foreyt, R.S. Reeves, et al. 1990. Effect of alcohol dose on plasma lipoprotein subfractions and lipolytic enzyme activity in active and inactive men. *Metabolism* 39: 81-86.

Hasler, C.M. 1996. Functional foods: The western perspective. *Nutrition Reviews* 54 (11 Part 2): S6-S10.

Hassmen, P., et al. 1994. Branched-chain amino acid supplementation during 30-km competitive run: Mood and cognitive performance. *Nutrition* 10: 405-410.

Haub, M.D., et al. 2002. Effect of protein source on resistive-training-induced changes in body composition and muscle size in older men. *American Journal of Clinical Nutrition* 76: 511-517.

Havemann, L., et al. 1985. Fat adaptation followed by carbohydrate loading compromises high-intensity sprint performance. *Journal of Applied Physiology* 100: 194-202.

Hawley, J.A., and Leckey, J.J. 2015. Carbohydrate dependence during prolonged, intense endurance exercise. *Sports Medicine* 45 (Suppl 1): S5-S12.

Health, M.K., ed. 1982. *Diet manual, including a vegetarian meal plan,* 6th ed. Loma Linda, CA: Seventh Day Adventist Dietetic Association.

Heaney, R.P. 1993. Protein intake and the calcium economy. *Journal of the American Dietetic Association* 93: 1259-1260.

Heaton, L.E., et al. 2017. Selected in-season nutritional strategies to enhance recovery for team sport athletes: A practical overview. *Sports Medicine* 47: 2201–2218.

Hegewald, M.G., et al. 1991. Ribose infusion accelerates thallium redistribution with early imaging compared with late 24-hour imaging without ribose. *Journal of the American College of Cardiology* 18: 1671-1681.

Heinonen, O.J. 1996. Carnitine and physical exercise. *Sports Medicine* 22: 109-132.

Hemila, H. 1996. Vitamin C and common cold incidence: A review of studies with subjects under heavy physical stress. *International Journal of Sports Medicine* 17: 379-383.

Henderson, S., et al. 2005. Effects of coleus forskohlii supplementation on body composition and hematological profiles in mildly overweight women. *Journal of the International Society of Sports Nutrition* 2: 54-62.

Herbert, V., and K.C. Dos. 1994. Folic acid and vitamin B$_{12}$. In *Modern nutrition in health and disease, ed.* M. Shils, J. Olson, and M. Shike, 1430-1435. Philadelphia: Lea & Febiger.

Hickson, J.F., et al. 1987. Nutritional intake from food sources of high school football athletes. *Journal of the American Dietetic Association* 87: 1656-1659.

Hitchins, S., et al. 1999. Glycerol hyperhydration improves cycle time trial performance in hot, humid conditions. *European Journal of Applied Physiology and Occupational Physiology* 80: 494-501.

Hodgson, A.B., et al. 2013. The metabolic and performance effects of caffeine compared to coffee during endurance exercise. *PLoS One* 8:e59561.

Hoffman, J.R., et al. 2004. Effects of beta-hydroxy beta-methylbutyrate on power performance and indices of muscle damage and stress during high-intensity training. *Journal of Strength and Conditioning Research* 1: 747-752.

Holt, S.H., et al. 1999. The effects of high-carbohydrate vs high-fat breakfasts on feelings of fullness and alertness, and subsequent food intake. *International Journal of Food Sciences and Nutrition* 50: 13-28.

Houltham, S.D., and Rowlands, D.S. 2014. A snapshot of nitrogen balance in endurance-trained women. *Applied Physiology, Nutrition, and Metabolism* 39: 219-225.

Hulmi, J.J., et al. 2005. Protein ingestion prior to strength exercise affects blood hormones and metabolism. *Medicine & Science in Sports & Exercise* 37: 1990-1997.

Hymowitz, T. 2007. History of soy. National Soybean Research Laboratory. www.nsrl.uiuc.edu/aboutsoy/history.html.

International Association for Dance Medicine & Science. 2016. www.dancescience.org.

Irving, B.A., et al. 2008. Effect of exercise training intensity on abdominal visceral fat and body composition. *Medicine & Science in Sports & Exercise* 40: 1863-1872.

Ivy, J.L. 2002. Early postexercise muscle glycogen recovery is enhanced with a carbohydrate- protein supplement. *Journal of Applied Physiology* 93: 1337-1344.

Ivy, J.L., et al. 1988. Muscle glycogen storage after different amounts of carbohydrate ingestion. *Journal of Applied Physiology* 65: 2018-2023.

Jackman, M., P. Wendling, D. Friars, et al. 1994. Caffeine ingestion and high-intensity intermittent exercise. Abstract. Personal communication with Larry Spriet, University of Guelph, Ontario, Canada.

Jacobsen, B.H. 1990. Effect of amino acids on growth hormone release. *The Physician and Sportsmedicine* 18: 68.

Jäger, R. et al. 2008. The effects of creatine pyruvate and creatine citrate on performance during high intensity exercise. *Journal of the International Society of Sports Nutrition* 5: 4.

Jamurtas, A.Z., et al. 2011. The effects of low and high glycemic index foods on exercise performance and beta-endorphin responses. *Journal of the International Society of Sports Nutrition* 8: 15.

Jennings, E. 1995. Folic acid as a cancer-preventing agent. *Medical Hypotheses* 45: 297-303.

Ji, L.L. 1996. Exercise, oxidative stress, and antioxidants. *The American Journal of Sports Medicine* 24: S20-S24.

Josse, A.R. et al. 2011. Increased consumption of dairy foods and protein during diet-and exercise-induced weight loss promotes fat mass loss and lean mass gain in overweight and obese premenopausal women. *Journal of Nutrition* 141:1626-1634.

Kalman, D., et al. 2012. Comparison of coconut water and a carbohydrate-electrolyte sport drink on measures of hydration and physical performance in exercise-trained men. *Journal of the International Society of Sports Nutrition* 9: 1.

Kanarek, R. 1997. Psychological effects of snacks and altered meal frequency. *British Journal of Nutrition* 77 (Suppl): S105-S118.

Kanter, M.M., et al. 1995. Antioxidants, carnitine and choline as putative ergogenic aids. *International Journal of Sport Nutrition* 5: S120-S131.

Kanter, M.M., L.A. Nolte, and J.O. Holloszy. 1993. Effects of an antioxidant vitamin mixture on lipid peroxidation at rest and postexercise. *Journal of Applied Physiology* 74: 965-969.

Kaplan, S.A., et al. 2004. A prospective, 1-year trial using saw palmetto versus finasteride in the treatment of category III prostatitis/chronic pelvic pain syndrome. *Journal of Urology* 171: 284-288.

Katz, D.L., et al. 2015. Effects of egg ingestion on endothelial function in adults with coronary artery disease: A randomized, controlled, crossover trial. *American Heart Journal* 169: 162-169.

Kelly, G.S. 2001. Conjugated linoleic acid: A review. *Alternative Medicine Review* 6: 367-382.

Keim, N.L., T.F Barbieri, M.D. Van Loan, and B.L. Anderson. 1990. Energy expenditure and physical performance in overweight women: Response to training with and without caloric restriction. *Metabolism* 39: 651-658.

Keim, N.L., A.Z. Belko, and T.F. Barbieri. 1996. Body fat percentage and gender: Associations with exercise energy expenditure, substrate utilization, and mechanical work efficiency. *International Journal of Sport Nutrition* 6: 356-369.

Keith, R.E., K.A. O'Keefe, D.L. Blessing, and G.D. Wilson. 1991. Alterations in dietary carbohydrate, protein, and fat intake and mood state in trained female cyclists. *Medicine & Science in Sports & Exercise* 2: 212-216.

Keller, U., et al. 2003. Effects of changes in hydration on protein, glucose and lipid metabolism in man: Impact on health. *European Journal of Clinical Nutrition* 57 (Suppl 2): S69-74.

Kendrick, Z.V., M.B. Affrime, and D.T. Lowenthal. 1993. Effect of ethanol on metabolic responses to treadmill running in well-trained men. *Journal of Clinical Pharmacology* 33: 136-139.

Kennedy A, et al. 2010. Antiobesity mechanisms of action of conjugated linoleic acid. *Journal of Nutritional Biochemistry* 21 (3): 171-179.

Kerksick, C., et al. 2001. Bovine colostrum supplementation on training adaptations II: Performance. Abstract presented at Federation of American Societies for Experimental Biology (FASEB) meeting, Orlando, FL, March 31-April 4.

Kim, S.H., et al. 2005. Effects of Panax ginseng extract on exercise-induced oxidative stress. *The Journal of Sports Medicine and Physical Fitness* 45: 178-182.

Kingsley, M.I., et al. 2005. Effects of phosphatidylserine on oxidative stress following intermittent running. *Medicine & Science in Sports & Exercise* 37: 1300-1306.

Kingsley, M.I., et al. 2006. Effects of phosphatidylserine on exercise capacity during cycling in active males. *Medicine & Science in Sports & Exercise* 38: 64-71.

Kirkendall, D.T. 1998. Fluid and electrolyte replacement in soccer. *Clinics in Sports Medicine* 17: 729-738.

Kleiner, S.M. 1991. Performance-enhancing aids in sport: Health consequences and nutritional alternatives. *Journal of the American College of Nutrition* 10: 163-176.

Kleiner, S.M. 1999. Water: An essential but overlooked nutrient. *Journal of the American Dietetic Association* 99: 200-206.

Kleiner, S.M. 2000. Bodybuilding. In *Sports nutrition: A guide for the professional working with active people*, 3rd ed., ed. C.A. Rosenbloom. Chicago: SCAN, American Dietetic Association.

Kleiner, S.M., et al. 1989. Dietary influences on cardiovascular disease risk in anabolic steroid-using and non-using bodybuilders. *Journal of the American College of Nutrition* 8: 109-119.

Kleiner, S.M., et al. 1990. Metabolic profiles, diet, and health practices of championship male and female bodybuilders. *Journal of the American Dietetic Association* 90: 962-967.

Kleiner, S.M., et al. 1994. Nutritional status of nationally ranked elite bodybuilders. *International Journal of Sport Nutrition* 1: 54-69.

Koopman, R., et al. 2009. Ingestion of a protein hydrolysate is accompanied by an accelerated in vivo digestion and absorption rate when compared with its intact protein. *American Journal of Clinical Nutrition* 90: 106-115.

Kraemer, W.J., et al. 1998. Hormonal responses to consecutive days of heavy-resistance exercise with or without nutritional supplementation. *Journal of Applied Physiology* 85: 1544-1555.

Kreider, R.B. 1999. Dietary supplements and the promotion of muscle growth. *Sports Medicine* 27: 97-110.

Kreider, R.B. 2001. Nutritional considerations of overtraining. In *Sport supplements: A complete guide to physique and athletic enhancement, ed* J.R. Stout and J. Antonio, 199-208. Baltimore, MD: Lippincott, Williams & Wilkins.

Krieder, R.B. 2003. Effects of creatine supplementation on performance and training adaptations. *Molecular and Cellular Biochemistry* 244: 89-94.

Krieder, R.B. 2007. Effects of ingesting protein with various forms of carbohydrate following resistance-exercise on substrate availability and markers of anabolism, catabolism, and immunity. *Journal of the International Society of Sports Nutrition* 4: 18.

Kreider, R.B., R. Klesges, K. Harmon, et al. 1996. Effects of ingesting supplements designed to promote lean tissue accretion on body composition during resistance training. *International Journal of Sport Nutrition* 6: 234-246.

Kreider, R.B., V. Miriel, and E. Bertun. 1993. Amino acid supplementation and exercise performance: Analysis of the proposed ergogenic value. *Sports Medicine* 16: 190-209.

Kreider, R.B., et al. 1998a. Effects of conjugated linoleic acid (CLA) supplementation during resistance training on bone mineral content, bone mineral density, and markers of immune stress. *FASEB Journal* 12: A244.

Kreider, R.B., et al. 1998b. Effects of creatine supplementation on body composition, strength, and sprint performance. *Medicine & Science in Sports & Exercise* 30: 73-82.

Kreider, R.B., et al., eds. 1998c. *Overtraining in sport.* Champaign, IL: Human Kinetics.

Kreider, R.B., et al. 1999a. Effects of calcium b-hydroxy b-methylbutyrate (HMB) supplementation during resistance-training on markers of catabolism, body composition and strength. *International Journal of Sports Medicine* 22: 1-7.

Kreider, R.B., et al. 1999b. Effects of protein and amino-acid supplementation on athletic performance. *Sportscience* 3. http://sportscie.org/jour/9901/rbk.html.

Kreider, R.B., et al. 2000. Nutrition in exercise and sport. In *Frontiers in nutrition, ed.* T. Wilson and N. Temple, 207-239. Totowa, NJ: Humana Press.

Kreider, R.B., et al. 2001. Bovine colostrum supplementation on training adaptations I: Body composition. Abstract presented at Federation of American Societies for Experimental Biology (FASEB) meeting, Orlando, FL, March 31-April 4.

Kreider, R.B., et al. 2007. Effects of ingesting protein with various forms of carbohydrate following resistance-exercise on substrate availability and markers of anabolism, catabolism, and immunity. *Journal of the International Society of Sports Nutrition* 4: 18.

Kreider, R.B., et al. 2017. *Journal of the International Society of Sports Nutrition* 14: 18.

Krieder, R.B., et al. 2010. Research and recommendations. *Journal of the International Society of Sports Nutrition* 7: 7.

Krochmal, R., et al. 2004. Phytochemical assays of commercial botanical dietary supplements. *Evidence-Based Complementary and Alternative Medicine* 1: 305-313.

Laaksonen, R., et al. 1995. Ubiquinone supplementation and exercise capacity in trained young and older men. *European Journal of Applied Physiology* 72: 95-100.

Lamb, D.R., K.F. Rinehardt, R.L. Bartels, et al. 1990. Dietary carbohydrate and intensity of interval swim training. *The American Journal of Clinical Nutrition* 52: 1058-1063.

Lambert, C.P., M.G. Flynn, J.B. Boone, et al. 1991. Effects of carbohydrate feeding on multiple-bout resistance exercise. *Journal of Applied Sport Science Research* 5: 192-197.

Lambert, C.P., et al. 2004. Macronutrient considerations for the sport of bodybuilding. *Sports Medicine* 34: 317-327.

Lambert, M.I., et al. 1993. Failure of commercial oral amino acid supplements to increase serum growth hormone concentrations in male bodybuilders. *International Journal of Sport Nutrition* 3: 298-305.

Lands, L.C., et al. 1999. Effect of supplementation with cysteine donor on muscular performance. *Journal of Applied Physiology* 87: 1381-1385.

Lane, L. 1999, September 17. Nutritionist calls for tighter regulation of supplements. CNN.com News.

Langfort, J., et al. 1997. The effect of a low-carbohydrate diet on performance, hormonal and metabolic responses to a 30-s bout of supramaximal exercise. *European Journal of Applied Physiology and Occupational Physiology* 76: 128-133.

Layman, D.K. 2002. Role of leucine in protein metabolism during exercise and recovery. *Canadian Journal of Applied Physiology* 27: 646-663.

Lee, E.C., et al. 2010. Ergogenic effects of betaine supplementation on strength and power performance. *Journal of the International Society of Sports Nutrition* 7: 27

Lefavi, R.G., R.A. Anderson, R.E. Keith, et al. 1992. Efficacy of chromium supplementation in athletes: Emphasis on anabolism. *International Journal of Sport Nutrition* 2: 111-122.

Leiper, J.B., et al. 2000. Improved gastric emptying rate in humans of a unique glucose polymer with gel-forming properties. *Scandinavian Journal of Gastroenterology* 35: 1143-1149.

Lemon, P.W.R. 1991. Effect of exercise on protein requirements. *Journal of Sports Sciences* 9: 53-70.

Lemon, P.W.R. 1994, November 11-12. Dietary protein and amino acids. Presented at Nutritional Ergogenic Aids Conference sponsored by the Gatorade Sports Institute, Chicago.

Lemon, P.W.R. 2000. Beyond the zone: Protein needs of active individuals. *Journal of the American College of Nutrition* 19: 513S-521S.

Lemon, P.W.R., et al. 1992. Protein requirements and muscle mass/strength changes during intensive training in novice bodybuilders. *Journal of Applied Physiology* 73: 767-775.

Lemon, P.W., et al. 2002. The role of protein and amino acid supplements in the athlete's diet: Does type or timing of ingestion matter? *Current Sports Medicine Reports* 1: 214-221.

Li, J.J., et al. 2008. Anti-obesity effects of conjugated linoleic acid, docosahexaenoic acid, and eicosapentaenoic acid. *Molecular Nutrition & Food Research* 52: 631-645.

Liang, M.T., et al. 2005. Panax notoginseng supplementation enhances physical performance during endurance exercise. *Journal of Strength and Conditioning Research* 19: 108-114.

Liberti, L.E., et al. 1978. Evaluation of commercial ginseng products. *Journal of Pharmaceutical Sciences* 67: 1487-1489.

Liese, A.D., et al. 2005. Dietary glycemic index and glycemic load, carbohydrate and fiber intake, and measures of insulin sensitivity, secretion, and adiposity in the Insulin Resistance Atherosclerosis Study. *Diabetes Care* 12: 2832-2838.

Lim, S., et al. 2011. Antioxidant enzymes induced by repeated intake of excess energy in the form of high-fat, high-carbohydrate meals are not sufficient to block oxidative stress in healthy lean individuals. *British Journal of Nutrition* 106: 1544-1551.

Linde, K., et al. 2006, January 25. Echinacea for preventing and treating the common cold. *Cochrane Database of Systematic Reviews*: CD000530.

Little, J.P., et al. 2010. A practical model of low-volume high-intensity interval training induces mitochondrial biogenesis in human skeletal muscle: Potential mechanisms. *Journal of Physiology* 588: 1011-1022.

Longland, T.M., et al. 2016. Higher compared with lower dietary protein during an energy deficit combined with intense exercise promotes greater lean mass gain and fat mass loss: A randomized trial. *American Journal of Clinical Nutrition* 103: 738–746.

Loucks, A.B. 2007. Low energy availability in the marathon and other endurance sports. *Sports Medicine* 37: 348-352.

Louis-Sylvestre, J., et al. 2003. Highlighting the positive impact of increasing feeding frequency on metabolism and weight management. *Forum of Nutrition* 56: 126-128.

Lowe, B. 2000. Powerful products. *Nutritional Outlook* 3: 37-43.

Lowery, L., et al. 2006. Protein and overtraining: Potential applications for free-living athletes. *Journal of the International Society of Sports Nutrition* 3: 42-50.

Lucas, L., et al. 2011. Molecular mechanisms of inflammation. Anti-inflammatory benefits of virgin olive oil and the phenolic compound oleocanthal. *Current Pharmaceutical Design* 17: 754-768.

Ludwig, D.S., et al. 2001. Relation between consumption of sugar-sweetened drinks and childhood obesity: A prospective, observational analysis. *Lancet* 357: 505-508.

Luhovyy, B.L., et al. 2007. Whey proteins in the regulation of food intake and satiety. *Journal of the American College of Nutrition* 26: 704S-712S.

Lukaski, H.C. 2000. Magnesium, zinc, and chromium nutriture and physical activity. *American Journal of Clinical Nutrition* 72 (Suppl. 2): 585S-593S.

Lukaszuk, J.M., et al. 2005. Effect of a defined lacto-ovo-vegetarian diet and oral creatine monohydrate supplementation on plasma creatine concentration. *Journal of Strength and Conditioning Research* 19: 735-740.

Lupton, J.R., et al. 2016. Nutrient reference value: Noncommunicable disease endpoints—A conference report. *European Journal of Nutrition* 55: (Suppl 1): S1–S10.

MacLean, D.B., and L.G. Luo. 2004. Increased ATP content/production in the hypothalamus may be a signal for energy-sensing of satiety: Studies of the anorectic mechanism of a plant steroidal glycoside. *Brain Research* 1020: 1-11.

Maki, K.C., et al. 2009. Green tea catechin consumption enhances exercise-induced abdominal fat loss in overweight and obese adults. *Journal of Nutrition* 139: 264-270.

Malm, C., et al. 1996. Supplementation with ubiquinone-10 causes cellular damage during intense exercise. *Acta Physiologica Scandinavica* 157: 511-512.

Manabe, I. 2011. Chronic inflammation links cardiovascular, metabolic and renal diseases. *Circulation Journal* 75: 2739-2748.

Mann, T.N., et al. 2017. Relationship between perceived exertion during exercise and subsequent recovery measurements. *Biology of Sport* 34: 3-9.

Manore, M.M. 2000a. Effect of physical activity on thiamine, riboflavin, and vitamin B-6 requirements. *American Journal of Clinical Nutrition* 72: 598S-606S.

Manore, M.M. 2000b. *Sports nutrition for health and performance*. Champaign, IL: Human Kinetics.

Manore, M.M., J. Thompson, and M. Russo. 1993. Diet and exercise strategies of a world-class bodybuilder. *International Journal of Sport Nutrition* 3: 76-86.

Manson, J.E., W.C. Willett, M.J. Stampfer, et al. 1994. Vegetable and fruit consumption and incidence of stroke in women. *Circulation* 89: 932.

Marette, A., et al. 2001. Prevention of skeletal muscle insulin resistance by dietary cod protein in high fat-fed rats. *American Journal of Physiology, Endocrinology, and Metabolism* 281: E62-E71.

Marquezi, M.L., et al. 2003. Effect of aspartate and asparagine supplementation on fatigue determinants in intense exercise. *International Journal of Sport Nutrition and Exercise Metabolism* 13: 65-75.

Matthan, N.R. 2007. Effect of soy protein from differently processed products on cardiovascular disease risk factors and vascular endothelial function in hypercholesterolemic subjects. *American Journal of Clinical Nutrition* 85: 960-966.

Maughan, R.J., and D.C. Poole. 1981. The effects of a glycogen-loading regimen on the capacity to perform anaerobic exercise. *European Journal of Applied Physiology* 46: 211-219.

Mazer, E. 1981, July. Biotin—The little known lifesaver. *Prevention*, 97-102.

McAfee, A.J., et al. 2011. Red meat from animals offered a grass diet increases plasma and platelet n-3 PUFA in healthy consumers. *British Journal of Nutrition* 105: 80-89.

McAnulty, S.R., et al. 2005. Effect of resistance exercise and carbohydrate ingestion on oxidative stress. *Free Radical Research* 39: 1219-1224.

McDermott, B.P., and Anderson, S.A. 2017. National Athletic Trainers' Association Position Statement: Fluid Replacement for the Physically Active. *Journal of Athletic Training* 52: 877–895.

McNaughton, L.R., et al. 1997. Neutralize acid to enhance performance. *Sportscience Training & Technology*. www.sportsci.org/traintech/buffer/lrm.htm.

McNulty, S.R., et al. 2005. Effect of alpha-tocopherol supplementation on plasma homocysteine and oxidative stress in highly trained athletes before and after exhaustive exercise. *The Journal of Nutritional Biochemistry* 16: 530-537.

Mekkes, et al. 2014. The development of probiotic treatment in obesity: a review. *Beneficial Microbes* 5: 19-28.

Mendel, R.W., et al. 2005. Effects of creatine on thermoregulatory responses while exercising in the heat. *Nutrition* 21: 301-307.

Mero, A. 1999. Leucine supplementation and intensive training. *Sports Medicine* 27: 347-358.

Mettler. S., et al. 2009. Development and validation of a food pyramid for Swiss athletes. *International Journal of Sport Nutrition and Exercise Metabolism* 19: 504-518.

Meydani, M., et al. 1993. Protective effect of vitamin E on exercise-induced oxidative damage in young and older adults. *American Journal of Physiology* 264 (5 Part 2): R992-998.

Miller, W.C., M.G. Niederpruem, J.P. Wallace, and A.K. Lindeman. 1994. Dietary fat, sugar, and fiber predict body fat content. *Journal of the American Dietetic Association* 94: 612-615.

Montain, S.N., et al. 2006. Exercise associated hyponatraemia: Quantitative analysis to understand the aetiology. *British Journal of Sports Medicine* 40: 98-106.

Morifuji, M., et al. 2005. Dietary whey protein downregulates fatty acid synthesis in the liver, but upregulates it in skeletal muscle of exercise-trained rats. *Nutrition* 21: 1052-1058.

Mosoni, L., et al. 2003. Type and timing of protein feeding to optimize anabolism. *Current Opinion in Clinical Nutrition and Metabolic Care* 6: 301-306.

Mountjoy, M., et al. 2014. The IOC consensus statement: Beyond the female athlete triad— Relative energy deficiency in sport. *British Journal of Sports Medicine* 48: 491–497.

Nagao, T., et al. 2005. Ingestion of a tea rich in catechins leads to a reduction in body fat and malondialdehyde-modified LDL in men. *American Journal of Clinical Nutrition* 81: 122-129.

National Cholesterol Education Program. 2006. *ATP III guidelines at-a-glance quick desk reference.* Washington, DC: USDHHS, Public Health Service, NIH, NHLBI.

National Research Council. 1989. *Diet and health: Implications for reducing chronic disease risk.* Washington, DC: National Academy Press.

National Research Council, Food and Nutrition Board. 1989. *Recommended dietary allowances,* 10th ed. Washington, DC: National Academy Press.

Nazar, K., et al. 1996. Phosphate supplementation prevents a decrease of triiodothyronine and increases resting metabolic rate during low energy diet. *Journal of Physiology and Pharmacology* 47: 373-383.

Nelson, G. 2001, September/October. American Heart Association calls for eating fish twice per week—What's a vegetarian to do? *Vegetarian Journal.* www.vrg.org/journal/vj2001sep/2001sepomega3.htm.

Nestle, M. 2012, June 19. Debunking the health claims of genetically modified foods. *The Atlantic Monthly.* www.theatlantic.com/health/archive/2012/06/debunking-the-health-claims-of-genetically-modified-foods/258665.

The new diet pills: Fairly but not completely safe. 1996. *Harvard Heart Letter* 7: 1-2.

Newhouse, I.J., et al. 2000. The effects of magnesium supplementation on exercise performance. *Clinical Journal of Sport Medicine* 10: 195-200.

Neychev, V.K. 2005. The aphrodisiac herb Tribulus terrestris does not influence the androgen production in young men. *Journal of Ethnopharmacology* 101: 319-323.

Nicholas, C.W., et al. 1999. Carbohydrate-electrolyte ingestion during intermittent high-intensity running. *Medicine & Science in Sports & Exercise* 31: 1280-1286.

Nielsen, F.H., et al. 2004. A moderately high intake compared to a low intake of zinc depresses magnesium balance and alters indices of bone turnover in postmenopausal women. *European Journal of Clinical Nutrition* 58: 703-710.

Nissen, S., R. Sharp, M. Ray, et al. 1996. Effect of leucine metabolite beta-hydroxy betamethylbutyrate on muscle metabolism during resistance-exercise training. *Journal of Applied Physiology* 81: 2095-2104.

Noakes, M., et al. 2004. Meal replacements are as effective as structured weight-loss diets for treating obesity in adults with features of metabolic syndrome. *Journal of Nutrition* 134: 1894-1899.

Noakes, T.D., et al. 2005. Three independent biological mechanisms cause exercise-associated hyponatremia: Evidence from 2,135 weighed competitive athletic performances. *Proceedings of the National Academy of Sciences of the United States* 102: 18550-18550.

Noble, E.E., at al. 2017. Gut to brain dysbiosis: mechanisms linking Western diet consumption, the microbiome, and cognitive impairment. *Frontiers in Behavioral Neuroscience* 11: 9.

Norris LE, et al. 2009. Comparison of dietary conjugated linoleic acid with safflower oil on body composition in obese postmenopausal women with type 2 diabetes mellitus. *American Journal of Clinical Nutrition* 90: 468-476.

Oakley, G.P., M.J. Adams, and C.M. Dickinson. 1996. More folic acid for everyone, now. *Journal of Nutrition* 126: 751S-755S.

O'Connor, D.M., et al. 2003. The effects of beta-hydroxy-beta-methylbutyrate (HMB) and HMB/creatine supplementation on indices of health in highly trained athletes. *International Journal of Sport Nutrition and Exercise Metabolism* 13: 184-197.

Olney, J. 1996, December 29. Transcript from *60 Minutes.* New York: CBS.

Palazon-Bru, A., et al. 2017. Screening tool to determine risk of having muscle dysmorphia symptoms in men who engage in weight training at a gym. *Clinical Journal of Sport Medicine* 2017, December 20: 1-6.

Parker, A.G., et al. 2011. The effects of IQPLUS Focus on cognitive function, mood and endocrine response before and following acute exercise. *Journal of the International Society of Sports Nutrition* 8: 16.

Parrott, S. 1999, October 14. Herbs said harmful before surgery. AOL News.

Peake, J., et al. 2004. Neutrophil activation, antioxidant supplements and exercise-induced oxidative stress. *Exercise Immunology Review* 10: 129-141.

Pedlar, C.R., et al. 2017. Iron balance and iron supplementation for the female athlete: A practical approach. *European Journal of Sport Science* 27:1-11.

Peeke, Pamela. 2005. Body for life for women: A woman's plan for physical and mental transformation. Emmaus, PA: Rodale.

Penry, J.T., and Manore, M.M. 2008. Choline: An important micronutrient for maximal endurance-exercise performance? *International Journal of Sport Nutrition and Exercise Metabolism* 18 (2): 191-203

Peyrot des Gachons, C., et al. 2011. Unusual pungency from extra-virgin olive oil is attributable to restricted spatial expression of the receptor of oleocanthal. *The Journal of Neuroscience* 31: 999-1009.

Phillips, S.M. 2009. The role of milk- and soy-based protein in support of muscle protein synthesis and muscle protein accretion in young and elderly persons. *Journal of the American College of Nutrition* 28: 343-354.

Phillips, S.M., et al. 2005. Dietary protein to support anabolism with resistance exercise in young men. *Journal of the American College of Nutrition* 24: 134S-139S.

Phillips, S.M., et al. 2009. Effects on mixed muscle protein synthesis at ingestion. *Journal of Applied Physiology* 107: 987-992.

Pieralisi, G. 1991. Effects of standardized ginseng extract combined with dimethylaminoethanol bitartrate, vitamins, minerals, and trace elements on physical performance during exercise. *Clinical Therapeutics* 13: 373-382.

Pline, K.A., et al. 2005. The effect of creatine intake on renal function. *The Annals of Pharmacotherapy* 39: 1093-1096.

Plourde M, et al. 2008. Conjugated linoleic acids: Why the discrepancy between animal and human studies? *Nutrition Reviews* 66 (7): 415-421.

Poortmans, J.R., et al. 2000. Do regular high protein diets have potential health risks on kidney function in athletes? *International Journal of Sport Nutrition and Exercise Metabolism* 10: 28-38.

Rains T.M., S. Agarwal, and K.C. Maki. Antiobesity effects of green tea catechins: A mechanistic review. *The Journal of Nutritional Biochemistry* 22 (1): 1-7.

Ramel, A., et al. 2008. Beneficial effects of long-chain n-3 fatty acids included in an energy-restricted diet on insulin resistance in overweight and obese European young adults. *Diabetologia* 51: 1261-1268.

Rankin, P., et al. 2018. The effect of milk on recovery from repeat-sprint cycling in female teamsport athletes. *Applied Physiology, Nutrition, and Metabolism* 43:113-122.

Rehrer, N.J. 2001. Fluid and electrolyte balance in ultra-endurance sport. *Sports Medicine* 31: 701-715.

Reilly, T. 1997. Energetics of high-intensity exercise (soccer) with particular reference to fatigue. *Journal of Sports Science* 15: 257-263.

Richards, J.B., et al. 2007. Higher serum vitamin D concentrations are associated with longer leukocyte telomere length in women. *American Journal of Clinical Nutrition* 86: 1420-1425.

Riserus, U., et al. 2001. Conjugated linoleic acid (CLA) reduced abdominal adipose tissue in obese middle-aged men with signs of the metabolic syndrome: A randomised controlled trial. *International Journal of Obesity and Related Metabolic Disorders* 25: 1129-1135.

Robergs, R.A. 1998. Glycerol hyperhydration to beat the heat? *Sportscience Training & Technology.* www.sportsci.org/traintech/glycerol/rar.htm.

Roberts, M.D., et al. 2011. Ingestion of a high-molecular-weight hydrothermally modified waxy maize starch alters metabolic responses to prolonged exercise in trained cyclists. *Nutrition* 27: 659-665.

Robinson, M.M., et al. 2017. Enhanced protein translation underlies improved metabolic and physical adaptations to different exercise training modes in young and old humans. *Cell Metabolism* 25: 581-592.

Rolls, BJ. 2009. The relationship between dietary energy density and energy intake. *Physiology & Behavior* 97 (5): 609-615.

Rolls, B.J., et al. 1988. The specificity of satiety: The influence of foods of different macronutrient content on the development of satiety. *Physiology and Behavior* 43: 145-153.

Rosse, A.R., et al. 2010. Effects of capsinoid ingestion on energy expenditure and lipid oxidation at rest and during exercise. *Nutrition & Metabolism* 7: 65.

Rossi, K.A. 2017. Nutritional aspects of the female athlete. *Clinics in Sports Medicine* 36: 627–653.

Rowlands, D.S., et al. 2011. Effect of high-protein feeding on performance and nitrogen balance in female cyclists. *Medicine & Science in Sports & Exercise* 43: 44-53.

Roy, B.D., et al. 2002. The influence of post-exercise macronutrient intake on energy balance and protein metabolism in active females participating in endurance training. *International Journal of Sport Nutrition and Exercise Metabolism* 12: 172-188.

Roy, B.D., et al. 2005. Creatine monohydrate supplementation does not improve functional recovery after total knee arthroplasty. *Archives of Physical Medicine and Rehabilitation* 86: 1293-1298.

Sachan, D.S., et al. 2005. Decreasing oxidative stress with choline and carnitine in women. *Journal of the American College of Nutrition* 24: 172-176.

Sacks, F.M. et al. 2014. Effects of high vs. low glycemic index of dietary carbohydrate on cardiovascular disease risk factors and insulin sensitivity: The OmniCarb Randomized Clinical Trial. *Journal of the American Medical Association* 312: 2531-2541.

Salter, J., et al. 2017. Low energy availability in exercising women: Historical perspectives and future directions. *Sports Medicine* 47: 207–220.

Sanchez, et al. 2014. Effect of Lactobacillus rhamnosus CGMCC1.3724 supplementation on weight loss and maintenance in obese men and women. *British Journal of Nutrition* 111: 1507-1519.

Sandsa, A.L., et al. 2009. Consumption of the slow-digesting waxy maize starch leads to blunted plasma glucose and insulin response but does not influence energy expenditure or appetite in humans. *Nutrition Research* 29: 383-390.

Sapone, A., et al. 2011. Divergence of gut permeability and mucosal immune gene expression in two gluten-associated conditions: celiac disease and gluten sensitivity. *BMC Medicine* 9: 23.

Sarubin, A. 2000. *The health professional's guide to popular dietary supplements.* Chicago: The American Dietetic Association, 184-188.

Saunders, M.J., et al. 2005. Effects of a carbohydrate/protein gel on exercise performance in male and female cyclists. *Journal of the International Society of Sports Nutrition* 2(1): 1-30.

Schabort, E.J., et al. 1999. The effect of a preexercise meal on time to fatigue during prolonged cycling exercise. *Medicine & Science in Sports & Exercise* 31: 464-471.

Schardt, D. 2006. Soyonara? *Nutrition Action Health Letter* 33: 1-7.

Schaun, G.Z., et al. 2017. Acute effects of highintensity interval training and moderateintensity continuous training sessions on cardiorespiratory parameters in healthy young men. *European Journal of Applied Physiology* 117: 1437-1444.

Schenk, S., et al. 2003. Different glycemic indexes of breakfast cereals are not due to glucose entry into blood but to glucose removal by tissue. *American Journal of Clinical Nutrition* 78: 742-748.

Schleppenbach, L., et al. 2017. Speed- and circuit-based high-intensity interval training on recovery oxygen consumption. *International Journal of Exercise Science* 10: 942-953.

Schoenfeld, B. 2011. Does cardio after an overnight fast maximize fat loss? *Journal of the National Strength and Conditioning Association* 33(1): 23-25.

Schwalfenberg, G.K. 2012. The alkaline diet: Is there evidence that an alkaline pH diet benefits health? *Journal of Environmental and Public Health* 727630.

Seaton, T.B., S.L. Welle, M.K. Warenko, and R.G. Campbell. 1986. Thermic effect of medium and long chain triglycerides in man. *The American Journal of Clinical Nutrition* 44: 630-634.

Seidle, R., et al. 2000. A taurine and caffeine-containing drink stimulates cognitive performance and well-being. *Amino Acids* 19: 635-642.

Shafer, K. 2009. Validity of segmental multiple-frequency bioelectrical impedance analysis to estimate body composition of adults across a range of body mass indexes. *William Nutrition* 25: 25–32.

Shaw, S.D., D. Brenner, M.L. Berger, D.O. Carpeter, C.S. Hong, and K. Kannan. 2006. PCBs,

PCDD/Fs, and organochlorine pesticides in farmed Atlantic salmon from Maine, eastern Canada, and Norway, and wild salmon from Alaska. *Environmental Science & Technology* 40 (17): 5347-5354.

Shugarman, A.E. 1999. Trends in the sports nutrition industry. *Nutraceuticals World* 2: 56-59.

Siekaniec, C., et al. The effects of alcohol on performance. *NSCA Coach*: 10-12, nsca.com.

Silk, D.B.A., et al. 2008. Clinical trial: The effects of a trans-galactooligosaccharide prebiotic on faecal microbiota and symptoms in irritable bowel syndrome. *Alimentary Pharmacology & Therapeutics* 29: 508-518.

Silva, M.R., and Paiva, T. 2014. Low energy availability and low body fat of female gymnasts before an international competition. *European Journal of Sport Science* 15: 591-599.

Simko, M.D., and J. Jarosz. 1990. Organic foods: Are they better? *Journal of the American Dietetic Association* 90: 367-370.

Singh, A., et al. 1994. Exercise-induced changes in immune function: Effects of zinc supplementation. *Journal of Applied Physiology* 76: 2298-2303.

Slavin, J.L. 1991. Assessing athletes' nutritional status. *The Physician and Sportsmedicine* 19: 79-94.

Smart waters. 2000. BevNet. www.bevnet.com/ reviews/smartwater/index/asp.

Snitker, S., et al. 2009. Effects of novel capsinoid treatment on fatness and energy metabolism in humans: Possible pharmacogenetic implications. *American Journal of Clinical Nutrition* 89: 45-50.

Somer, E. 1996, May. Maximum energy: How to eat and exercise for it. *Working Woman*, 72-76.

Speechly, D.P., et al. 1999. Greater appetite control associated with an increased frequency of eating in lean males. *Appetite* 33: 285-297.

Spriet, L.L. 1995. Caffeine and performance. *International Journal of Sport Nutrition* 5: S84-S99.

Spriet, L.L., et al. 2004. Nutritional strategies to influence adaptations to training. *Journal of Sports Sciences* 22: 127-141.

St-Onge, M-P. 2005. Dietary fats, teas, dairy, and nuts: Potential functional foods for weight control. *American Journal of Clinical Nutrition* 81: 7-15.

St-Onge, M-P., and Bosarge, A. 2008. Weight-loss diet that includes consumption of medium-chain triacylglycerol oil leads to a greater rate of weight and fat mass loss than does olive oil. *American Journal of Clinical Nutrition* 87: 621-626.

St-Onge, M-P., et al. 2007. Supplementation with soy-protein-rich foods does not enhance weight loss. *Journal of the American Dietetic Association* 107: 500-505.

Stanko, R.T., et al. 1996. Inhibition of regain in body weight and fat with addition of 3-carbon compounds to the diet with hyperenergetic refeeding after weight reduction. *International Journal of Obesity Related Metabolic Disorders* 20: 925-930.

Steinmetz, K.A., et al. 1996. Vegetables, fruit, and cancer prevention: A review. *Journal of the American Dietetic Association* 96: 1027-1039.

Stephens, F.B., et al. 2006a. An acute increase in skeletal muscle carnitine content alters fuel metabolism in resting human skeletal muscle. *The Journal of Clinical Endocrinology & Metabolism* 91: 5013-5018.

Stephens, F.B., et al. 2006b. Insulin stimulates L-carnitine accumulation in human skeletal muscle. *The FASEB Journal* 20: 377-379.

Stephens, F.B., et al. 2007a. Carbohydrate ingestion augments L-carnitine retention in humans. *Journal of Applied Physiology* 102: 1065-1070.

Stephens, F.B., et al. 2007b. New insights concerning the role of carnitine in the regulation of fuel metabolism in skeletal muscle. *Journal of Physiology* 581: 431-444.

Stephens, F.B., et al. 2007c. A threshold exists for the stimulatory effect of insulin on plasma L-carnitine clearance in humans. *American Journal of Physiology, Endocrinology and Metabolism* 292: E637-E641.

Stewart, A.M. 1999. Amino acids and athletic performance: A mini-conference in Oxford. *Sportscience Training & Technology.* www.sportsci.org/jour/9902/ams.html.

Stofilova, J. et al. 2015. Co-administration of a probiotic strain Lactobacillus plantarum LS/07 CCM7766 with prebiotic inulin alleviates the intestinal inflammation in rats exposed to N,N-dimethylhydrazine. *Internal Immunopharmacology* 24: 361-368.

Stone, N. 1996. AHA medical/scientific statement on fish consumption, fish oil, lipids, and coronary heart disease. www.americanheart.org.

Stout, J.R., et al. 2001. Effects of resistance exercise and creatine supplementation on myasthenia gravis: A case study. *Medicine & Science in Sports & Exercise* 33: 869-872.

Stout, J.R., et al. 2006. Effects of 28 days of beta-alanine and creatine monohydrate supplementation on physical working capacity at neuromuscular fatigue threshold. *The Journal of Strength and Conditioning* 20(4): 1550-2783.

Stuessi, C., et al. 2005. L -Carnitine and the recovery from exhaustive endurance exercise: A randomised, double-blind, placebo-controlled trial. *European Journal of Applied Physiology* 95: 431-435.

Szlyk, P.C., R.P. Francesconi, M.S. Rose, et al. 1991. Incidence of hypohydration when consuming carbohydrate-electrolyte solutions during field training. *Military Medicine* 156: 399-402.

Tagliabue, A., et al. 2017. Short-term impact of a classical ketogenic diet on gut microbiota in GLUT1 Deficiency Syndrome: A 3-month prospective observational study. *Clinical Nutrition* 17: 33-37.

Taku, K., et al. 2007. Soy isoflavones lower serum total and LDL cholesterol in humans: A meta-analysis of 11 randomized controlled trials. *American Journal of Clinical Nutrition* 85: 1148-1156.

Talanian, J.I., et al. 2007. Two weeks of high-intensity aerobic interval training increases the capacity for fat oxidation during exercise in women. *Journal of Applied Physiology* 102: 1439-1447.

Tarnopolsky, M.A. 1998. Influence of differing macronutrient intakes on muscle glycogen resynthesis after resistance training. *Journal of Applied Physiology* 84: 890-896.

Tarnopolsky, M.A., et al. 1992. Evaluation of protein requirements for trained strength athletes. *Journal of Applied Physiology* 73: 1986-1995.

Tarnopolsky, M.A., et al. 1997. Postexercise protein-carbohydrate supplements increase muscle glycogen in men and women. *Journal of Applied Physiology* 83: 1877-1883.

Thomas, D.E., et al. 1991. Carbohydrate feeding before exercise: Effect of glycemic index. *International Journal of Sports Medicine* 12: 180-186.

Thomas, D.T., et al. 2016. Position of the Academy of Nutrition and Dietetics, Dietitians of Canada, and the American College of Sports Medicine: Nutrition and Athletic Performance. *Journal of the Academy of Nutrition and Dietetics* 116: 501-528.

Thornton, J.S. 1990. How can you tell when an athlete is too thin? *The Physician and Sportsmedicine* 18: 124-133.

Tiidus, P.M., et al. 1995. Vitamin E status and response to exercise training. *Sports Medicine* 20: 12-23.

The triad. 2006. www.femaleathletetriad.org.

Trimmer, R., et al. 2005. Effects of two naturally occurring aromatase inhibitors on male hormonal and blood chemistry profiles. *Journal of the International Society of Sports Nutrition* 2: 14.

Trumbo, P., et al. 2001. Dietary reference intakes. *Journal of the American Dietetic Association* 101 (3): 294-301.

Tsang. G. 2006. Which sweeteners are safe? www.healthcastle.com/sweeteners.shtml.

Tsuji, K., et al. Effects of short-lasting supra-maximal-intensity exercise on diet-induced increase in oxygen uptake. *Physiological Reports* 5: e13506.

Tullson, P.C., et al. 1991. Adenine nucleotide synthesis in exercising and endurance-trained skeletal muscle. *American Journal of Physiology* 261 (2 Part 1): C342-347.

Tyler, V.E. 1987. *The new honest herbal: A sensible guide to the use of herbs and related remedies.* Philadelphia: George F. Stickley Co.

U.S. Department of Agriculture. 1998, August 11. USDA urges consumers to use food thermometer when cooking ground beef patties. Washington, DC: USDA.

U.S. Department of Agriculture and U.S. Department of Health and Human Services. 1995. Nutrition and your health: Dietary guidelines for Americans. Washington, DC: Government Printing Office.

Van Someren, K.A., et al. 2005. Supplementation with beta-hydroxy-beta-methylbutyrate (HMB) and alpha-ketoisocaproic acid (KIC) reduces signs and symptoms of exercise-induced muscle damage in man. *International Journal of Sport Nutrition and Exercise Metabolism* 15: 413-424.

Van Zyl, C.G., et al. 1996. Effects of medium-chain triglyceride ingestion on fuel metabolism and cycling performance. *Journal of Applied Physiology* 80: 2217-2225.

Vanhatalo, A., et al. 2010. Acute and chronic effects of dietary nitrate supplementation on blood pressure and the physiological responses to moderate-intensity and incremental exercise. *American Journal of Physiology—Regulatory, Integrative and Comparative Physiology* 299: R1121–R1131.

Vanheesti, J.L., et al. 2014. Ovarian suppression impairs sport performance in junior elite female swimmers. *Medicine and Science in Sports and Exercise* 46: 156-166.

Vieira, A.T., et al. 2013. The role of probiotics and prebiotics in inducing gut immunity. *Frontiers in Immunology* 4: 445.

Viitala, P.E., et al. 2004a. The effects of antioxidant vitamin supplementation on resistance exercise induced lipid peroxidation in trained and untrained participants. *Lipids in Health and Disease* 3: 14.

Viitala, P.E., et al. 2004b. Vitamin E supplementation, exercise and lipid peroxidation in human participants. *European Journal of Applied Physiology* 93: 108-115.

Vikoren, L.A., et al. 2013. A randomised study on the effects of fish protein supplement on glucose tolerance, lipids and body composition in overweight adults. *British Journal of Nutrition* 109: 648-657.

Vitamin drink. 2000. *Nutritional Outlook* 3: 70.

Vitamin E pills: Now it's thumbs down. 2005. Consumer Reports. 70(7): 55.

Volek, J.S., et al. 2006. Nutritional aspects of women strength athletes. *British Journal of Sports Medicine* 40: 742–748.

Volpe, S.L., et al. 2001. Effect of chromium supplementation and exercise on body composition, resting metabolic rate and selected biochemical parameters in moderately obese women following an exercise program. *Journal of the American College of Nutrition* 20: 293-306.

Wagner, D.R. 1999. Hyperhydrating with glycerol: Implications for athletic performance. *Journal of the American Dietetic Association* 99: 207-212.

Wagner, D.R., et al. 1992. Effects of oral ribose on muscle metabolism during bicycle ergometer exercise in AMPD-deficient patients. *Annals of Nutrition and Metabolism* 35: 297-302.

Wagner, J.C. 1991. Enhancement of athletic performance with drugs: An overview. *Sports Medicine* 12: 250-265.

Walberg, J.L., et al. 1988. Macronutrient content of a hypoenergy diet affects nitrogen retention and muscle function in weight lifters. *International Journal of Sports Medicine* 9: 261-266.

Walberg-Rankin, J.L. 1994, November 11-12. Ergogenic effects of carbohydrate intake during long- and short-term exercise. Presented at Nutritional Ergogenic Aids Conference sponsored by the Gatorade Sports Institute, Chicago.

Walberg-Rankin, J.L. 1995. Dietary carbohydrate as an ergogenic aid for prolonged and brief competitions in sport. *International Journal of Sport Nutrition* 5: S13-S28.

Walberg-Rankin, J.L., et al. 1994. The effect of oral arginine during energy restriction in male weight lifters. *Journal of Strength and Conditioning Research* 8: 170-177.

Wall, B.T., et al. 2011. Chronic oral ingestion of L-carnitine and carbohydrate increases muscle carnitine content and alters muscle fuel metabolism during exercise in humans. *Journal of Physiology 589*: 963-973.

Walton, R.G., R. Hudak, and R.J. Green-Waite. 1993. Adverse reactions to aspartame: Double-blind challenge in patients from a vulnerable population. *Biological Psychiatry* 34: 13-17.

Ward, R.J., et al. 1999. Changes in plasma taurine levels after different endurance events. *Amino Acids* 16 (1): 71-77.

Wardlaw, G.M., P.M. Insel, and M.F. Seyler. 1994. *Contemporary nutrition.* St. Louis: Mosby-Year Book, Inc.

Washington State Department of Agriculture. 1995. Organic food standards. Organic Food Program, Food Safety and Animal Health Division.

Watras, A.C., et al. 2007. The role of conjugated linoleic acid in reducing body fat and preventing holiday weight gain. *International Journal of Obesity* 31: 481-487.

Watson S. 2006. Diet pills: What you need to know. http://health.howstuffworks.com/diet-pill.htm.

Wein, D., et al. 2011. To eat or not to eat: the truth behind exercising on an empty stomach. *National Strength and Conditioning Association's Performance Training Journal* 10: 25-26.

Wesson, M., L. McNaughton, P. Davies, and S. Tristram. 1988. Effects of oral administration of aspartic acid salts on the endurance capacity of trained athletes. *Research Quarterly for Exercise and Sport* 59: 234-239.

Wilborn, C.D., et al. 2004a. Effects of methoxyisoflavone, ecdysterone, and sulfopolysaccharide (CSP3) supplementation during training on body composition and training adaptations.

White paper from Exercise and Sport Nutrition Laboratory, Texas A&M University, Waco.

Wilborn, C.D., et al. 2004b. Effects of zinc magnesium aspartate (ZMA) supplementation on training adaptations and markers and anabolism and catabolism. *Journal of the International Society of Sports Nutrition* 1: 12-20.

Williams, C. 1995. Macronutrients and performance. *Journal of Sports Sciences* 13: S1- S10.

Williams, M.B., et al. 2003. Effects of recovery beverages on glycogen restoration and endurance exercise performance. *Journal of Strength and Conditioning Research* 17: 12-19.

Williams, M.H. 1989. Vitamin supplementation and athletic performance. *International Journal for Vitamin and Nutrition Research* (Suppl.) 30: 163-191.

Williams, M.H., et al. 1998. *The ergogenics edge.* Champaign, IL: Human Kinetics.

Williams, M.H., et al. 1999. *Creatine: The power supplement.* Champaign, IL: Human Kinetics.

Williams, M.H. 2005. Dietary supplements and sports performance: Minerals. *Journal of the International Society of Sports Nutrition* 2: 43-49.

Wilmore, J.H., and D.L. Costill. 1994. *Physiology of sport and exercise.* Champaign, IL: Human Kinetics, 392-395.

Winters, L.R., R.S. Yoon, H.J. Kalkwarf, J.C. Davies, et al. 1992. Riboflavin requirements and exercise adaption in older women. *The American Journal of Clinical Nutrition* 56: 526-532.

Woolf, K., et al. 2009. Iron status in highly active and sedentary young women. *International Journal of Sport Nutrition and Exercise Metabolism* 19: 519-535.

Wu, C-L., et al. 2010. Sodium bicarbonate supplementation prevents skilled tennis performance decline after a simulated match. *Nutrition* 7: 33.

Xu, Q., et al. 2009. Multivitamin use and telomere length in women. *American Journal of Clinical Nutrition* 89: 1857-1863.

Yaspelkis, B.B., et al. 1999. The effect of a carbohydrate-arginine supplement on postexercise carbohydrate metabolism. *International Journal of Sports Nutrition* 9: 241-250.

Yates, D. 2007, May 16. Soy estrogens and breast cancer: Research offers overview. News Bureau, University of Illinois. www.news.uiuc.edu/news/07/0516helferich.html.

Youl Kang, H., et al. 2002. Effects of ginseng ingestion on growth hormone, testosterone, cortisol, and insulin-like growth factor 1 responses to acute resistance exercise. *Journal of Strength and Conditioning Research* 16: 179-183.

Zarratti, et al. 2014. Effects of probiotic yogurt on fat distribution and gene expression of proinflammatory factors in peripheral blood mononuclear cells in overweight and obese people with or without weight-loss diet. *Journal of the American College of Nutrition* 33: 417-425.

Zawadzki, K.M., B.B. Yaselkis, and J.L. Ivy. 1992. Carbohydrate-protein complex increases the rate of muscle glycogen storage after exercise. *Journal of Applied Physiology* 72: 1854-1859.

Zeisel, S.H., and da Costa, K.A. 2009. Choline: an essential nutrient for public health. *Nutrition Reviews* 67: 615–623.

Zhang, M., et al. 2004. Role of taurine supplementation to prevent exercise-induced oxidative stress in healthy young men. *Amino Acids* 26: 203-207.

Zhou, S., et al. 2005. Muscle and plasma coenzyme Q10 concentration, aerobic power and exercise economy of healthy men in response to four weeks of supplementation. *The Journal of Sports Medicine and Physical Fitness* 45: 337-346.

Ziegenfuss, T.N., et al. 2006. Safety and efficacy of a commercially available, naturally occurring aromatase inhibitor in healthy men. *Journal of the International Society of Sports Nutrition* 2: 28.

Index

About the Authors

Susan M. Kleiner, PhD, RD, is a titan in sports nutrition. Her seminal research on male and female bodybuilders studied the nutritional needs of muscle building, power, and strength. Her expertise and research have expanded to hydration, and she is passionate about the nutritional needs of athletic women and girls. She is the founder and owner of the internationally recognized consulting firm High Performance Nutrition, LLC. The author of six other popular books, she has written numerous academic

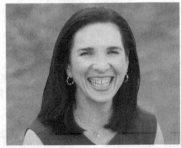

Courtesy of Katie M. Simmons Photography.

chapters and peer-reviewed scientific journal articles, as well as featured columns in all forms of media.

Kleiner has consulted with professional athletes and teams, Olympians, and elite athletes in countless sports. She is currently the high-performance nutritionist for the Seattle Storm and previously served that role for the Seattle Reign FC, the Seattle Seahawks, the Seattle Supersonics, the Miami Heat, the Cleveland Cavaliers, and the Cleveland Browns. She is a cofounder and fellow of the International Society of Sports Nutrition, a fellow of the American College of Nutrition, and a member of both the American College of Sports Medicine and the National Strength and Conditioning Association. Kleiner is a frequent invited speaker at national and international conferences and is a regular expert presence in online, print, and broadcast media.

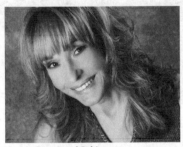

Maggie Greenwood-Robinson.

Maggie Greenwood-Robinson, PhD, is a leading health and medical writer in the United States. She has authored or coauthored more than 65 books on nutrition, exercise, weight loss, psychological health, and other health-related issues, among them *The Biggest Loser*, a New York Times best seller that was the official diet and fitness book for NBC's hit reality show of the same name. Through her many collaborations, she has had 12 other New York Times best sellers, including *20/20 Thinking, Good Carbs vs. Bad Carbs*, and *Foods That Combat Cancer*. Greenwood-Robinson has appeared on numerous television and radio shows, including *Dr. Phil* and NBC's *Dateline*. She has also written articles that have appeared in the magazines *Shape, Let's Live, Great Life, American Health, Physical, Muscle & Fitness*, and *MuscleMag International*. Greenwood-Robinson resides in Flower Mound, Texas.

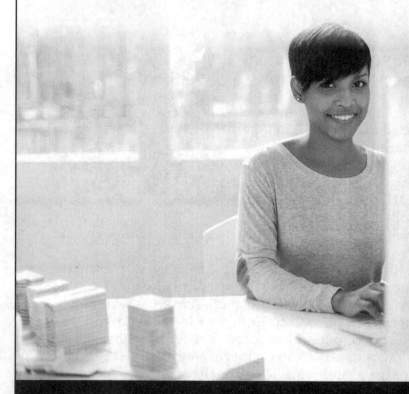
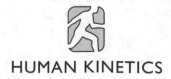